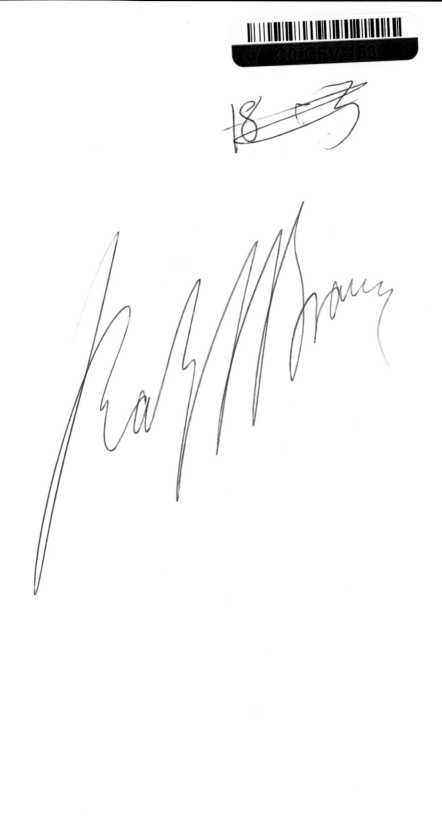

Chemoreceptors and Reflexes in Breathing

CHEMORECEPTORS AND REFLEXES IN BREATHING

Cellular and Molecular Aspects

The Julius H. Comroe Memorial Volume

Edited by

Sukhamay Lahiri
Robert E. Forster, II
Richard O. Davies
Allan I. Pack

University of Pennsylvania School of Medicine
Philadelphia, Pennsylvania

New York   Oxford
OXFORD UNIVERSITY PRESS
1989

Oxford University Press

Oxford   New York   Toronto
Delhi   Bombay   Calcutta   Madras   Karachi
Petaling Jaya   Singapore   Hong Kong   Tokyo
Nairobi   Dar es Salaam   Cape Town
Melbourne   Auckland

and associated companies in
Berlin   Ibadan

Copyright © 1989 by Oxford University Press, Inc.

Published by Oxford University Press, Inc.,
200 Madison Avenue, New York, New York 10016

Oxford is a registered trademark of Oxford University Press

Library of Congress Cataloging-in-Publication Data
Julius H. Comroe Memorial Symposium (1987 : University of Pennsylvania)
   Chemoreceptors and reflexes in breathing : cellular and molecular aspects :
the Julius H. Comroe Memorial Symposium volume /
edited by S. Lahiri . . . [et al.].   p.   cm.
   Papers from a symposium held at University of Pennsylvania, Mar. 1987.
   Includes bibliographies and index.   ISBN 0-19-505227-7
   1. Respiration—Regulation—Congresses. 2. Chemoreceptors—Congresses.
3. Reflexes—Congresses. 4. Comroe, Julius H. (Julius Hiram), 1911—Congresses.
I. Lahiri, Sukhamay. II. Comroe, Julius H.
(Julius Hiram), 1911– III. Title.
   [DNLM: 1. Chemoreceptors—physiology—congresses. 2. Reflex—physiology—congresses.
3. Respiration—congresses.
WF 102 J94c 1987]   QP123.J84 1987   599′.012—dc19
DNLM/DLC for Library of Congress   88-9894   CIP

9 8 7 6 5 4 3 2 1

Printed in the United States of America

Preface

The idea for holding a symposium to honor Julius H. Comroe, Jr. originated several years ago in the Department of Physiology at a meeting of the Respiratory Journal Club founded by Comroe in 1951. As the idea developed further, organizing and program committees were formed that advised the symposium chairman and contributed to many other aspects of the meeting.

The symposium was held at the University of Pennsylvania where Comroe spent a major part of his life, first as a student and subsequently as a teacher in the School of Medicine and Graduate School of Medicine. The actual proceedings took place in a lecture room often used by Dr. Comroe, now newly renovated, in the old medical school building.

The theme of the symposium, chemoreceptors and reflexes in breathing, was deliberately chosen to coincide with the personal investigations of Comroe, but it was clear that the task was a difficult one because his contributions covered many current research areas. Thus, while we tried to develop this theme and stay with it, we succeeded only partially. The topics covered, from molecules to cells and systems, focused on mechanisms of oxygen sensing and transduction processes. It was clear that the knowledge of the mechanisms of oxygen chemoreception is incomplete despite a great deal of active interest in the field over a span of half a century. On the other hand, the symposium generated new ideas and exciting expectations. The effects of hypoxia on brain energy and neurotransmitter metabolism in relation to integrative respiratory control was discussed at length. The state-of-the-art of mechanisms of airway regulation was highlighted in a brief session. Another objective of the symposium was to bring together established and new scientists and to generate discussions among these participants; in this we were quite successful.

The symposium was inaugurated at an evening session on March 26, 1986. The opening lecture, "Central Asian Odyssey: In Search of the Great Ice Mountain," by Thomas F. Hornbein set the high standard for the scientific sessions that were to follow during the next two days.

The book begins with the tributes to Julius Comroe by Seymour S. Kety and John C. G. Coleridge which were given at the symposium banquet on March 27 at the University Museum. Among those who also spoke were Robert E. Forster, Suzanne Hurd, George B. Koelle, Brian B. Lloyd, Robert L. Mayock, J. A. Nadel, Elizabeth K. Rose, and Norman C. Staub. The ceremonial function at the symposium banquet was climaxed by a brief video presentation of Julius Comroe delivering the Herstein Memorial Lecture in 1976. Thus, the published tributes exemplify the spirit of respect for Dr. Comroe's achievements and contributions shared by the participants; our written words capture only part of this ambiance. This commemorative book includes 27 papers based on all the oral presentations given and 9 of the 25 papers presented in the poster sessions. We regret that space limitations prevent us from publishing a paper from every presentation. Although the discussions on the symposium floor were exciting and illuminating, we could not include the proceedings in this volume because of space and resource limitations.

The decision to publish the commemorative volume was taken for two reasons: to reach those interested in the subject matter but who could not participate, and to record a memorable event held in honor of this man who made such an enduring contribution to medical science and education. The publication will have been justified if the objectives are met and the book inspires new ideas and stimulates decisive future experiments.

Acknowledgments

The initial planning of the symposium was given critical momentum by a generous grant from the Barra Foundation. Dr. George H. Acheson, Dr. Albert J. Berger, Dr. Robert S. Fitzgerald, Dr. Robert L. McNeil, Jr., Dr. Robert L. Mayock, Dr. Jay A. Nadel, and Dr. Edward J. Stemmler gave valuable help in seeking support.

We owe special thanks to the National Heart, Lung and Blood Institute; Rorer Group Inc; Boehringer Ingelheim Pharmaceuticals, Inc.; the Council for Tobacco Research; SmithKline Beckman; the Johns Hopkins Medical Institutions; the American Physiological Society; the School of Medicine, University of Pennsylvania; the Respiratory Group, University of Pennsylvania; and anonymous donors.

Many individuals were instrumental in making this event a success, for which we are grateful. Dr. Susanna J. Dodgson compiled the abstracts; Ms. Roberta C. Metelits orchestrated logistics; Mrs. Jean Wyeth supervised the arrangements for the Reception Banquet; Dr. Neil J. Smatresk recorded the proceedings on video; Dr. Machiko Shirahata, Mr. Anil Mokashi, and others were always in attendance to help. Mr. Daniel C. Barrett, Mrs. Esther Cramer, and Ms. Terri Jeffries provided secretarial assistance. The editing of the volume was assisted by Dr. Eileen M. Mulligan.

We would like to acknowledge the fact that we received enthusiastic letters from many participants regarding the success of the symposium. The experience was most gratifying for us.

We are grateful to the publishers and authors for permission to reproduce the previously published material.

Contents

Part III. Oxygen-Sensing Mechanisms

Part IV. Peripheral Chemoreceptors: Adaptation

Part V. Central Effects of Hypoxia

Part VI. Airway Mechanisms

Part VII. Central Mechanisms and Effectors

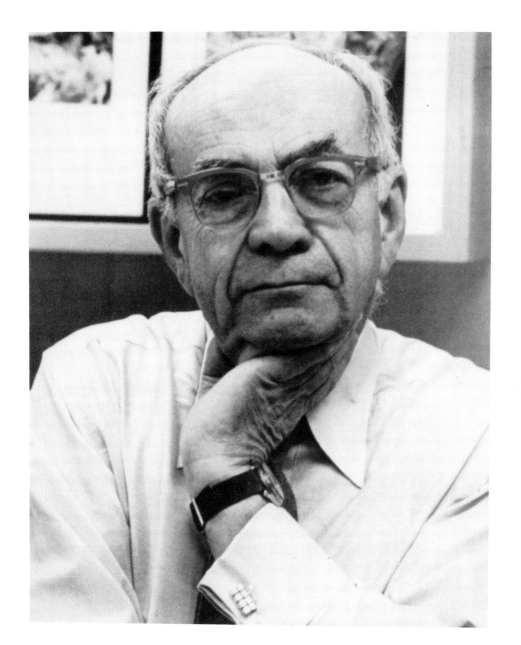

Julius H. Comroe, Jr.

SEYMOUR S. KETY

This year is the golden anniversary of my knowledge and admiration of Julius Comroe whom I first got to know when I was a second year student at the Medical School of the University of Pennsylvania, entering the course in pharmacology, probably the most intellectually challenging one in both the preclinical and clinical years. At a time when pharmacology in most other schools was an advanced course in *materia medica* and ten years before the first edition of Goodman and Gilman, the faculty in pharmacology at Penn taught the "physiological basis of therapeutics." A. N. Richards had recently retired as chairman, to be succeeded by Carl Schmidt and the men associated with him: Earl Walker and Hugh Montgomery. Isaac Starr gave a course in experimental therapeutics and Robert Dripps lectured on anesthetic agents. Comroe, who had joined the faculty a year before after a brilliant record at the Medical School and Hospital, was, even at that tender age, giving the most lucid and interesting lectures of any we received in any course. He used to claim with ingenuous and erroneous humility that if his lectures were as lucid as people asserted them to be, it was merely that he himself was simple-minded and had to figure out a simple exposition of complex processes before he could understand them! Although he was undoubtedly sincere, that was, in fact, the first of his jokes that I remember. A few years later I joined that department and from that time forward became a friend and colleague.

Comroe's lectures were brilliant—crisp, clear, peppered with inimitable wit, always conveying an important message: humility regarding the limited knowlege we had, the need for new knowledge, but, at the same time, a healthy skepticism in respect of new claims. I remember particularly his series of lectures on what used to be called *materia medica,* which were given when I was a student by a gentleman of the old school who taught us how to write Latin prescriptions for complicated, evil-smelling, or bad-tasting concoctions which I am sure were largely placebos. When Julius took over that course, he dragged it into the middle of the twentieth century, making it not only an experimental science, but also great fun. Since pharmacy had by then moved from pill rolling and the preparation of infusions to the transfer of tablets from the manufacturer's bottle to the druggist's vial, he taught how to read critically the lessons in the postgraduate education of physicians, which consisted at that time of the advertisements and brochures of the pharmaceutical industry, and to evaluate the results of the clinical trial. I remember one of his lectures in which he listed some twenty-five herbals or drugs which had been used "successfully" in the treatment of essential hypertension, pointing out that if any were really successful, the list would be considerably shorter. One of these was garlic and he had found an advertisement in one of the current medical journals promoting some proprietary preparation of garlic for the treatment of hypertension which actually cited four references. He then took the trouble to look up those references. I am not sure that I remember the nature of all four, but I believe that one was to a botanical textbook describing the plant, another to an ancient pharmacopeia, a third to a current textbook of pharmacology which indicated that it had no therapeutic value, and the last was a reference to the same advertisement in another journal! He had the students sampling some of the drugs they would be prescribing and learning empirically how best to improve the taste of the more unpleasant ones. I will never forget the actual demonstration of the effectiveness of syrup of chocolate in disguising the bitter taste of quinine.

There was an episode much later in his career, reminiscent of his criticism of the claims for garlic in the treatment of hypertension. In 1978, while he was on the editorial board of the *Proceedings of the National Academy of Sciences,* the board was seized with a major problem. A distinguished member had submitted a paper on the treatment of cancer with large doses of vitamin C which was inadequately controlled and should have been rejected, except for a long-honored rule of the *PNAS* that papers by members must be published. The member was not disposed to withdraw the paper and so it was published. But the *PNAS* also published an immediately succeeding paper, written by Comroe, and probably one of the shortest papers in the scientific literature. Entitled "Experimental Studies Designed to Evaluate the Management of Patients with Incurable Cancer," it consisted of three paragraphs on less than half a page, listing six requirements for a well-controlled clinical trial.

The members of the department used to bring their lunch to school in brown paper bags. There was no faculty club at the time, and few of us could have afforded it if there had been one. Carrying the paper bags, however, bothered some of us, and Julius had solved the problem by carrying his lunch in a hollowed-out old textbook. That custom also gave the world a great anesthesiologist, for after spending several years in the Department of Pharmacology, Bob Dripps moved into the Department of Anesthesiology stating that he could not bear the thought of carrying a brown paper bag to work for the rest of his career. Bob and Julius remained close friends even after they were separated by 3,000 miles and, together, initiated their monumental and scientific demonstration of the importance of basic research to the significant advances which clinical medicine and surgery had made. I still remember the party that Julius and Jeannette threw for Bob Dripps when he left the department and the amusing "gifts" which the various members gave to Bob to help him in his new career as an anesthesiologist. The most amusing, of course, was Julius's, which was a large wooden mallet bearing the inscription, "WHEN ALL ELSE FAILS."

In 1947 or thereabouts, Julius took over the antiquated Department of Physiology and Pharmacology in the Graduate School of Medicine at Pennsylvania and did for that department and for medical education generally what he had done for the course in materia medica but with a far greater impact. He organized a course in the preclinical sciences for graduate physicians most of whom had not learned or appreciated as medical students the importance to clinical medicine of the growing knowledge in fundamental science. He recruited a faculty in the basic sciences: William Ehrich for pathology, David Drabkin for biochemistry, John Flick for microbiology, and myself to complement him in physiology and pharmacology, and infused all of us with his enthusiasm.

That was probably the first course in this country to integrate the basic sciences with the discussion of a series of important clinical problems. Although he brought together an excellent faculty and an innovative curriculum, it was *his* lectures that were responsible for the immense popularity of that course and that attracted students from the entire country and a number of foreign countries as well. The large auditorium was always full, many commuting regularly from New York and other centers within a radius of 100 miles. As always, his lectures were full of wit and sparkle. I remember one comment vividly. In a lecture on the blood gases, he illustrated Henry's Law by what happens with the release of pressure on a gas over a liquid and with the bubbles of gas that arise "when you open a bottle of ginger ale or, in the case of surgeons, champagne"!

He carried his aim of bringing fundamental science to clinicians in a highly successful series of courses he organized for the American College of Physicians. He was able to attract as lecturers some of the most distinguished scientists of the time, and his introduction of them were highly original and surprising. I remember his introduction of Alfred Gilman whose landmark volume with Goodman had revolutionized the teaching of pharmacology. He mentioned the great impact of the book and the fact that it had been translated into many languages, concluding with the Spanish edition whose authorship he read as: "Goodman. *why* Gilman?"

The Cardiovascular Research Institute of the University of California at San Francisco was really organized in the basement laboratories of physiology and pharmacology at the Graduate School of Medicine at Penn. With his remarkable ability for recognizing young and talented scientists, intellectually stimulating them, cultivating their individual efforts and collaborations, and earning their admiration and loyalty, he recruited a small but excellent permanent faculty and a large number of postdoctoral fellows from all over the world who later became leaders in their fields. When the University of California was wise enough to choose him in 1957 as the top candidate for the chairmanship of physiology in San Francisco, he apparently sold them instead on his directing the Cardiovascular Research Institute which he eventually made the greatest of its kind in the world. It was there also that he accomplished the third metamorphosis of his career, this time involving not merely a course in materia media or even in the preclinical sciences but an entire medical school and what was soon to become a great medical center as well.

That was not easy, because the University of California was laboring under the thickest and most impenetrable bureaucracy imagineable. I was invited there for a month in 1945 to start a group in cerebral circulation research. By the end of the month I left with the task hardly begun; it had taken more than three weeks to order the few pieces of equipment we needed from local suppliers who had them in stock! I had been told before I came that they were cutting the red tape. In fact, they must have been cutting it lengthwise.

Julius told me an interesting tale about the processing of grant applications by the University. I had persuaded him to accept appointment to the National Advisory Mental Health Council (I am not sure why I did or he did) not too long after his move to UCSF. At each meeting the members were presented with a huge pile of grant applications from every school in the country. Julius noticed that the time between completion of the application by the investigator and its submission to the NIH by the University of California was unduly long, so he plotted the distribution of delay times for all of the applications. The frequency curve started up at 1 day, peaked at 4 days, and trailed to zero by 10 days. But a second distribution began at 65 days and went to 100 days with a peak at 80 days, and these were all from UC. Julius mailed a copy of his graph with appropriate explanation to Clark Kerr whom UC was fortunate to have as president at that time and who promptly removed enough of the bureaucratic accretions to permit applications to go out in one or two days.

Julius built a great research institute, but that was not enough. He wanted the medical school that housed it to raise its sights as well. He convinced the regents to delegate more responsibility to the faculty and convinced the faculty to change some of its time-worn ideas and throw off its complacency. A succession of outstanding scientific leaders were recruited as department chairpersons, and gradually the school rose from mediocrity to a position of preeminence. There were good reasons why Holly Smith, the distinguished chairman of medicine,, would speak of Comroe as the "architect of the renaissance of the School of Medicine."

Comroe's wisdom influenced more than the UCSF Medical Center. A consummate clinical physiologist who made important contributions to the diagnosis and treatment of lung disease, he was also a basic scientist and was keenly aware of the importance of basic research to ultimate practical accomplishments. He exhibited this awareness early on at the Graduate School of Medicine at Penn where he taught the basic principles on which clinical medicine depends, argued persuasively for basic research in his service as a member of presidential biomedical research panels, and made it the crucial thesis of his regular "retrospectroscope" series in the *American Review of Respiratory Disease.* His most significant contribution to this important mission was the exhaustive study he carried out with Robert Dripps on the factors that operated to bring about the ten most practical clinical advances in circulatory and pulmonary disease. In an admirable design to ensure their own objectivity, they polled a large number of clinicians to learn which were the most practical and highly regarded advances in the field. They then went to the literature to make an exhaustive search for the antecedent discoveries that were crucial in the chain of knowledge leading to the final result. They found that fully half of these papers would not have been considered 'relevant" at the time they were published; in fact, in most instances, the authors did not realize the important contribution to diagnosis, prevention, or treatment that would eventually result from their findings. In their own words:

> We believe that the first priority should be to earmark a generous portion of the nation's biomedical research dollars to identify and then to provide long-term for creative scientists whose main goal is to learn how living organisms function, without regard to the immediate relation of their research to specific human diseases—i.e., those who are most apt to produce the next generation of key discoveries. We believe that this *finding* function of the NIH is as important as its *funding* function.

Christopher Wren lies buried in the great cathedral in London which was his crowning achievement. No monument marks his grave. His son, however, installed an inscription on the wall nearby which reads: *"Si monumentam requiris, circumspice"*—"if you need a monument, look around you." We could say the same for Julius. Although there is a new chair endowed in his name at the UCSF School of Medicine, that is not his major memorial. There is the Cardiovascular Research Institute there, his major scientific and teaching contributions at Penn, the students and fellows he trained here and in California, many of whom are now distinguished scientists, and the unassailable evidence he amassed while speaking eloquently for the importance of basic research. Julius Comroe will not quickly be forgotten.

The Retrospectroscopist Retrospectroscoped: Memories of Julius Comroe

JOHN C. G. COLERIDGE

First, the official record: Julius H. Comroe, Jr., M.D., a world-famous researcher and teacher in heart and lung physiology, came to University of California San Francisco in 1957 to head the newly formed Cardiovascular Research Institute (CVRI). In his sixteen brilliant years as director, he built the institute into a model center for multidisciplinary research on diseases of the cardiovascular and pulmonary systems, and made it a unique training ground for a generation of doctors and medical scientists.

Postdoctoral fellows in the CVRI often ask, "What was Julius Comroe really like? I've heard a lot about him—I once saw him at the end of the corridor, but I never met him. What was he like?" What does one remember about Julius? Many remember him most vividly in the lecture room: Julius as teacher.

Imagine if you will, a morning in early July in the Cardiovascular Research Institute in San Francisco, some 20 years or so ago. It is the first day of the orientation program for the new batch of postdoctoral research fellows and visiting scientists. The lecture room is filling up. Down at the podium, a stocky man of rather less than medium height, his shoulders slightly hunched, his head tilted to one side, a high forehead, of sunburnt appearance, with creased, pleated facial skin, is busy "casing the joint." To the end of his days in the CVRI, Julius always "cased the joint" before his lecture. Chalk, blackboard duster, podium light, pointer, microphone. Having checked that everything is in order, he sits in the front row of seats for all of ten seconds. His timing was always precise and calculated to best advantage.

On the stroke of nine he goes to the podium and introduces himself, in that distinctive, attractively gravelly voice, once heard never forgotten: "My name is Julius Comroe, I am the director of the Cardiovascular Research Institute. In the CVRI, 9 am is always 9 am, we don't observe the academic ten minutes past the hour; we start punctually on the hour."

He then launches into his introductory talk about the University of California and the Cardiovascular Research Institute. In finely balanced proportion, he mixes science, gossip, history, biography, a good measure of anecdote, all leavened with humor—a humor that ranges from atrocious puns tauntingly told to the fine cutting edge of his distinctive wit. He projects a refreshing sense of irony, a rare element in the heavily dedicated world of modern biomedical academia. As in his more formal presentations on scientific topics, he does not overwhelm his audience with ponderous thoughts, nor does he talk down to them. He sails through his talk with an assurance, a generosity of spirit, a freshness, and a good humor that rule out any possibility of boredom.

The new fellows, who previously were slumped and slouched in their seats, displaying a carefully studied nonchalance verging on insolence, begin to sit up and take notice. Those who had managed to win the struggle for the backmost seats in the lecture room, begin to wish they had opted for the front. It is obvious that they have begun to feel elated. They have, in fact, succumbed to the theatrical presence and the magnetic personality projected by the old magician. They have succumbed to his enthusiasm, his timing, his riveting stage presence, his infectious optimism, and above all to his sense of fun.

The subsequent speakers in the three-day orientation program are rather an anticlimax. The associate director—a worthy soul—drones on about the details of the research training program. Speakers drawn from the various laboratory groups in the institute pass in endless procession before the audience: Enthusiastically they describe their individual research projects; with even greater enthusiasm they project innumerable slides. The fellows doodle on their yellow pads. By the end of the third day, the new fellows begin to feel like old fellows. They will soon forget most of what they have heard during these three days. But they will remember Julius Comroe, and they will do so for the rest of their lives.

Most will remember that they felt strangely excited—that they had been put into a receptive mood. A few, a small few, may also remember entertaining a slight suspicion that perhaps they had been sold the Brooklyn Bridge—and immediately they will be cross with themselves for feeling so. But all would agree that they had been subject to the wily siren song of one of physiology's great teachers.

One remembers Julius the campaigner. Julius was always campaigning, plotting on behalf of the CVRI. His schemes for territorial aggrandizement were notorious. He had a continually roving eye for space. Other people's space. "Coleridge," he would say, "you know that room at the end of the Department of Y____'s corridor; if we took out the wash basin and the toilet, it would make a perfect centrifuge room." "But Julius . . ." "Don't worry, if Y____ makes a fuss, we could always take the janitor's broom and bucket out of the small closet next door, and put the toilet there." Look out, Y____, with a compliant dean (and deans were usually compliant in Julius's hands), anything is possible!

One remembers, with affection, Julius the inconsistent. In one of the first science writing courses in which I took part, Julius talked about the pernicious habit of bibliographical inflation: "No one over the age of twenty-eight should include abstracts in his bibliography." Afterward, I teased him with the fact that he included in his bibliography an abstract of his work with Addison on the aortic body. Julius seemed cross: I had overstepped the mark. "Who the hell said I should be consistent!" he growled. "Yes," I replied, "consistency is the hobgoblin of small minds." Julius roared with laughter—and to the end the abstract remained in his bibliography.

One remembers Julius the director, the arranger, bringing people, ideas, and funds together for a voyage on the ship of research. Julius had an unerring eye for what was possible and a consummate ability to make it happen. He had impeccable political judgment; he did his homework and he rarely fought battles he could not win. He was a guiding spirit. He had a deep sense of responsibility, and he assumed responsibility as a matter of course.

One remembers Julius the optimist. He had a truly nineteenth-century sense of optimism. Something could always be done. Things could always be improved by hard work, by knowledge, by education. He was constantly striving to bring scientific knowledge to bear on practical problems of disease. When he came across something he did not like, he did not lament but set about to determine what could be done—and did it. He was a prodigious worker. His optimism about things was tempered by a pessimism about human fallibility, about the absurdities of human affairs.

One remembers Julius the man. The most warmhearted and generous of men. The most loyal of colleagues—indeed, his loyalty was sometimes his undoing. He was unfailingly kind. Occasionally he would allow himself a comment about senior university administrators that was perceptively near the mark—even near the bone—but one never heard a seriously unkind or malicious word about a colleague.

One remembers Julius beavering away, with his tongue in his cheek and that characteristic half smile on his face, beavering away at his image of crusty, feisty curmudgeon. He was undoubtedly what the British call a *card*—a collector's item. If pushed he would, I think, admit to a smidgen of vanity in his makeup. Vain perhaps, but endearingly so, and never, never, self-important. He detested pretentiousness in others. He appeared to find surgeons hard to take. He had a rich vein of humor, which, though often manifest in anecdote, stemmed from a deep sense of life's absurdities. He delighted in telling jokes against himself, although he did not invariably delight in listening to jokes against himself. The temperature always rose several degrees when Julius entered the room, and once in the room he would proceed, effortlessly, to charm the birds out of the trees.

For the sixteen years of his directorship, Uncle Julius, the old magician, the Wizard of Oz, pulling the levers behind the curtain in his minuscule office, made the Cardiovascular Research Institute in San Francisco a very special place.

Symposium Introduction

C. J. LAMBERTSEN

I had the good fortune of once being a student of Julius Comroe, and since then doing scholarly work during a period in our present civilization when research has become widely popular and broadly accepted as an occupation. Over that period, while investigators seem not to have changed at all in their fine dedication and astuteness, their circumstances have changed dramatically.

During these years, from the time Heymans so directly unveiled the carotid arterial chemoreceptors, and firm concepts of electrical synaptic transmission grudgingly gave way to chemical transmission, there have been almost inconceivable engineering instrumentation developments that have allowed multiform attacks upon the sensible questions posed from the very beginning of chemoreceptor research: What are the sensors in the glomus? What stimulates them to fire? What is their role?

The extensive offerings of instrumentation have given all investigators massive armaments to replace the early simple weapons of respirometer and, for a few, the vacuum tube amplifier. The newer armaments include the electron microscope in all its forms, exquisite histochemistry, solid-state electronic recorders and frequency analyzers, gas analyzers, and pH controllers, and computers for calculating and even plotting results. The many hundred man-years of imaginative work represented by this symposium alone provide formidable amounts of important detail. The questions remaining to be discussed are: What are the sensors? What stimulates them to fire? What is their role? Their overall roles in the animal being have become clearer.

It is logical for me to conceive of the chemoreceptors as having, not one role in respiratory control, but at least two. One that is still valid is the early accepted view of its ultimate support of and substitution for the direct drive of a central system, when—for reason of drug, disease, or hostile environment—the central system is not able to sustain pulmonary ventilation appropriate to its own survival. However, that occasional powerful role of the glomus, in failing respiration or extreme environments, is not its sole function. There is clearly another more sensitive and continuous role in normal respiration in sea-level atmosphere, in which "temporal fine adjustment" by the arterial chemoreceptor provides almost breath-by-breath modulation of the normal central system. This receptor function is aided by the beautifully rapid, normal time constant of only a few seconds which its human circulatory anatomy has endowed it with, for sensing both oxygen and carbon dioxide effects. Such a concept of multiple, overlapping functional roles does not require a common "stimulus" of hydrogen ion or some as yet unknown local consequence of hypoxia. The functional stimulus mechanism can also be a dual one, and any such different elements can be interacting.

It has also seemed necessary, in light of the persistent searching, to question again whether there is an "hypoxic stimulus" at all. When we consider that the lack of something is hardly a "stimulus," it is worth restating that the lowering or raising of oxygen partial pressure is just as easily defined as the lowering or raising of a "suppressor" of intrinsic excitability and the resultant discharge generation. If so, there is no hypoxic stimulus to look for, either for the respiratory "support" role of the chemoreceptor in respiratory insufficiency, or for the respiratory "driving" role in an hypoxic atmosphere. Whereas the effects of $CO_2/[H^+]$ are proportional to elevation or lowering of a stimulus, the role of the chemoreflex as well as the central effects of CO_2 in normal respiration in rest or work at sea level appears negative, more related to sustaining respiration than to driving it—or more related to countering excess ventilation.

In the face of such considerations, why was it sensible to make measurements of blood flow and oxygen consumption of the carotid body? The reason was that in the earliest days of this research, there was a confluence of interest in Neil's observation of chemoreceptor activation by a decrease in arterial pressure, and in the emergence of attention to measurements of human brain blood flow and oxygen consumption. It seemed logical to approach the single carotid body as a small and relatively simple "brain," capable of sensing and responding, and to examine the primary factors in its oxygenation and, possibly, its self-activation. Regardless of why it seemed appropriate to study the carotid body, blood flow through this organ was high—a property that fit its temporal role but was not at all essential for its support role. Regardless of interpretation, its arteriovenous oxygen removal, and therefore oxygen consumption rate was also large as compared to mean rates for other organs. However, not many—if any—mean measurements for a selected 2-mg mass of brain or other organ have been made for comparison, and furthermore, the mean for an organ a million times larger is not relevant.

Tasks still remaining include consideration of whether a high rate of oxygen metabolism is coincidental or has any functional significance for either a central respiratory system support role of the chemoreceptor or a continuously sensitive temporal adjustment role in maintaining arteriolar and central neuronal carbon dioxide tension and $[H^+]$ at the levels optimal for the functioning and self-interest of the respiratory centers and their arterioles, and, possibly, the internal acid–base environment of the brain. Despite all the attention given to the roles of a hypoxic "stimulus," it may be that the influence of the latter occurs through the influence of carbon dioxide. This book should offer new insights into these and more current considerations.

Contributors

ACKER, H.	Max-Plank-Institut für Systemphysiologie, Rheinlanddamm 201, 4600 Dortmund 1, F.R.G.
ALBERTINE, K.	Department of Physiology, University of Pennsylvania School of Medicine, Philadelphia, PA 19104, U.S.A.
ALMARAZ, L.	Departamento de Fisiologia y Bioquimica, Facultad de Medicina, Universidad de Valladolid, Valladolid, Spain.
ANDERSON, S. J.	Department of Biometrics, University of Colorado Medical School, Denver, CO 80266, U.S.A.
ASHCROFT, F. M.	Department of Physiology, Oxford University, Oxford OX1 3PT, U.K.
BALLANTYNE, D.	Physiologisches Institut, Universität Heidelberg, D-6900 Heidelberg 1, F.R.G.
BANNIGAN, J.	Department of Anatomy, University College, Earlsfort Terrace, Dublin 2, Ireland.
BARNARD, P.	Department of Physiology, University of Pennsylvania School of Medicine, Philadelphia, PA 19104, U.S.A.
BARNETT, S.	Department of Physiology, University of Pennsylvania School of Medicine, Philadelphia, PA 19104, U.S.A.
BAUER, C.	Physiologisches Institut der Universität Zürich, 8057 Zürich, Switzerland.
BERGER, A. J.	Department of Physiology and Biophysics, University of Washington School of Medicine, Seattle, WA 98195, U.S.A.
BISGARD, G. E.	Department of Comparative Biosciences, School of Veterinary Medicine, University of Wisconsin, Madison, WI 53706, U.S.A.
BROWN, H. F.	Department of Physiology, Oxford University, Oxford, OX1 3PT, U.K.

CHANCE, B.   Department of Biochemistry and Biophysics,
                           University of Pennsylvania School of Medicine,
                           Philadelphia, PA 19104, U.S.A.

CHERNIACK, N. S.   Department of Medicine, Case Western Reserve
                           University School of Medicine, Cleveland, OH
                           44106, U.S.A.

CHIANG, C.-H.   Pulmonary Unit, Department of Medicine
                           Massachusetts General Hospital and Harvard
                           Medical School, Boston, MA 02114 WA

COBURN, R. F.   Department of Physiology, University of
                           Pennsylvania School of Medicine, Philadelphia, PA
                           19104, U.S.A.

COHEN, H. L.   Department of Physiology, State University of New
                           York—Downstate Medical Center, Brooklyn, NY
                           11202, U.S.A.

COLERIDGE, H. M.   Cardiovascular Research Institute, University of
                           California, San Francisco School of Medicine, San
                           Francisco, CA 94143, U.S.A.

COLERIDGE, J.C.G.   Cardiovascular Research Institute, University of
                           California, San Francisco School of Medicine, San
                           Francisco, CA 94143, U.S.A.

DARISTOTLE, L.   Department of Comparative Biosciences, School of
                           Veterinary Medicine, University of Wisconsin,
                           Madison, WI 53706, U.S.A.

DATA, P. G.   Institute of Physiological Sciences, University of
                           Chisti, Chisti, Italy.

DAVIES, R. O.   Department of Animal Biology, University of
                           Pennsylvania School of Veterinary Medicine,
                           Philadelphia, PA 19104, U.S.A.

DELPIANO, M. A.   Max-Planck-Institut für Systemphysiologie,
                           Rheinlanddamm 201, 4600 Dortmund, F.R.G.

DICK, T. E.   Pulmonary Division, Department of Medicine, Case
                           Western Reserve University School of Medicine,
                           Cleveland, OH 44106, U.S.A.

DINGER, B. G.   Department of Physiology, University of Utah
                           School of Medicine, Salt Lake City, UT 84108,
                           U.S.A.

EDELMAN, N. H.   Departments of Physiology and Medicine,
                           University of Medicine and Dentistry of New Jersey
                           - Rutgers Medical School, New Brunswick, NJ
                           08903, U.S.A.

EDEN, G. J.   Department of Physiology and Biochemistry,
                           University of Reading, Whiteknights, Reading RG6
                           2AJ, U.K.

ELDRIDGE, F. L.   Departments of Medicine and Physiology,
                       University of North Carolina School of Medicine,
                       Chapel Hill, NC 27514, U.S.A.

ENGWALL, M.   Department of Comparative Biosciences, University
                       of Wisconsin, School of Medicine, Madison, WI
                       53706, U.S.A.

ENNIS, S.   Department of Physiology, University College,
                       Earlsfort Terrace, Dublin 2, Ireland.

EYZAGUIRRE, C.   Department of Physiology, University of Utah
                       School of Medicine, Salt Lake City, UT 84108,
                       U.S.A.

FIDONE, S. J.   Department of Physiology, University of Utah
                       School of Medicine, Salt Lake City, UT 84108,
                       U.S.A.

FITZGERALD, R. S.   Department of Environmental Health Sciences, The
                       Johns Hopkins University School of Medicine,
                       Baltimore, MD 21205, U.S.A.

FORSTER, H. V.   Department of Physiology, Medical College of
                       Wisconsin, Milwaukee, WI 53226, U.S.A.

FORSTER, R. E.   Department of Physiology, University of
                       Pennsylvania School of Medicine, Philadelphia, PA
                       19104, U.S.A.

GALLMAN, E. A.   Department of Physiology, University of North
                       Carolina at Chapel Hill School of Medicine, Chapel
                       Hill, NC 27514, U.S.A.

GONZALEZ, C.   Departamento de Fisiologia y Bioquimica, Facultad
                       de Medicina, Universidad de Valladolid, Valladolid,
                       Spain.

GOOTMAN, P. M.   Department of Physiology, State University of New
                       York Health Science Center at Brooklyn College of
                       Medicine, Brooklyn, NY 11203, U.S.A.

GREEN, T. J.   Department of Biochemistry and Biophysics,
                       University of Pennsylvania School of Medicine,
                       Philadelphia, PA 19104, U.S.A.

HANSEN, J. T.   Department of Neurobiology and Anatomy,
                       University of Rochester School of Medicine and
                       Dentistry, Rochester, NY 14642, U.S.A.

HANSON, G.   Department of Physiology, University of Utah
                       School of Medicine, Salt Lake City, UT 84108,
                       U.S.A.

HANSON, M. A.   Department of Physiology and Biochemistry,
                       University of Reading, Whiteknights, Reading RG6
                       2AJ, U.K.

HAZEKI, O.   Biophysics Division, Research Institute of Applied
                     Electricity, Hokkaido University, Sapporo, Japan.

HERBERT, D. A.   Department of Anesthesia, University of California,
                     San Francisco School of Medicine, San Francisco,
                     CA 94143, U.S.A.

HITZIG, B. M.   Pulmonary Unit, Medical Services, Massachusetts
                     General Hospital, and Departments of Medicine
                     and Physiology, Harvard Medical School, Boston,
                     MA 02114, U.S.A.

HOOP, B.   Pulmonary Unit, Medical Services, Massachusetts
                     General Hospital and Department of Medicine,
                     Harvard Medical School, Boston, MA 02114,
                     U.S.A.

JODKOWSKI, J. S.   Department of Physiology and Biophysics,
                     University of Washington School of Medicine,
                     Seattle, WA 98195, U.S.A.

KAZEMI, H.   Pulmonary Unit, Department of Medicine,
                     Massachusetts General Hospital, and Harvard
                     Medical School, Boston, MA 02114, U.S.A.

KENNEDY, M.   Department of Physiology, University College,
                     Earlsfort Terrace, Dublin 2, Ireland.

KETY, S. S.   National Institutes of Health (Bldg. 10), Bethesda,
                     Maryland 20892, U.S.A.

LAHIRI, S.   Department of Physiology, University of
                     Pennsylvania School of Medicine, Philadelphia, PA
                     19104, U.S.A.

LALLEY, P. M.   Physiologisches Institut, Universität Heidelberg, D-
                     6900 Heidelberg 1, F.R.G.

LAMBERTSEN, C. J.   Department of Pharmacology and Institute for
                     Environmental Medicine, University of
                     Pennsylvania School of Medicine, Philadelphia, PA
                     19104, U.S.A.

LAWSON, E. E.   Physiologisches Institut, Universität Heidelberg, D-
                     6900 Heidelberg 1, F.R.G.

LLOYD, B. B.   High Wall, 1 Pullens Lane, Oxford, OX3 0BX, U.K.

MCDONALD, D. M.   Cardiovascular Research Institute and Department
                     of Anatomy, University of California, San Francisco
                     School of Medicine, San Francisco, CA 94143,
                     U.S.A.

MELTON, J. E.   Department of Medicine, University of Medicine
                     and Dentistry of New Jersey - Robert Wood
                     Johnson Medical School, New Brunswick, NJ
                     08903, U.S.A.

MILLHORN, D. E.   Department of Physiology, University of North Carolina at Chapel Hill School of Medicine, Chapel Hill, NC 27514, U.S.A.

MITCHELL, R. A.   Department of Anesthesia, and Cardiovascular Research Institute, University of California, San Francisco School of Medicine, San Francisco 94143, U.S.A.

MOKASHI, A.   Department of Physiology, University of Pennsylvania School of Medicine, Philadelphia, PA 19104, U.S.A.

MOORE, P. J.   Department of Physiology and Biochemistry, University of Reading, Whiteknights, Reading RG6 2AJ, U.K.

MULLIGAN, E.   Department of Physiology, Temple University School of Medicine, Philadelphia, PA 19122, U.S.A.

NADEL, J. A.   Departments of Medicine and Physiology, and Cardiovascular Research Institute, University of California, San Francisco School of Medicine, San Francisco, CA 94143, U.S.A.

NEUBAUER, J. A.   Department of Medicine, University of Medicine and Dentistry of New Jersey - Robert Wood Johnson Medical School, New Brunswick, NJ 08903, U.S.A.

NIELSEN, A.   Department of Comparative Biosciences, University of Wisconsin School of Medicine, Madison, WI 53706

NIJHUIS, J. G.   Department of Physiology and Biochemistry, University of Reading, Whiteknights, Reading, RG6 2AJ, U.K.

NIOKA, S.   Departments of Physiology and Biochemistry and Biophysics, University of Pennsylvania School of Medicine, Philadelphia, PA 19104, U.S.A.

NYE, P.C.G.   Department of Physiology, Oxford University, Oxford OX1 3PT, U.K.

OBESO, A.   Departamento de Fisiologia y Bioquimica, Facultad de Medicina, Universidad de Valladolid, Valladolid, Spain.

O'DONNELL, J.M.M.   Department of Physiology, Oxford University, Oxford OX1 3PT, U.K.

O'REGAN, R. G.   Department of Physiology, University College, Earlsfort Terrace, Dublin 2, Ireland.

PACK, A. I. — Cardiovascular-Pulmonary Division,, Department of Medicine, University of Pennsylvania School of Medicine, Philadelpia, PA 19104, U.S.A.

PIETRUSCHKA, F. — Max-Planck-Institut für Systemphysiologie, Rheinlanddamm 201, 4600 Dortmund, F.R.G.

POKORSKI, M. — Department of Physiology, University of Pennsylvania School of Medicine, Philadelphia, PA 19104, U.S.A.

PRABHAKAR, N. R. — Pulmonary Division, Department of Medicine, Case Western Reserve University School of Medicine, Cleveland, OH 44106, U.S.A.

REYNAFARJE, B. — Department of Biological Chemistry, The Johns Hopkins University School of Medicine, Baltimore, MD 21205, U.S.A.

RICHARDSON, C. A. — Cardiovascular Research Institute, University of California, San Francisco School of Medicine, San Francisco, CA 94143, U.S.A.

RICHTER, D. W. — Physiologisches Institut, Universität Heidelberg, D-6900 Heidelberg 1, F.R.G.

RIGUAL, R. — Departamento de Fisiologia y Bioquimica, Facultad de Medicina, Universidad de Valladolid, Valladolid, Spain.

ROBIOLO, M. — Department of Biochemistry and Biophysics, University of Pennsylvania School of Medicine, Philadelphia, PA 19104, U.S.A.

RUMSEY, W. L. — Department of Biochemistry and Biophysics, University of Pennsylvania School of Medicine, Philadelphia, PA 19104, U.S.A.

SHIRAHATA, M. — Department of Physiology, University of Pennsylvania School of Medicine, Philadelphia, PA 19104, U.S.A.

SICA, A. L. — Long Island Jewish Hillside Medical Center, Schneider Children's Hospital Research Center, New Hyde Park, NY 11042, U.S.A.

SMATRESK, N. J. — Physiology Section, Department of Biology, University of Texas, Arlington, TX 76019, U.S.A.

SMITH, D. S. — Department of Anesthesia, University of Pennsylvania School of Medicine, Philadelphia, PA 19104, U.S.A.

SPYER, K. M.	Department of Physiology, Royal Free Hospital School of Medicine, London, NW3 2PF, U.K.
STEELE, A. M.	Department of Physiology, State University of New York at Stony Brook School of Medicine, Stony Brook, NY 11794, U.S.A.
SWANSON, G. D.	Department of Anesthesiology, University of Colorado Medical School, Denver, CO 80266, U.S.A.
TALLMAN, R. D., JR.	School of Allied Medical Professions and Department of Physiology, Ohio State University College of Medicine, Columbus, OH 43210, U.S.A.
TAMURA, M.	Biophysics Division, Research Institute of Applied Electricity, Hokkaido University, Sapporo, Japan.
TORBATI, D.	Department of Physiology, University of Pennsylvania School of Medicine, Philadelphia, PA 19104, U.S.A.
TRZEBSKI, A. M.	Department of Physiology, Institute of Physiological Sciences, Warsaw Medical Academy, PL-00927, Warsaw, Poland.
VANDERKOOI, J. M.	Department of Biochemistry and Biophysics, University of Pennsylvania School of Medicine, Philadelphia, PA 19104, U.S.A.
VIANA, F.	Department of Physiology and Biophysics, University of Washington School of Medicine, Seattle, WA 98195, U.S.A.
VIDRUK, E.	Department of Preventive Medicine, University of Wisconsin School of Medicine, Madison, WI 53706,U.S.A.
VIZEK, M.	Cardiovascular Pulmonary Research Laboratory, University of Colorado Health Sciences Center, Denver, CO 80262, U.S.A.
WAGERLE, L. C.	Department of Physiology, University of Pennsylvania School of Medicine, Philadelphia, PA 19104, U.S.A.
WEIL, J. V.	Cardiovascular Pulmonary Research Laboratory, University of Colorado Health Sciences Center, Denver, CO 80262, U.S.A.
WILSON, D. F.	Department of Biochemistry and Biophysics, University of Pennsylvania School of Medicine, Philadelphia, PA 19104, U.S.A.

Introduction

S. LAHIRI

The peripheral chemoreceptor responses to natural stimuli are dependent on their blood flow; arterial blood carries exogenous stimuli to and endogenous stimuli away from the chemoreceptors. The control of blood flow and hence the tissue stimulus levels are still not clearly understood. The observations on carotid body are controversial, and little is reported on aortic bodies. Also, the vasculature of chemoreceptor tissue is of special interest because of its extraordinary characteristics. These blood vessels themselves are chemosensitive just as the parenchyma of the carotid and aortic bodies. Accordingly the first section is devoted particularly to the topic.

Mulligan, using microsphere technique, gives evidence in favor of high blood flow as was first reported by Daly, Lambertsen, and Schweitzer, unlike the recent reports by Acker and O'Regan.

O'Regan, using large latex sphere (28–52 μm), presents evidence for a significant amount of arteriovenous shunts within the carotid body tissues, suggesting that the total blood flow would be significantly greater than the flow reported by Mulligan. The high blood flow is consistent with the extreme vascularity of the carotid body tissue and its blood gas monitoring function. McDonald discusses the question of distribution of the blood. He suggests that the terminal arterioles and arteriovenous anastomoses are critical in determining the flow through the capillaries. What determines this regulation is unclear. The sympathetic innervation is a candidate but there is little compelling evidence for its role during normal physiological condition.

Comparative physiology of arterial chemoreflex functions were presented in two papers—Tallman in the bird and Smatresk in the fish.

Hansen, Gonzalez, Obeso, Dinger, and Fidone report that the sympathetic superior cervical ganglia responds to acute hypoxia by releasing neuropeptides like substance P, thus mimicking carotid body responses. They concluded that the locally secreted neurochemicals modulate postganglionic activity, a conclusion consistent with the stimulatory effect of hypoxia independently of the peripheral chemoreceptors.

Aging of carotid body is considered by Hansen. He shows a significant structural change in the aged primate, indicating a declining function of the carotid body with aging.

1

Routes for Blood Flow Through the Rat Carotid Body

D. M. McDONALD

The carotid body's distinctive vasculature may be responsible for some of the chemoreceptor's unusual functional characteristics. It is known, for example, that the chemoreceptors are comparatively unresponsive to conditions such as carboxyhemoglobinemia (3,9) and anemia (5,8) which reduce the oxygen content of blood without lowering the partial pressure of oxygen (Po_2). This phenomenon may be due to the carotid body's enormous blood flow—as much as 2000 ml/100g/min (4). Blood flow in the carotid body is so high that the Po_2 of this organ's venous blood is almost as high as it is in arterial blood (4). However, the Po_2 of carotid body tissues is comparatively low (1). Furthermore, sympathetic nerve stimulation diminishes the carotid body's total blood flow but does not change the tissue Po_2 or the local blood flow to the chemoreceptive tissue (2). These findings would suggest that there are at least two routes for blood flow through the carotid body, one permitting most of the blood entering the carotid body to bypass the chemoreceptive tissue, and the other directing the remainder of the blood to the chemoreceptive tissue.

Can the carotid body's vasculature explain these phenomena? The answer to this question is not known, but the organ's blood vessels have long been recognized as one of its most distinctive morphological features. In particular, the capillary-like blood vessels next to the chemoreceptive tissue are conspicuously larger, more tortuous, and more closely packed than are capillaries in most other organs (6). Further, there are reports of arteriovenous (AV) anastomoses in the carotid body that could shunt blood away from the chemoreceptive tissue, but other reports claim that shunt vessels do not exist (see ref. 10 for a review).

Why have studies of the carotid body not revealed the significance of the unusual blood vessels with respect to the high blood flow, insensitivity to anemia, and low tissue Po_2? Part of the problem results from not having a clear understanding of the anatomical routes by which blood flows through the carotid body under various conditions. This problem does not exist because the morphology of the vasculature of the carotid body has not been studied. Indeed, experiments involving light and electron microscopy, reconstruction of serial sections, and vascular casts have documented the abundance, tortuosity, branching, and close packing of the blood vessels (see ref. 10 for a review). Rather it is the complexity of the vascular architecture that has frustrated these efforts. Yet knowledge of the pathways for blood flow is essential for testing hypotheses regarding how the carotid body functions as a chemoreceptor.

TWO APPROACHES WE HAVE USED TO IDENTIFY ROUTES FOR BLOOD FLOW

We have used two different approaches to obtain a more complete understanding of the anatomical routes for blood flow through the carotid body of the rat. We chose this species for the studies because its carotid body is comparatively small, and therefore the vasculature readily lends itself to morphological analysis. The first approach involved the use of transmission electron microscopy to analyze the morphology of various types of blood vessels in carotid bodies, scanning electron

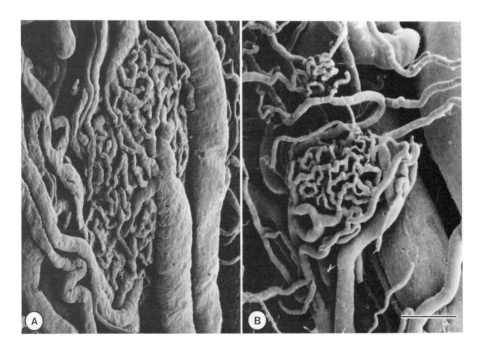

Fig. 1.1 Scanning electron micrographs of methacrylate vascular casts of the rat carotid body **(A)** and superior laryngeal nerve paraganglion **(B),** which are shown at the same magnification to compare the sizes of the two organs. Most vessels visible in these casts are tortuous type I capillaries and venules located at the surface of the organs. Scale marker = 100 μm.

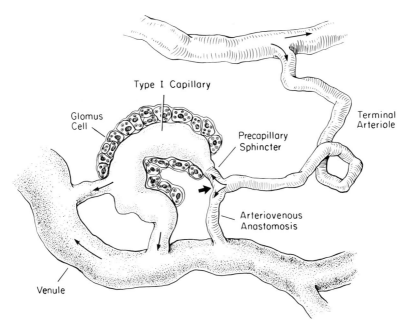

Type I Capillary

Glomus
Cell

Terminal
Arteriole

Precapillary
Sphincter

Arteriovenous
Anastomosis

Venule

Fig. 1.2 Diagram summarizing the major routes for blood flow that we identified in the carotid body and superior laryngeal nerve paraganglion of the rat. Arrows show the presumed directions of blood flow. A distinctive feature of blood vessels in both organs is that terminal arterioles divide (bold arrow) near glomus cell clusters. One branch of each arteriole supplies the large type I capillaries next to the glomus cells, whereas the other branch is an arteriovenous anastomosis that bypasses these cells.

microscopy to examine vascular casts of carotid bodies, and light microscopy to reconstruct the connections between arterioles, capillaries, and venules in serial 0.5-μm sections of carotid bodies (11,13,15). Each of these methods provided a different view of the carotid body's vasculature, and from these views we developed a model of the vascular architecture. The second approach was to test this model by doing corresponding studies on superior laryngeal nerve (SLN) paraganglia in the rat (14). These paraganglia were studied because they are anatomically similar to the carotid body but are even smaller (12). Because of their tiny size, these paraganglia are comparatively easy to analyze in serial sections and vascular casts (compare Fig. 1.1A and 1.1B).

ROUTES FOR BLOOD FLOW THROUGH THE CAROTID BODY

Our anatomical studies revealed that there were four separate routes for blood flow through the rat carotid body (11,13,15). The first route was through type I capillaries (Fig. 1.2). These were tortuous, large-diameter (12–24 μm), thin-walled vessels that were one of the most conspicuous features of the carotid body. Type I capillaries were the vessels most closely associated with glomus cells. These capillaries were supplied by small, densely innervated terminal arterioles. Type I capillaries had multiple connections with venules, which formed an elaborate plexus throughout the carotid body and were particularly large and numerous at the surface.

The second route for blood flow was through AV anastomoses (Fig. 1.2). These vessels were short branches of terminal arterioles that joined venules directly. The AV anastomoses did not differ in size (10 μm in diameter) or wall morphology (one thin layer of smooth muscle cells or pericyte-like cells) from terminal arterioles; they were, therefore, identifiable only by their direct connection to venules. Because of this connection, these vessels provided a route for blood to bypass the type I capillaries.

The third route was through type II capillaries, which were comparatively uncommon vessels that resembled in size (less than 10 μm in diameter), shape, and wall structure the capillaries of skeletal muscle and many other organs. Type II capillaries were supplied by the same terminal arterioles and drained by the same venules as were the type I capillaries, but they were distinguished from type I capillaries by their smaller size and lack of a consistently close association with glomus cells.

The fourth route for blood flow was through branches of the carotid body artery that passed through the carotid body en route to adjacent organs. These arteries had no connections with capillaries or venules in the carotid body and therefore did not contribute to the organ's blood supply, but their presence and location would ensure a high velocity of blood flow through the arterioles that supply the carotid body.

ROUTES FOR BLOOD FLOW THROUGH SLN PARAGANGLIA

The vascular architecture of SLN paraganglia was similar but not identical to that of the carotid body (14). An obvious similarity was the presence of type I capillaries next to glomus cells. These capillaries were supplied by arterioles that divided when they reached the surface of the paraganglia. One branch of each arteriole joined the network of type I capillaries. The other branch was an AV anastomosis that formed a route bypassing the type I capillaries (Fig. 1.2). However, SLN paraganglia—unlike the carotid body—had no arterioles inside their capsule because all arterioles made their connections at the surface of the paraganglia. In this respect, the vasculature of SLN paraganglia resembled that of a single lobule of the carotid body rather than that of the entire carotid body.

REGULATION OF BLOOD FLOW THROUGH TYPE I CAPILLARIES

Our studies have shown that the distinctive appearance of the vasculature of the carotid body and SLN paraganglia is due mainly to the unusually large size and tortuosity of type I capillaries that supply the glomus tissue. This feature has been recognized also by Seidl (18) and Taguchi (19). Because of their location, type I capillaries are likely to be the principal route for blood to reach the chemoreceptive tissue.

The carotid body's high blood flow could result from the large diameter and low resistance of type I capillaries. However, because the terminal arterioles that supply type I capillaries are small and densely innervated, these arterioles are likely to be more important in the control of blood flow to the chemoreceptive tissue than are the large type I capillaries.

Terminal arterioles are not the only vessels that have a strategic location within the carotid body for influencing blood flow to the chemoreceptive tissue. Arteriovenous anastomoses that arise from the same terminal arterioles as supply type I capillaries could divert blood away from the glomus tissue when the resistance to flow through the anastomoses is lower than that through the type I capillaries.

ARE ARTERIOVENOUS ANASTOMOSES ACTUALLY PRESENT?

The issue regarding whether AV anastomoses exist in the carotid body has been debated in the literature for decades. There are two major reasons why previous morphological studies that have dealt with this issue have not resolved it. First, articles reporting the existence or lack of existence of such anastomotic vessels have not provided sufficient documentation to justify their conclusions. Second, the criteria used to identify AV anastomoses have varied from study to study; therefore, the vessels designated AV anastomoses by some investigators have been disregarded as such by others.

De Castro (6) reported that AV anastomoses are a characteristic feature of the cat carotid body. The vessels he identified as AV anastomoses invariably had thick walls containing smooth muscle cells and myoepithelial cells, had narrow lumens, and were located in the connective tissue at the surface of the organ. Schafer et al. (17) reported that AV anastomoses with this morphology were present in a quarter of the cat carotid bodies they examined in serial sections, but Niedorf (16) and Seidl (18) found none in the cat carotid bodies they studied. Habeck et al. (7) found such anastomoses in serial sections of only 2 of 12 rat carotid bodies.

Taguchi (19) concluded that no AV anastomoses were present in vascular casts of rat carotid bodies examined by scanning electron microscopy. Such casts can be successfully used to identify the type of AV anastomosis described by De Castro but are not so useful for finding AV anastomoses within the carotid body. The problem is that methacrylate vascular casts lack the landmarks of such tissues as glomus cells, because these tissues are corroded away during preparation to expose the cast of the blood vessels. Without knowing the location of the glomus cells, one cannot distinguish type I capillaries from small venules. If small venules are misinterpreted as type I capillaries, then AV anastomoses would be misinterpreted as arterioles that join these type I capillaries.

Despite these reports, I conclude from our observations that AV anastomoses are present in the rat carotid body. The morphology of these AV anastomoses is not, however, as described by De Castro; they are not large and conspicuous vessels, they do not have thick walls containing myoepithelial cells, and they are not located at the surface of the carotid body. Our studies indicate instead that AV anastomoses in the rat carotid body are branches of typical terminal arterioles, have a diameter of about 10 μm, and join small venules located in the interior of the carotid body. Arteriovenous anastomoses in SLN paraganglia are identical in morphology to those in the carotid body, and the relative simplicity of the vasculature of SLN paraganglia makes their AV anastomoses easy to identify.

CONCLUSIONS

The extreme vascularity of the carotid body is a clue to the organ's high total blood flow, but it is not a clue to how this blood flow is distributed within the organ. Our morphological studies indicate that at least three types of vessels must be considered in attempting to understand the routes by which blood traverses the carotid body and the factors that influence the flow to the chemoreceptive tissue: terminal arterioles, AV anastomoses, and type I capillaries.

Terminal arterioles and AV anastomoses are likely to be key vessels in regulating not only the total blood flow of the carotid body but also the distribution of blood flow. The resistance of these vessels, under the control of autonomic nerves and no doubt other factors, would determine the amount and proportion of the total blood flow that goes to type I capillaries—and thereby supplies the chemoreceptive tissue—and would also govern the amount and proportion of blood flow that bypasses the chemoreceptive tissue. If the resistance of terminal arterioles that supply type I capillaries is regulated separately from that of AV anastomoses, blood flow to the chemoreceptive tissue could be controlled independently of the carotid body's total blood flow.

ACKNOWLEDGMENTS
    I thank Ms. Amy Haskell for helping with the experiments described in this paper. This research was supported in part by NIH Pulmonary Program Project Grant HL-24136.

REFERENCES

1. Acker, H., and D. W. Lübbers. The meaning of the tissue Po_2 of the carotid body for the chemoreceptive process. In: *The Peripheral Arterial Chemoreceptors,* ed. M. J. Purves. Cambridge: Cambridge University Press, 1975, pp. 325–343.
2. Acker, H., and R. G. O'Regan. The effects of stimulation of autonomic nerves on carotid body blood flow in the cat. *J. Physiol. (Lond.) 315:* 99–110, 1981.
3. Comroe, J. H., and C. F. Schmidt. The part played by reflexes from the carotid body in the chemical regulation of respiration in the dog. *Am. J. Physiol. 121:* 75–97, 1938.
4. Daly, M. de B., C. J. Lambertsen, and A. Schweitzer. Observations on volume of blood flow and oxygen utilization of the carotid body in the cat. *J. Physiol. (Lond.) 125:* 67–89, 1954.

5. Davies, R. O., T. Nishino, and S. Lahiri. Sympathectomy does not alter the response of carotid chemoreceptors to hypoxemia during carboxyhemoglobinemia or anemia. *Neurosci. Lett. 21:* 159–163, 1981.

6. De Castro, F. Sur la structure de la synapse dans les chemocepteurs: leur mécanisme d'excitation et rôle dans la circulation sanguine locale. *Acta Physiol. Scand. 22:* 14–43, 1951.

7. Habeck, J. O., A. Honig, C. Huckstorf, and C. Pfeiffer. Arteriovenous anastomoses at the carotid bodies of rats. *Anat. Anz. 156:* 209–215, 1984.

8. Hatcher, J. D., L. K. Chiu, and D. B. Jennings. Anemia as a stimulus to aortic and carotid chemoreceptors in the cat. *J. Appl. Physiol. 44:* 696–702, 1978.

9. Lahiri, S., E. Mulligan, T. Nishino, A. Mokashi, and R. O. Davies. Relative responses of aortic body and carotid body chemoreceptors to carboxyhemoglobinemia. *J. Appl. Physiol. 50:* 580–586, 1981.

10. McDonald, D. M. Peripheral chemoreceptors: structure–function relationships of the carotid body. In: *Regulation of Breathing,* Part 1, ed. T. F. Hornbein. New York: Marcel Dekker, 1981, pp. 105–319.

11. McDonald, D. M. A morphometric analysis of blood vessels and perivascular nerves in the rat carotid body. *J. Neurocytol. 12:* 155–199, 1983.

12. McDonald, D. M., and R. W. Blewett. Location and size of carotid bodylike organs (paraganglia) revealed in rats by the permeability of their blood vessels to Evans blue dye. *J. Neurocytol. 10:* 607–643, 1981.

13. McDonald, D. M., and A. Haskell. Morphology of connections between arterioles and capillaries in the rat carotid body analyzed by reconstructing serial sections. In: *The Peripheral Arterial Chemoreceptors,* ed. D. J. Pallot. London: Croom Helm, 1984, pp. 195–206.

14. McDonald, D. M., and A. Haskell. Vascular geometry of arterial chemoreceptors: learning about the carotid body by studying paraganglia of the superior laryngeal nerve. In: *Chemoreceptors in Respiratory Control,* ed. J. A. Ribeiro and D. J. Pallot. London: Croom Helm, 1987, pp. 39–49.

15. McDonald, D. M., and D. T. Larue. The ultrastructure and connections of blood vessels supplying the rat carotid body and carotid sinus. *J. Neurocytol. 12:* 117–153, 1983.

16. Neidorf, H. R. Die normale und pathologische Anatomie des Glomus caroticum. *Med. Welt 21:* 251–257, 1970.

17. Schäfer, D., E. Seidl, H. Acker, H. P. Keller, and D. W. Lübbers. Arteriovenous anastomoses in the cat carotid body. *Z. Zellforsch. 142:* 515–524, 1973.

18. Seidl, E. On the morphology of the vascular system of the carotid body of cat and rabbit and its relation to the glomus type I cells. In: *The Peripheral Arterial Chemoreceptors,* ed. M. J. Purves. Cambridge: Cambridge University Press, 1975, pp. 293–299.

19. Taguchi, T. Blood vascular organization of the rat carotid body: a scanning electron microscopic study of corrosion casts. *Arch. Histol. Jpn. 49:* 243–254, 1986.

2

Assessment of the Diameter of Blood Vessels Linking the Arterial and Venous Systems in the Carotid Body of the Anesthetized Cat

R. G. O'REGAN, S. ENNIS, M. KENNEDY, AND J. BANNIGAN

The carotid body has an extensive and complex vasculature (13), in keeping with its enormous rate of blood perfusion (8). Based on a venous outflow from the carotid body of 38 μl/min and a carotid body wet weight of 1.8 mg, the organ's perfusion rate in the cat has been estimated to be 2 l/100g/min (8). However, a recent study involving morphological analysis of serial histological sections (7) indicates that the weight of the cat carotid body is considerably less than 1.8 mg and that the organ's perfusion rate is more likely to be 5 rather than 2 l/100g/min. Regardless of its true value, the carotid body perfusion rate is well in excess of that required to satisfy O_2 needs so that the organ's arteriovenous difference in O_2 content is trivial (8,17).

An unresolved problem concerning the control of blood flow in the carotid body is why tissue P_{O_2} values measured by electrodes inserted into the organ are substantially lower than those present in the venous blood draining the organ (3,22). Another puzzling feature is that carotid body tissue P_{O_2} and local flow, as measured by H_2 clearance electrodes, remain unaffected by hypercapnia (2), alterations in inflow perfusion pressure (2), and activation of autonomic nerves supplying the organ (4), although total blood flow as determined by measurement of the organ's venous outflow undergoes appropriate changes in these conditions (4,8,15,17). Moreover, despite changes in carotid body total blood flow during steady-state changes in systemic arterial blood pressure (BP), sinus nerve chemosensory activity remains unaltered (6,12) indicating autoregulation of blood flow in the capillary network of the specific chemoreceptor tissue of the organ.

A possible explanation for the lower P_{O_2} levels in tissue versus venous blood and the different responses of total versus local flow in the carotid body could be the presence of shunt pathways linking the arterial and venous systems either on or within the organ. Such pathways would contribute arterial blood to the veins draining the capillary network of the specific tissue of the carotid body, would be under the control of the autonomic nervous system, and would alter their caliber in response to hypercapnia and changes in BP. On the basis of histological studies and microscopic examination of the carotid body vasculature during hypercapnia, hypoxia, hyperoxia, and changes in BP, De Castro (9) reported that superficially located arteriovenous anastomoses are a constant feature of the organ's circulation. Subsequent investigations, however, have been equivocal in that some workers have described arteriovenous anastomoses on the surface of the carotid body whereas others have denied it (see refs. 13,16). As an example of this uncertainty, Seidl (19) reported that serial reconstructions of thin sections of 14 cat carotid bodies showed no arteriovenous anastomoses, yet the same worker together with other coauthors (18) reported that these vessels could be demonstrated in at least some resin cast models of the carotid body of the same species. Direct connections between arterioles and venules within, rather than on, the carotid body have recently been demonstrated (14) and could account for shunt channels in the organ. Alternatively, shunt pathways could be wide capillaries in the microcirculation of the carotid body specific tissue, as have been described by various investigators (10,14).

Another explanation for the lower Po_2 levels of the carotid body versus the venous drainage is that plasma skimming causes a reduction in hematocrit and, therefore, oxygen delivery in the blood perfusing the capillaries of the specific tissue of the organ (1). This proposal of variable hematocrit of carotid body capillary blood has not received experimental support (21).

In order to supplement morphological studies on the carotid body vasculature, we injected inelastic latex spheres of varying diameters into the arterial supply of the carotid body in in vivo experiments and examined the venous drainage of the organ for their presence, in order to elucidate the maximum diameter of latex spheres traversing the carotid body circulation. At the end of the experiments, the organs were fixed and then processed for light and electron microscopy to determine vascular lodgment sites of the latex spheres.

METHODS

Experiments were carried out on nine spontaneously breathing adult cats (1.9–3.0 kg) anesthetized with pentobarbitone sodium (induction, 42–48 mg/kg, i.p.; maintenance, 6–12 mg, i.v. as required). Cannulae were inserted into a femoral vein, a femoral artery, and the trachea low in the neck. The blood pressure was continuously monitored (Statham P23A transducer; Grass Models 7DAC, 7PIA amplifiers) and recorded on an ink writing oscillograph (Grass Model 7WC 12 PA). Arterial blood samples were withdrawn periodically for determination of gas tensions and pH (Radiometer). Nonrespiratory acidosis was corrected by i.v. administration of sodium bicarbonate (1–5 mmol/kg). The rectal temperature was continuously monitored and maintained at 37°C by use of a thermostatically controlled electric blanket (Harvard Apparatus Ltd.). Heparin (1000 i.v./kg) was periodically administered throughout the experiments. Midline structures in the neck, including parts of the trachea, larynx, pharynx, and esophagus, were reflected cranially to expose the right carotid bifurcation.

Collection and Measurement of the Venous Outflow from the Carotid Bifurcation

The technique used for this procedure has been described in detail elsewhere (15). In summary, a venous segment (usually the transverse pharyngeal vein) that received the venous drainage from the right carotid bifurcation (mainly the carotid body) and that was sufficiently large for the insertion of a siliconed glass capillary tube was vascularly isolated from all neighboring structures apart from the carotid bifurcation. Tributaries of the carotid bifurcation vein or veins were tied. Blood flowing from the capillary tube inserted into the isolated venous segment was led to a collecting pipette by polyethylene (Polythene) tubing. The volume of the capillary and polyethylene tubing was 0.12 ml. The rates of venous outflow from the carotid bifurcation were obtained by timing the advancing column of blood in the collecting pipettes over distances corresponding to volumes of 5–20 μl.

Administration of Latex Spheres

A thin cannula, inserted into the right lingual artery and pushed caudally into the common carotid artery until its tip lay in this vessel low in the neck, was used to inject large inelastic latex spheres having a mean diameter (in μm) of 25.7 $\pm$ 5.8 SD (21 trials). In three further trials, latex spheres with a mean diameter of 45.0 μm (no data available on SD) were injected intracarotidly (i.c.). After the i.c. injection of latex spheres of known size and concentration (4.15×10^3–11.1×10^5/ml) in 0.5-ml doses, the venous outflow of the carotid bifurcation was measured and collected in 0.1-ml samples. Smears obtained from the venous blood samples were systematically examined for the presence or absence of latex spheres with a light microscope. All latex spheres located were counted and their diameters measured. In initial experiments, some difficulties were encountered in locating the colorless latex spheres in the blood smears, and it was decided to color the interior of the particles with Sudan Black, an oil-soluble dye, using a technique described elsewhere (5). As discrete purple-to-black particles, the latex spheres were more readily identified in the blood smears. Where doubt existed, verification that spheres were indeed latex was obtained by use of a polarizing microscope.

Histological Techniques

At the end of each experiment, the carotid bifurcation, including the carotid body, was dissected from the animal and then fixed by immersion in a buffered 2% glutaraldehyde solution. Because of the presence of latex spheres lodged in carotid body blood vessels, it was not feasible to fix the organ by perfusion. The specimen was processed for light and electron microscopy with the use of conventional techniques. For light microscopy, semithin sections (1–2 μm) were cut, mounted, and

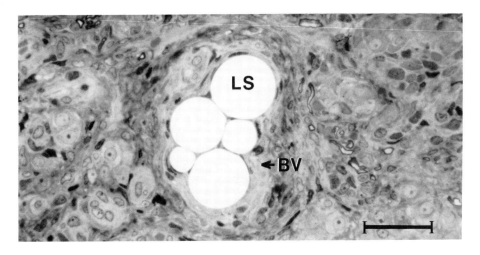

Fig. 2.1 Light micrograph of a carotid body section (thickness, 1.0 μm) showing a small muscular blood vessel (BV; diameter, 70.0 μm) containing aggregated latex spheres (LS; diameter, 10.0–30.0 μm). Bar = 30.0 μm.

stained with 1% toluidine blue in a 1% borax solution. These sections were used for the location and measurement of latex spheres within the carotid body vasculature and also for orientation purposes prior to ultrathin sectioning. Ultrathin sections, stained with uranyl acetate and lead citrate, were viewed in a Phillips 201C electron microscope and then photographed. Because sections randomly obtained from carotid bodies did not always show latex spheres, we decided to examine complete carotid bodies by using serial sectioning. When located, dyed latex spheres were found to be pale in color in both semithin and ultrathin sections, a circumstance that could be explained by either the thinness of the section or the leakage of dye from the sectioned spheres during processing.

RESULTS

Prior to i.c. injections of latex spheres, venous outflows from the carotid bifurcation varied considerably among experiments, having a mean value (± SD) of 36.1 ± 27.1 μl/min (range, 7–120 μl/min).

In the first experiment, an i.c. injection of 5.55×10^5 latex spheres (mean diameter, 25.7 μm) was associated with a gross reduction of venous outflow to 1.3 μl/min from a control level of 30 μl/min, and no spheres were located in the venous blood. As shown in Fig. 2.1, light microscopy (and also electron microscopy, not shown) revealed aggregates of latex spheres lodged in muscular vessels in the carotid body, and these lodgments were obviously responsible for the impairment of blood flow. Administration of smaller numbers of latex spheres (2.075–8.300 × 10^3 i.c.) induced a variable but lesser reduction in venous outflow. Thus, after i.c.

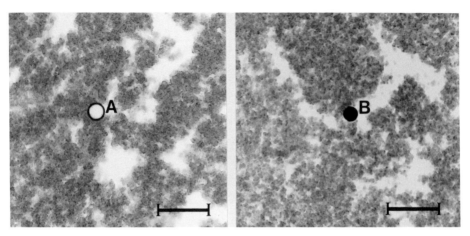

Fig. 2.2 Blood smears showing undyed (**A**) and dyed (**B**) latex spheres present in the venous outflow of the carotid bifurcation. Bar = 100.0 μm.

injections of these numbers of latex spheres having mean diameters of 25.7 μm (20 trials) and 45.0 μm (3 trials), venous outflows showed reductions of 26.7 $\pm$ 20.5% (range, 0–68%). In 15 out of 23 trials following these injections, latex spheres were found in the venous effluent of the carotid bifurcation. Overall, 56 latex spheres with a mean diameter ($\pm$ SD) of 28.1 $\pm$ 8.7 μm (range, 10.0–52.5 μm) were located. Examples of undyed and dyed latex spheres as found in the venous blood can be seen in Fig. 2.2.

Latex spheres did appear in samples of venous blood taken soon after the i.c. injections, indicating a relatively unrestricted passage through vessels linking arteries and veins in the carotid bifurcation. However, a sizable number of spheres took some considerable time to appear in the venous effluent, reflecting a degree of restriction of their passage through those linkage vessels. A major aim of this study was to ascertain if conditions such as hypoxia, hypercapnia, and activation of autonomic efferent nerves supplying the carotid body could modify the passage of microspheres through the organ. Of necessity this assessment involved comparison of successive trials in the same experiment. The slow appearance of microspheres in the venous blood samples after their i.c. administration, however, renders successive trials useless for this purpose. The difficulties in the interpretation of results obtained in successive trials is well illustrated in Figure 2.3. This figure shows the numbers of latex spheres located in successive 0.1-ml samples after two i.c. injections of these spheres. Spheres were observed in the third venous sample after the first injection. This finding indicates a reasonably rapid passage of the latex spheres through linkage vessels, especially when one considers that the volume of the collecting cannulae was 0.12-ml. Latex spheres found in subsequent venous samples suffered restriction of passage as judged by their latency of appearance. Three latex spheres appeared in the first sample obtained after the second i.c. injection. Because of the volume of the collecting cannulae, these spheres could not have resulted

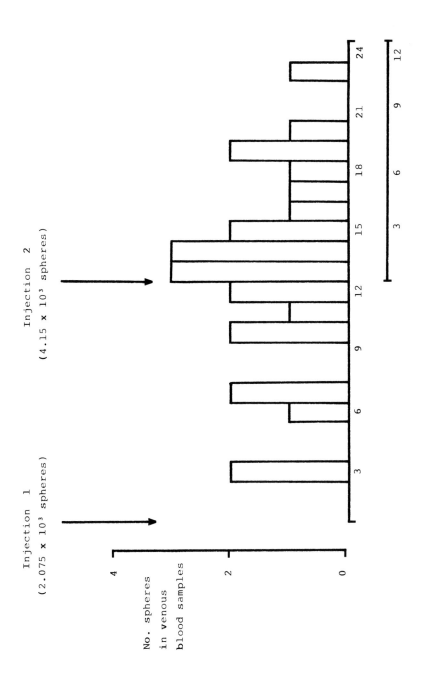

Fig. 2.3 Quantities of latex spheres appearing in sequential (numbered on *x* axis) 0.1-ml samples of carotid bifurcation venous blood. The times of the i.c. injections of latex spheres are indicated by the arrows (see text).

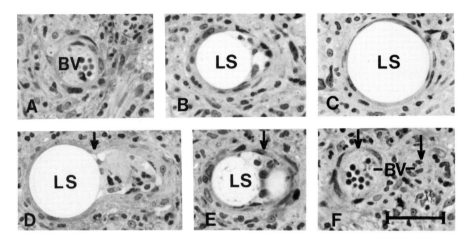

Fig. 2.4 Selected micrographs of a serially sectioned muscular blood vessel (BV) within the carotid body, showing the appearance and subsequent disappearance of a latex sphere (LS). **(A)** Section taken prior to appearance of the sphere; **(B–E)** sections through the latex sphere; **(F)** section taken after disappearance of the latex sphere. During D, E, and F, the blood vessel bifurcates (see arrows). For further information, consult text. Bar = 30.0 μm.

from this injection; rather, they were the consequence of a slow passage through linkage vessels after their i.c. administration in the first injection. Thereafter, spheres were present in all of the seven venous samples taken after the second injection, but whether they were derived from this or the first injection is conjectural.

Light microscopic examination of serial sections of carotid bodies removed at the end of the experiment showed latex spheres at locations throughout the extent of the organ with substantial numbers of the spheres (range, 5–45 μm; mean diameter, 28.0 ± 10.7 μm) located inside muscular vessels, mainly within, but sometimes outside, the specific tissue of the organ. Occasionally, these vessels contained trains of latex spheres. Figure 2.4 illustrates the appearance and subsequent disappearance of a latex sphere in selected sections of a series of 50 serial sections (1.0 μm in thickness) of a muscular vessel centrally located within the carotid body. This example was taken after three i.c. injections of latex spheres, the last of which contained spheres having a mean diameter of 45.0 μm. Figure 2.4A, a section taken before the appearance of the latex sphere, shows the muscular vessel (12.8 μm in diameter) containing blood. The sixth section of the series (Fig. 2.4B) shows a latex sphere located in the same vessel, which now has a diameter of 28.8 μm. The sphere at its maximum diameter (45.0 μm) can be seen in Fig. 2.4C; its size is such that it greatly dilates the blood vessel, causing a marked attenuation of its wall; this section was 25th in the series. In the next two sections (36th and 46th in the series), the sphere is decreasing in diameter in the vessel, which is in the process of branching in an oblique fashion (Fig. 2.4D,E). In the final section (50th in the series), the sphere has disappeared and the vessel diameter has decreased to 17.6 μm (Fig. 2.4F). The branch of this vessel can be seen alongside (see arrows).

DISCUSSION

The investigation shows that uniform inelastic latex spheres of up to 52.5-μm diameter can pass from the arterial to the venous systems of the carotid bifurcation in anesthetized cats. In histological studies, latex spheres, of much the same diameter as those appearing in the venous effluent of the carotid bifurcation, were found in small muscular blood vessels in the specific tissue of the carotid body. On the other hand, few latex spheres were located outside the carotid body tissue. It should be noted that structures apart from the carotid body make a trivial contribution to the venous effluent of the carotid bifurcation (8). On the basis of these observations we can assume that most, if not all, of the latex spheres traversed the carotid body circulation before they appeared in the venous outflow of the carotid bifurcation.

A major snag in morphological studies designed to determine diameters of blood vessels in fixed specimens of the carotid body concerns the inaccuracies introduced by variable shrinkage of tissues during processing procedures. The experiments we conducted in vivo do not suffer from this disadvantage and, consequently, should more accurately assess the diameters of arteriovenous linkage vessels which are, in this preparation, capable in themselves of both active and passive alterations in caliber. In this context, we noted that some latex spheres appeared in samples of venous blood obtained soon after their i.c. administration, indicating a relatively free passage through the carotid body circulation. However, other latex spheres, especially those of the largest size, took some considerable time to traverse the circulation of the organ before eventually entering the venous outflow of the carotid bifurcation. This reflects a restriction of their passage in the organ's circulation. In light microscopic studies of serial sections of carotid bodies, latex spheres, sometimes in trains, were found to be lodged in muscular blood vessels within the specific tissue of the organ. It is probable, therefore, that the slow passage of spheres through arteriovenous linkage vessels in the carotid body stems from their gradual propulsion, either actively (smooth muscle contraction) or passively (blood pressure), through these vessels to appear eventually in the venous outflow. Nonetheless, the diameter of the latex spheres that did reach the venous effluent may reflect the caliber that these vessels are capable of achieving in normal circumstances.

A question posed by this investigation concerns the category and location of arteriovenous linkage vessels that permit the passage of latex spheres of such substantial size. Passage through arteriovenous anastomoses located on the surface of the carotid body is a distinct possibility, but, as previously mentioned, the occurrence of these vessels is debatable. Injection of specimens with Indian ink or colored gelatine, perfusion of organs with latex, and corrosion cast models have been the usual techniques employed for locating arteriovenous anastomoses on the surface of the carotid body (see ref. 13). However, when these techniques are employed, it is difficult to accurately distinguish true arteriovenous anastomoses from junctions that in reality represent vessels crossing each other or from loci where extravasation of material may have produced artificial junctions. Nonetheless, scanning electron microscopy of resin casts of the carotid body vasculature has successfully demonstrated these vessels situated on the surface of the organ

(18). Because of its considerable depth of focus and the possibility of viewing the casts at various perspectives, the scanning electron microscope should permit a precise evaluation of the surface vasculature of the carotid body. When superficially located arteriovenous anastomoses have been described, they take two distinct forms (18). The first form consists of short noncapillary vascular links which resemble a bridge between artery and vein; these are consequently designated "bridge anastomoses." The second variety are much longer, are coiled, and display modified cells in the arterial wall. It must be stressed, however, that reconstruction of blood vessels observed in serial sections of the carotid body has failed to demonstrate superficially situated arteriovenous anastomoses in either the cat (19) or the rat (14). In the current investigation, latex spheres were found mainly in muscular vessels within the specific tissue of the carotid body. Further investigation is needed to determine if spheres in blood vessels outside the carotid body were in arteriovenous anastomoses or in small arteries destined to supply either this organ or adjacent structures.

Latex spheres could have traversed short connections directly linking arterioles and venules in the carotid body. However, although these connections have been described in the rat carotid body (14), they are of small diameter (ca. 10.0 μm) and their presence in the cat carotid body has not been demonstrated (19). In the investigation reported here, the muscular vessels where latex spheres lodged could have been the arteriolar portion of arteriolar–venular connecting vessels. Further investigation of serial sections of carotid bodies will be needed to investigate this possibility.

Thoroughfare channels in the form of wide capillaries in the microcirculation of the carotid body are further possibilities to explain the passage of latex spheres from the arterial to the venous systems of this organ. In the cat, De Castro and Rubio (10) have described convoluted capillaries 14–28 μm in diameter, and these vessels may represent preferential pathways traversed by latex spheres. Other capillaries described by De Castro and Rubio (10) are short, but of a smaller diameter (6–12 μm). Wide capillaries similar to those described in the cat have been demonstrated also in the rat (14,20), but their caliber varies considerably throughout the long course through the specific tissue of the carotid body. In our investigation, latex spheres were never found in carotid body blood vessels lacking a muscular coat. We would have expected some spheres to be lodged in capillaries if these vessels were those that permitted the slow passage of spheres through the circulation of the organ. From our studies to date, which are admittedly not complete, we would consider arteriovenous or arteriolar–venular anastomoses within the carotid body as the most likely vessels permitting the passage of the latex spheres that we found in the venous drainage of the carotid bifurcation.

Intracarotid injection of approximately a million latex spheres was followed by a gross reduction in the venous outflow from the carotid bifurcation; furthermore, in this circumstance, aggregates of spheres were found to be lodged in muscular blood vessels in the carotid body. This embolization of carotid body vasculature by latex spheres resembles the results obtained when lycopodium spores are used to abolish carotid chemoreceptor reflexes while at the same time keeping baroreceptor function in the neighboring carotid sinus intact (see ref. 11). This investigation provides evidence that i.c. injection of particles can successfully produce virtually total carotid body ischemia and, therefore, abolition of carotid chemoreceptor function. However, because the major blood supply to the carotid sinus is derived from the same artery as that supplying the carotid body (14), there must be some likelihood of impairment of baroreceptor function during such embolization procedures. Recording of sinus nerve chemosensory and barosensory discharges after i.c. injections of high concentrations of latex spheres could be of benefit in exploring this possibility.

A puzzling feature of our investigation is that, in some trials, i.c. injections of a few thousand latex spheres did not induce much reduction in the venous outflow of the carotid bifurcation, although spheres were subsequently found to be lodged in muscular blood vessels in the carotid body. It is possible that anastomotic connections between carotid body blood vessels may permit an effective compensation even when there is widespread embolization within the organ. Once more it would be of interest to assess this possibility by recording the effects on sinus nerve chemosensory activity of an i.c. injection of the smaller concentration of latex spheres.

As previously pointed out, total blood flow through the carotid body appears to represent two fractions, one of which (local flow) is unaffected by changes in blood pressure and hypercapnia (2) as well as by activation of autonomic efferent nerves supplying the organ (4). The other fraction, presumed to represent flow through shunt pathways, undergoes appropriate alterations in the above circumstances (see ref. 16). Another feature that distinguishes local from total flow is the finding that hypoxic hypoxia decreases local flow (2,4) while at the same time accentuates total flow (17). It would be of interest therefore, to ascertain if the passage of latex spheres through arteriovenous linkage vessels in the carotid body is affected by activation of autonomic nerves supplying the organ (sympathetic, vasoconstrictor; parasympathetic, vasodilator), close arterial infusion of vasoactive agents, alterations in inflow perfusion pressure, hypoxia, and hypercapnia. Although such an investigation could give more information on the control of so-called shunt flow in the carotid body, our experience to date indicates some experimental difficulties arising from the considerable intertrial variability in the recovery of latex spheres in the venous outflow from the carotid bifurcation after their i.c. injection. It is obvious that this variability could prevent meaningful quantitative analysis.

CONCLUSIONS

Latex spheres of a mean diameter of 28.1 μm and up to a diameter of 52.5 μm were shown to be capable of passing from the common carotid artery to the venous drainage of the carotid body. Some latex spheres appeared in the venous blood soon after their injection into the common carotid artery, indicating a relatively free passage through the carotid body circulation. Other spheres lodged in muscular blood vessels in the carotid body and were then gradually propelled through the circulation to enter the venous outflow of the organ. After intracarotid injections, latex spheres did not lodge in carotid body capillaries. We conclude that the latex spheres reached the venous drainage of the carotid body by traversing arteriovenous or arteriolar–venular anastomoses mainly located within the specific tissue of the organ.

REFERENCES

1. Acker, H., and D. W. Lübbers. The kinetics of local tissue Po_2 decrease after perfusion stop within the carotid body of the cat in vivo and in vitro. *Pflügers Arch. 369:* 135–140, 1977.
2. Acker, H., D. W. Lübbers, and H. Durst. The relationship between local and total flow of the cat carotid body at changes of blood pressure, arterial Po_2 and Pco_2. *Bibl. Anat. 15:* 395–398, 1977.
3. Acker, H., D. W. Lübbers, and M. J. Purves. Local oxygen tension field in the glomus caroticum of the cat and its change at changing arterial Po_2. *Pflügers Arch. 329:* 136–155, 1971.
4. Acker, H., and R. G. O'Regan. The effects of stimulation of autonomic nerves on carotid body blood flow in the cat. *J. Physiol. (Lond.) 315:* 99–110, 1981.
5. Bangs, L. B. *Uniform Latex Particles.* Indianapolis: Seragen Diagnostics Inc., 1985, p. 40.
6. Biscoe, T. J., G. W. Bradley, and M. J. Purves. The relation between carotid body chemoreceptor discharge, carotid sinus pressure and carotid body venous flow. *J. Physiol. (Lond.) 208:* 99–120, 1970.
7. Clarke, J. A., M. de B. Daly, and H. W. Ead. Dimensions and volume of the carotid body in the adult cat, and their relation to the specific blood flow through the organ. *Acta Anat. 126:* 84–86, 1986.
8. Daly, M. de B., C. J. Lambertsen, and A. Schweitzer. Observations on the volume of blood flow and oxygen utilization of the carotid body in the cat. *J. Physiol. (Lond.) 125:* 67–89, 1954.
9. De Castro, F. Sur la structure de la synapse dans les chémocepteurs: leur mécanisme d'excitation et rôle dans la circulation sanguine locale. *Acta Physiol. Scand. 22:* 14–43, 1951.
10. De Castro, F., and M. Rubio. The anatomy and innervation of the blood vessels of the carotid body and the role of chemoreceptive reactions in the autoregulation of the blood flow. In: *Wates Foundation Symposium on Arterial Chemoreceptors,* ed. R. W. Torrance. Oxford: Blackwell Scientific, 1968, pp. 267–277.
11. Heymans, C., and E. Neil. *Reflexogenic Areas of the Cardiovascular System.* London: Churchill, 1958, pp. 135–136.
12. Lahiri, S., T. Nishino, A. Mokashi, and E. Mulligan. Relative responses of aortic body and carotid body chemoreceptors to hypotension. *J. Appl. Physiol. 48:* 781–788, 1980.
13. McDonald, D. M. Peripheral chemoreceptors: structure–function relationships of the carotid body. In: *The Regulation of Breathing,* Part 1, ed. T. F. Hornbein. New York: Marcel Dekker, 1981, pp. 105–319.
14. McDonald, D. M., and D. T. Larue. The ultrastructure and connections of blood vessels supplying the rat carotid body and carotid sinus. *J. Neurocytol. 12:* 117–153, 1983.
15. Neil E., and R. G. O'Regan. The effects of electrical stimulation of the distal end of the cut sinus and aortic nerves on peripheral arterial chemoreceptor activity in the cat. *J. Physiol. (Lond.) 215:* 15–32, 1971.
16. O'Regan, R. G., and S. Majcherczyk. Control of peripheral chemoreceptors by efferent nerves. In: *Physiology of the Peripheral Arterial Chemoreceptors,* ed. H. Acker and R. G. O'Regan. Amsterdam: Elsevier, 1983, pp. 257–298.

17. Purves, M. J. The effect of hypoxia, hypercapnia and hypotension upon carotid body blood flow and oxygen consumption in the cat. *J. Physiol. (Lond.)* 209: 395–416, 1970.
18. Schäfer, D., E. Seidl, H. Acker, H. P. Keller, and D. W. Lübbers. Arteriovenous anastomoses in the cat carotid body. *Z. Zellforsch.* 142: 515–524, 1973.
19. Seidl, E. On the variability of form and vascularization of the cat carotid body. *Anat. Embryol.* 149: 79–86, 1976.
20. Taguchi, T. Blood vascular organization of the rat carotid body: a scanning electron microscopic study of corrosion casts. *Arch. Histol. Jpn.* 49: 243–254, 1986.
21. Verna, A. The carotid body blood supply: evidence against plasma skimming. In: *Arterial Chemoreceptors,* ed. C. Belmonte, D. J. Pallot, H. Acker, and R. W. Torrance. Leicester, UK: Leicester University Press, 1981, pp. 336–340.
22. Whalen, W. J., J. Savoca, and P. Nair. Oxygen tension measurements in carotid body of the cat. *Am. J. Physiol.* 225: 986–991, 1973.

3

New Evidence for High Blood Flow in the Carotid Body

E. MULLIGAN, S. BARNETT, L. C. WAGERLE, AND S. LAHIRI

The carotid body rapidly senses changes in arterial Po_2 and Pco_2 and the resulting chemoreflex affects the appropriate changes in ventilation. Carotid body blood flow measured by direct venous effluent measurement has been reported to be of the order of 2000 ml/(100g · min) (4), which is the highest flow reported for any organ in the body. This measurement was made by collecting the venous effluent from the carotid body area. The carotid body is difficult to isolate vascularly. Collection of venous effluent therefore potentially overestimates carotid body blood flow because of the possibility of collecting flow from tissues other than the carotid body or flow from vessels that course around the carotid body. Also, any flow through large arteriovenous (AV) shunts that may be present in the carotid body vasculature (5) would be included in the measurement of venous effluent.

We therefore decided to use the radioactive microsphere technique (7,10) to measure carotid body blood flow. This technique is noninvasive with respect to the carotid body, as it does not involve vascular isolation of the carotid body and does not require any surgery in the vicinity of the carotid body. This method measures flow only to the carotid body tissue and, with selection of the appropriate size microsphere, avoids measurement of flow through large AV shunts. The microsphere method also offers the advantage that flow to many tissues can be measured simultaneously. Thus the blood flow to the carotid body can be compared to that of other tissues in the same animal.

METHODS

The radioactive microsphere technique was used to measure carotid body flow as well as blood flow to other tissues in the cat (7,10). Thirteen cats were anesthetized with sodium pentobarbital (25 mg/kg, i.p.). The animals were tracheostomized, paralyzed with gallamine triethiodide (3 mg/kg/h, i.v.) and mechanically ventilated with air or air plus O_2 (P_aO_2 = 101 ± 5.6 torr, P_aCO_2 = 28.4 ± 0.8 torr, pH_a = 7.371 ± 0.013). Catheters were placed in a femoral vein, in both femoral arteries for continuous monitoring of blood pressure and for reference blood withdrawal for the microsphere technique, and in the left brachial artery also for reference blood withdrawal. A catheter placed in the left atrium was used for injection of radioactive microspheres. This was performed by exposing the heart through an incision in the fifth intercostal space and collapsing a lobe of the left lung with saline-soaked gauze. After the catheter was placed, the lung was reinflated. The cats were heparinized. Tracheal tidal PCO_2 was monitored continuously (Beckman LB-2), and arterial blood gases were measured (Radiometer) before and after microsphere injection.

The microsphere technique was used to measure tissue blood flow (7,10). Radioactive microspheres of known diameters (25 μm, 15 μm, and 9 μm; labeled with ^{141}Ce, ^{95}Sr, and ^{46}Sc, respectively) were injected into the left atrium. During, and for 1 min following the injection, reference blood samples were withdrawn from the brachial and femoral arteries at a known flow rate (0.388 ml/min). The animal was then killed and the tissues were removed, weighed, and placed into counting vials for determination of radioactivity due to entrapped microspheres. The tissues removed for blood flow determination included the heart, the left and right kidneys, both adrenal glands, the pancreas, a lobe of the liver, the superior cervical ganglia, a portion of the left and right carotid arteries, and the carotid bodies. The carotid bodies were carefully dissected free from the carotid bifurcations and other surrounding tissue under a dissecting microscope.

The tissues and reference blood samples were counted for radioactivity in a gamma counter using standard techniques for radionuclide separation (7). Blood flow to the various tissues was calculated using the formula $Q = A_t \cdot Q_r/A_r$, where Q is the blood flow to the tissue (in ml/min), A_t and A_r are the activities (in counts/min) in the tissue and reference blood sample, respectively, and Q_r is the rate of withdrawal of the reference blood sample (ml/min). The brachial reference blood samples were used for this calculation because of the proximity of the brachial artery to the carotid body. There was always good agreement between the brachial and femoral blood samples. Blood flows are expressed as flow per 100 g of tissue (ml/(100g · min). The number of microspheres in each tissue sample could be calculated from the specific activity of the spheres.

In order to validate the method for the carotid body, experiments were performed to determine the appropriate size and number of microspheres for injection. For a ± 10% statistical accuracy using the microsphere method, Buckberg et al. (2) calculated that at least 400 microspheres must be entrapped within a tissue sample. In pilot experiments, we determined that measurement of blood flow with an injection of 5 million microspheres allowed a sufficient number of microspheres to be entrapped within the carotid bodies.

The microsphere method is useful in making serial measurements of tissue blood flow in the same animal. Because the carotid body is a small mass of tissue, experiments were performed to determine if serial measurements of blood flow could be made in the carotid body without seriously impeding its blood flow. To do this, we gave three consecutive injections of 5 million each of differently labeled

15-μm microspheres under the same blood gas conditions and compared the flows calculated for each injection.

RESULTS

Initially, three different sizes of microspheres (25, 15, and 9 μm) were injected simultaneously for blood flow measurements. When the 25-μm microspheres were used, either the animal died or the simultaneous measurement of blood flow with the other sizes of microspheres was very low or very variable. Further experimentation was therefore carried out using only the 15-μm and 9-μm microspheres.

Figure 3.1 shows the results of experiments in which blood flow to various tissues was determined via simultaneous injection of 9-μm and 15-μm microspheres. For most tissues, the blood flow calculated using the 9-μm microspheres was slightly less than that calculated using the 15-μm microspheres. For the liver, it was slightly greater. However, for the carotid bodies and the adrenal gland, the blood flow values using the 9-μm microspheres were about half of those calculated using the 15-μm microspheres. The blood flow to the carotid bodies was greater than the flow to any other organ measured.

Because the flow measurement for the carotid bodies was much lower when the 9-μm microspheres were used, further experiments were performed using the 15-μm microspheres. Figure 3.2 shows the results for the carotid bodies from experiments in which three consecutive determinations of blood flow were made using three consecutive injections of differently labeled 15-μm microspheres under the same blood gas conditions ($P_aO_2 = 101 \pm 5.6$ torr, $P_aCO_2 = 28.4 \pm 0.8$ torr, pH$_a$

Fig. 3.1 Comparison of tissue blood flows using 9-μm and 15-μm microspheres. Tissued: LK, left kidney; RK, right kidney; LVR, liver; PAN, pancreas; HRT, heart; ADR, adrenal glands; SCG, superior cervical ganglia; CBS, both carotid bodies; LCB, left carotid body; RCB, right carotid body. Flows are expressed as mean $\pm$ SE ($n = 4$).

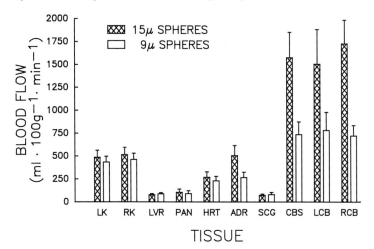

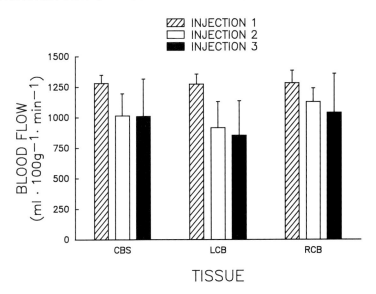

Fig. 3.2 Serial measurements of carotid body blood flow using 15-μm microspheres. Tissue abbreviations are as in Fig. 3.1. Mean $\pm$ SE (LCB, $n = 4$; RCB, $n = 3$; CBS, $n = 3$).

= 7.371 $\pm$ 0.013). The results show that mean carotid body blood flow decreased by about 20% after the first injection and that the variability of mean blood flow increased with each injection. The blood flow measured to other organs did not show this pattern.

The results for tissue blood flow determination using the 15-μm microspheres from the first group of cats and the results from the first injection of 15-μm microspheres from the second group of cats are combined in Fig. 3.3. The carotid bodies have the highest blood flow of any organ measured [1417 $\pm$ 143 ml/(100g $\cdot$ min)]. This is in stark contrast to the low flow of the carotid artery wall (Fig. 3.3) upon which or near which the carotid bodies lie.

DISCUSSION

In this study we determined that the radioactive microsphere technique could be used to measure cat carotid body blood flow and that the carotid bodies had the highest flow of any organ measured. This was true, for the data obtained with the 15-μm microspheres (Figs. 3.1 and 3.3) as well as the 9-μm microspheres (Fig. 3.1), although the carotid body flow measured using the 9-μm microspheres [Q_9; 736 $\pm$ 139 ml/(100g $\cdot$ min)] was only about half of that measured using the 15-μm microspheres (Q_{15}; 1417 $\pm$ 143 ml/100g/min). For most tissues, there was good agreement between the flows determined using the two microsphere sizes, with the 9-μm microspheres yielding a value slightly lower than the 15-μm microspheres (Fig. 3.1). This small difference occurs because a small amount of the 9-μm microspheres pass through the microcirculation of the tissues, resulting in an underestimation of tis-

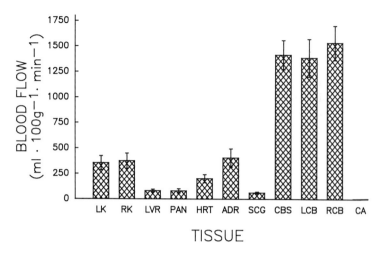

Fig. 3.3 Tissue blood flows using 15-μm microspheres. CA, carotid artery wall. Other tissues are as in Fig. 3.1. Mean $\pm$ SE ($n = 8$ for all tissues except RCB, $n = 7$; and CBS, $n = 7$). Carotid bodies have the highest flow.

sue blood flow by Q_9. The microvasculature in the carotid body and the adrenal glands must allow many more 9-μm microspheres to pass through because Q_9 is so much lower than Q_{15} in these tissues. Despite this, Q_9 to the carotid bodies is still higher than any other measured tissue blood flow. In agreement with Fan et al. (6), the liver shows a slightly higher Q_9 than Q_{15} (Fig. 3.1), because the small intestines do not effectively trap all of the 9-μm microspheres; they then pass into the portal vein and are entrapped in the liver (6).

The value of carotid body blood flow measured using the microsphere technique potentially underestimates the carotid body flow for the following reasons. Anatomically, the carotid body is surrounded by nervous and connective tissue and can be situated near or upon the wall of the carotid artery or occipitopharyngeal trunk (3,9). In dissecting the carotid bodies, every effort was made to completely remove all extraneous tissue. However, if any was left on the carotid bodies, this extra tissue with low flow (see Fig. 3.3 for carotid artery wall flow) would add to the weight of the carotid bodies without adding to the flow and would therefore result in an underestimation of carotid body flow.

The mean value of carotid body blood flow in this study was 1417 $\pm$ 143 ml/ (100g $\cdot$ min). This is somewhat less than the value of 2000 ml/(100g $\cdot$ min) reported by Daly et al. (4) and others (1,8), which was obtained by collecting the venous effluent, but it is still by far the highest blood flow measured for any tissue (Fig. 3.3). This high flow is consistent with the rapid responses of the carotid body chemoreceptors to changes in blood gas parameters and to blood-borne stimuli. If the AV shunts in the cat carotid body are large (5), then this high flow perfuses the specific tissue of the carotid body. If the AV shunts in the cat carotid body are not large, as has been reported for the rat carotid body by McDonald (Chap. 1, this volume), then the measurement of carotid body blood flow by the microsphere technique does not distinguish between flow to the specific tissue and shunt flow in the carotid body. Further analysis of this phenomenon awaits further microanatomical information on the cat carotid body. The results using the microsphere technique do, however, confirm that flow through the cat carotid body itself is high and that the bulk of the high flow measured by venous effluent collection (1,4,8) is not due to flow through vessels which course around the carotid body.

One of the advantages of the microsphere method is that for most tissues it can be used to make multiple sequential measurements of the blood flow to a tissue in the same animal (10). This possibility was examined for the carotid bodies by performing three consecutive blood flow determinations under the same blood gas conditions (Fig. 3.2). Because mean carotid body blood flow decreased by about 20% after the first injection, and because the variability of the flow determinations for the carotid bodies increased greatly, we concluded that multiple blood flow measurements using the microsphere technique were probably not appropriate for the carotid body since it comprises such a small amount of tissue. The other tissues examined did not show such decreases in mean blood flow with multiple flow measurements.

In summary, the radioactive microsphere technique, a new method for measuring blood flow that is noninvasive with respect to the carotid body, has been applied to the study of this organ and has provided new evidence indicating that this structure has the highest blood flow of any organ in the body.

ACKNOWLEDGMENTS

The authors are grateful to Dr. Stella Andronikou, Mark Alsberge, Joshua Madden, and Russell Roth for their valuable assistance. This work was supported in part by NIH grants HL-19737 (S.L.), NS-21068 (S.L.), HL-35339 (E.M.), and NS-19762 (L.C.W.).

REFERENCES

1. Acker, H., and R. G. O'Regan. The effects of stimulation of autonomic nerves on carotid body blood flow in the cat. *J. Physiol. (Lond.) 315:* 99–110, 1981.

2. Buckberg, G. D., J. C. Luck, D. B. Payne, J.I.E. Hoffman, J. P. Archie, and D. E. Fixler. Some sources of error in measuring regional blood flow with radioactive microspheres. *J. Appl. Physiol. 31:* 598–604, 1971.

3. Chungcharoen, D., M. de B. Daly, and A. Schweitzer. The blood supply of the carotid body in cats, dogs and rabbits. *J. Physiol. (Lond.) 117:* 347–358, 1952.

4. Daly, M. de B., C. J. Lambertsen, and A. Schweitzer. Observations on the volume of blood flow and oxygen utilization of the carotid body in the cat. *J. Physiol. (Lond.) 125:* 67–89, 1954.

5. De Castro, F., and M. Rubio. The anatomy and innervation of the blood vessels of the carotid body and the role of chemoreceptive reactions in the autoregulation of the blood flow. In: *Arterial Chemoreceptors,* ed. R. W. Torrance. Oxford: Blackwell Scientific, 1968, pp. 267–277.

6. Fan, F. C., G. B. Schuessler, R.Y.Z. Chen, and S. Chien. Determinations of blood flow and shunting of 9- and 15-μm spheres in regional beds. *Am. J. Physiol. 237 (Heart Circ. Physiol. 6):* H25–H33, 1979.

7. Heymann, M. A., B. D. Payne, J.I.E. Hoffman, and A. M. Rudolph. Blood flow measurements with radionuclide-labeled particles. *Prog. Cardiovasc. Dis. 20:* 55–79, 1977.

8. Purves, M. J. The effect of hypoxia, hypercapnia and hypotension upon carotid body blood flow and oxygen consumption in the cat. *J. Physiol. (Lond.) 209:* 395–416, 1970.

9. Verna, A. Ultrastructure of the carotid body in mammals. *Int. Rev. Cytol. 60:* 271–330, 1979.

10. Wagerle, L. C., T. M. Heffernan, L. M. Sacks, and M. Delivoria-Papadopoulos. Sympathetic effect on cerebral blood flow regulation in hypoxic newborn lambs. *Am. J. Physiol. 245 (Heart Circ. Physiol. 14):* H487–H494, 1983.

4

Morphology of the Carotid Body Chemoreceptor in Aged Primates

J. T. HANSEN

The monkey carotid body chemoreceptor possesses many of the morphological features typical of this organ in other mammalian species studied thus far (4). Numerous studies have documented the fine structure of the mammalian carotid body under normal and a variety of experimental conditions in an effort to understand structure–function relationships during chemoreception (see refs. 3,6,7). However, little is known about the fine structure of this organ in aged mammals, and how carotid body morphology in older species may contribute to respiratory reflexes. Therefore, in an effort to understand better how carotid body morphology may be influenced by the natural aging process, the following study was undertaken to examine this chemoreceptor in a select group of aged primates.

MATERIALS AND METHODS

Six female rhesus monkeys *(Macaca mulatta),* each weighing over 5 kg and between 20 and 23 years old, were obtained from the National Institutes of Health (NICHD) for various studies related to aging. All animals were anesthetized with sodium pentobarbital (35 mg/kg, i.v.) prior to tissue collection and sacrifice. Carotid bodies from two of the monkeys were processed for catecholamine histofluorescence using the glyoxylic acid technique of de la Torre (2). Carotid bodies from the remaining four primates were processed for electron microscopy, after intracardiac perfusion with a fixative containing 4% paraformaldehyde. The carotid bodies were quickly removed and immersion-fixed for an additional 24 h in 3% glutaraldehyde, 2% paraformaldehyde in 0.1 M cacodylate buffer. The tissues then were routinely processed for electron microscopy, including post-fixation in osmium tetroxide. Because a variety of other studies were being carried out on these valuable animals, initial perfusion fixation did not include glutaraldehyde. Nevertheless, tissue preservation was excellent, and the occurrence of "dark" cells indicative of poor fixation and tissue anoxia were not observed.

RESULTS

Light and Fluorescence Microscopy

The carotid body of the aged monkey no longer resembled a well-encapsulated, discretely defined organ, as is more typical of the younger primate organ (Fig. 4.1a). Glomus cells still were organized into small lobules of cells, but the number of cells comprising each lobule numbered only three or four in any single cross section. The glomus cells exhibited a bright catecholamine-induced fluorescence, although some lobules were less fluorescent than others (Fig. 4.1b). Connective tissue elements formed a meshwork around and between the isolated lobules of cells. Most lobules were separated from one another by interstitial spaces that measured from 5 to 20 μm or more.

Electron Microscopy

The diffuse nature of the glomus cell lobules was evident in low-power electron micrograhs (Fig. 4.1c). Characteristically, several glomus cells, ensheathed by their supporting cells and penetrated by one or several unmyelinated nerve fibers, comprised each lobule. The glomus cells possessed dense-core vesicles and other organelles typical of all mammalian glomus cells. Subtypes of glomus cells based upon dense-core vesicle size and numerical density were evident (Fig. 4.1d). Approximately one in 20 glomus cells demonstrated some signs of degeneration, including the presence of numerous cytoplasmic filaments, myelin figures, and aggregates of small electron-lucent vesicles (Fig. 4.2a). Glomus cells possessing a darker-staining cytoplasm and referred to as "dark" cells were not observed in any of the samples.

Interspersed among the lobules of glomus cells were numerous capillaries, fibroblasts, loosely organized collagenous fibers, and nerve fiber profiles surrounded by supporting or Schwann cell cytoplasmic processes (Figs. 4.1c and 4.2b).

Fig. 4.1 (a) Light micrograph showing several glomus cell lobules. The lobules are diffuse and lie within a tangle of connective tissue elements and small capillaries. The carotid body did not constitute a distinct encapsulated organ in the aged primate. v, blood vessel. Bar = 50 μm. (b) Micrograph showing the intense catecholamine histofluorescence of the glomus cells. Note the abundance of connective tissue and the dispersion of glomus cells into small lobules of 3 or 4 cells. Bar = 100 μm. (c) Electron micrograph showing a portion of one glomus cell lobule, several glomus cell processes (gp), and the large interstitial space filled with unmyelinated axons (a), collagen (co), and capillaries (c). Axons are numerous throughout the interstitium and in contact with glomus cells. Bar = 10 μm. (d) Two different types of glomus cells based upon the size and number of their dense-core vesicles. Glomus cells with a similar appearance are present in younger primate carotid bodies. Bar = 1 μm.

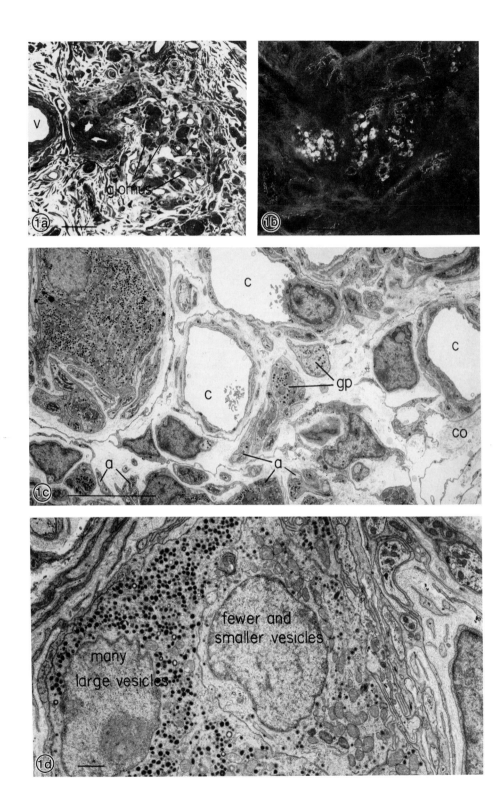

33

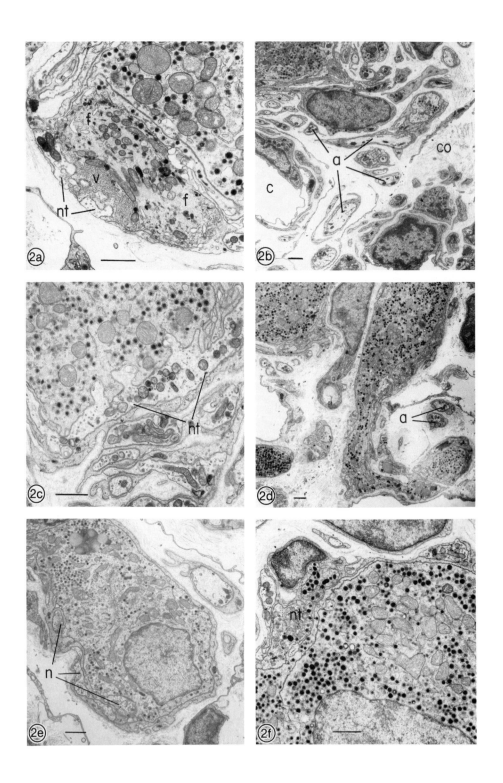

Small groups of several unmyelinated axons ensheathed by cytoplasmic processes were very common in the interstitium between the glomus cell lobules and capillaries.

Numerous unmyelinated axons were observed either directly in contact with the glomus cells or separated from the cells by a thin supporting cell cytoplasmic sheath (Fig. 4.2c–f). In any cross section, at least one axonal profile usually was in contact with a glomus cell, and in many instances several axons made contact. However, examination of over 200 axonal profiles in contact with glomus cells revealed not a single membrane specialization or junction indicative of a synaptic active zone. In all other respects, the axon terminals appeared normal.

DISCUSSION

This study represents the first ultrastructural analysis of the carotid body in aged primates. The general morphology of the glomus cells and nerve endings is similar to that described previously in younger primates (1,4). However, three significant differences exist which were present in all of the carotid bodies examined. First, the number of glomus cells that comprise each lobule is smaller, with only 3 or 4 cells per lobule in the older animals, compared to as many as eight cells in younger primate lobules (4). Second, glomus cell lobules in older primates are widely scattered, with large interstitial spaces filled with capillaries, fibroblasts, and groups of unmyelinated axonal profiles. Finally, although nerve endings directly adjacent to glomus cells are common, membrane specializations resembling synaptic contacts (synaptic active zones) are not observed.

Recently, Hurst et al. (5) reported on several histological changes in the human carotid body based upon necropsy material from 47 subjects, aged 14 to 100. They found a gradual decrease in the percentage of glomic tissue and a progressive fibrosis, perhaps due to the conversion of supporting cells to fibrocytes (5). These findings in humans agree with the present observations in the aged primate, although it cannot be determined from this study whether fibroblasts are derived from the carotid body supporting cells. Perhaps of greater significance is the observation of

←
_____

Fig. 4.2 (a) Portion of a glomus cell that may be undergoing degeneration. Note the abundance of cytoplasmic filaments (f), and the large number of small electron-lucent vesicles (v). Two nerve terminals make contact with this cell (nt). Bar = 1 μm. (b) Carotid body interstitial space filled with small axons (a) ensheathed in Schwann cell cytoplasm, capillaries (c), and collagen (co). These large areas of interstitium devoid of glomus cells are unique to the aged primate. Bar = 1 μm. (c) Nerve terminal (nt) which makes extensive contact with a glomus cell. Although nerves frequently contact glomus cells, membrane specializations typical of synaptic active zones are not observed. Bar = 1 μm. (d) Glomus cell, and its process adjacent to a capillary (at bottom of micrograph). Axons (a) are present both in the interstitial space and in contact with the glomus cell. Bar = 1 μm. (e) Glomus cell lobule with several nerves (n) either ensheathed in supporting cell cytoplasm or in contact with the glomus cell. No synaptic active zones are visible. Bar = 1 μm. (f) Portions of several glomus cells with a nerve terminal (nt). Synaptic active zones are not visible. Bar = 1 μm.

numerous axonal profiles, surrounded by Schwann cell sheaths, in these spaces. These axonal profiles may persist after the degeneration of glomus cells. Their presence in the interstitial compartment may be all that remains of a once functional glomus–nerve unit. Moreover, the nerve endings that are adjacent to the glomus cells do not possess membrane specializations reminiscent of synaptic active zones. Therefore, in addition to a decrease in glomic tissue, the aged carotid body also may become gradually denervated. This phenomenon could have implications with regard to ventilatory drive. A reduction in the innervation of the glomus cells in older individuals could mean a reduction in the chemoreflexes linked to ventilatory drive. Further physiological testing will be necessary to determine if there is a correlation between carotid body innervation in older animals and a decrease in the chemoreflex.

ACKNOWLEDGMENTS

Excellent technical assistance was provided by Mr. Andrew Howell. This research was supported by American Heart Association grant 86 733, PHS grants S7RR05403-25 and NS-22511, and the PEW Charitable Trust.

REFERENCES

1. Al-Lami, F., and R. G. Murray. Fine structure of the carotid body of *Macaca mulatta* monkey. *J. Ultrastruct. Res. 24:* 465–478, 1968.
2. de la Torre, J. C. An improved approach to histofluorescence using the SPG method for tissue monoamines. *J. Neurosci. Methods 3:* 1–15, 1980.
3. Fidone, S. J., and C. Gonzalez. Initiation and control of chemoreceptor activity in the carotid body. In: *Handbook of Physiology,* Sec. 3: *The Respiratory System,* Vol. 2: *Control of Breathing,* ed. N. S. Cherniack and J. G. Widdicombe. Bethesda: Am. Physiol. Soc., 1986, pp. 247–312.
4. Hansen, J. T. Ultrastructure of the primate carotid body: a morphometric study of the glomus cells and nerve endings in the monkey *(Macaca fascicularis). J. Neurocytol. 14:* 13–32, 1985.
5. Hurst, G., D. Heath, and P. Smith. Histological changes associated with aging of the human carotid body. *J. Pathol. 147:* 181–187, 1985.
6. McDonald, D. M. Peripheral chemoreceptors: structure–function relationships of the carotid body. In: *Regulation of Breathing,* Vol. 17, Part 1: *Lung Biology in Health and Disease,* ed. T. F. Hornbein. New York: Marcel Dekker, 1981, pp. 105–319.
7. Verna, A. Ultrastructure of the carotid body in the mammals. *Int. Rev. Cytol. 60:* 271–330, 1979.

5

Local Regulation of Sympathetic Ganglionic Activity During Acute Hypoxia

G. HANSON, C. GONZALEZ, A. OBESO, B. DINGER, AND S. FIDONE

Postganglionic sympathetic activity is essential for the mediation of homeostatic and behavioral responses of diverse neuroeffector organs in the periphery. An implicit postulate of sympathetic nervous system physiology is that postganglionic neuronal activity is controlled principally by central preganglionic neurons, whose cell bodies lie in the central nervous system. Among the variety of stimuli to which the sympathetic nervous system responds, one of the more important is systemic hypoxia, which significantly augments the neural output of the superior cervical sympathetic ganglion (SCG; ref. 19) and evokes prominent changes in heart rate and blood pressure. In the present study, we have tested the hypothesis that sympathetic ganglia—in particular, the superior cervical ganglion (SCG)—contain intrinsic mechanisms that respond locally to certain physiological stimuli, independently of central nervous system regulation. Our data show that hypoxia, at a level that activates the chemoreceptor response of the carotid body but fails to affect the metabolism of other nervous tissues, produces significant changes in neuropeptide (substance P and met-enkephalin) content and metabolism (2-deoxyglucose uptake) of isolated rabbit SCG. The results suggest that such stimuli, acting locally, may influence neurotransmission in the ganglion, as well as the interaction of postganglionic neurons with their neuroeffector organs.

METHODS

The experiments were conducted on adult New Zealand rabbits (2–2.5 kg). The animals used for the studies of ganglionic neuropeptides received unilateral sections of SCG preganglionic fibers and contralateral sham operations. Two weeks following surgery, the unanesthetized animals were placed singly in a clear Lucite chamber continuously flushed (4 l/min) with either room air or 5% O_2 in N_2 (certified gas mixture, $\pm 0.5\%$ of rated purity, IAP, Portland, OR) for two 30-min periods, with a 20-min interim. The animals were then anesthetized with sodium pentobarbital and respired with the appropriate gas mixture during surgical removal of the SCG. The ganglia were quickly cleaned of surrounding connective tissue in a bath of ice-cold modified Tyrode's medium (in mM: NaCl, 112; KCl, 4.7; $CaCl_2$, 2.2; $MgCl$, 1.1; sodium glutamate, 42; Hepes, 5; glucose, 5.6) equilibrated with either room air or 5% O_2 in N_2, and immediately frozen to $-20°C$ and stored at $-70°C$. Frozen ganglia were thawed and homogenized in 0.01 N HCl in preparation for radioimmunoassay. An aliquot was removed from each sample, and the protein content was measured according to Bradford (1). The remaining homogenate was heated in boiling water for 10 min to denature proteases, after which the samples were centrifuged and the resultant supernatant was removed and lyophilized. Samples were reconstituted with phosphate-buffered saline, pH 7.4, containing 0.1% gelatin. The reconstituted samples were halved and assayed for either substance P-like immunoreactivity (SPLI) or met-enkephalin-like immunoreactivity (MELI). The SPLI analysis has been described in detail by Hanson and Lovenberg (8). The SP antiserum used in this study could reliably detect 10 pg of synthetic bovine hypothalamic SP at a 1:200,000 dilution and displayed less than 2% cross-reactivity with neurokinin A, eledoisin, and physalaemin, three peptides structurally similar to SP. Analysis for MELI was done in a manner similar to that for SPLI except that after the additions of ^{125}I-labeled met-enkephalin (ME) and the ME antiserum, the samples were allowed to incubate at 4°C for 48 h, after which the charcoal separation was performed. The antiserum for MELI (Immunonuclear Corporation, Stillwater, MN, 55082) could reliably detect 10 pg of MELI and displayed less than 3% cross-reactivity with leu-enkephalin.

Glucose consumption was determined in vitro in normoxic (100% O_2) and hypoxic (20% O_2) media. The ganglia were removed, cleaned, and preincubated for 25 min (37°C) in 4 ml of Tyrode's solution equilibrated with 100% O_2 (pH = 7.4) and containing 3 mM glucose. After preincubation, the tissue samples were transferred to minivials containing 750 μl of Tyrode's incubation media with 3 mM glucose and 2 μM 2-[^3H]deoxyglucose ([^3H]2DG; 28 Ci/mmol, ICN) in accordance with the method described by Mata et al. (21). The experimental incubation media were equilibrated with 20% O_2 in N_2 gas. The incubation period was 5 min, and was followed by a 2-min wash (0–4°C) to remove extracellular [^3H]2DG. The reaction was terminated in 100 μl of ice-cold 0.4 N perchloric acid (PCA), and the tissues were weighed, homogenized in 250 μl of 0.4 N PCA, and centrifuged. A 200-μl volume of supernatant was combined with 55 μl of 0.8 M K_2CO_3 to precipitate $KClO_4$. The vials were recentrifuged, and 200 μl of supernatant was removed for analysis (of which 10 μl was directly counted). The separation of the phosphorylated and nonphosphorylated [^3H]2DG was achieved by ion-exchange chromatography as described by Gonzalez and Garcia-Sancho (5). The eluate contained 2-[^3H]deoxyglucose-6-phosphate ([^3H]2DG-6-P) which was counted; it contained less than 0.01% contamination by nonphosphorylated [^3H]2DG and had an overall recovery of [^3H]2DG-6-P of approximately 45%.

Table 5.1 Effects of Hypoxic Stress on SPLI and MELI in Rabbit SCG

	SPLI		MELI	
Condition	Sham-operated	Pregang. section	Sham-operated	Pregang. section
Air	340 ± 61 (5)	322 ± 51 (6)	1196 ± 108 (6)	174 ± 33 (6)
5% O_2 + 95% N_2	†216 ± 29 (6)	‡190 ± 10 (6)	‡811 ± 89 (5)	*190 ± 27 (5)

Note: Values (means ± SEM) are given in pg/mg protein; *n* values are shown in parentheses.

*$p < .4$, †$p < .05$, ‡$p < .025$, for breathing air as compared to 5% O_2/95% N_2 (*t*-test).

RESULTS

Table 5.1 shows the effects of hypoxia on the SP-like immunoreactivity (SPLI) and ME-like immunoreactivity (MELI) in normal and decentralized SCG. When compared with ganglia from animals exposed only to air ($\sim$20% O_2), hypoxia (5% O_2) reduced SPLI both in ganglia with intact preganglionic axons (36%), and in ganglia chronically isolated from the CNS by decentralization (41%). The 36% reduction in SPLI in sham-operated ganglia agrees with the reduction we previously observed in ganglia from unoperated animals which were similarly exposed to hypoxia (7). Decentralization alone did not alter the levels of SPLI in rabbit SCG. This latter observation confirms the findings of Robinson et al. (27), and substantiates the conclusion of Kessler and colleagues (14,15) that SP is associated with parenchymal elements within the ganglion. However, after decentralization, MELI in the ganglia was dramatically reduced to 15% of control, which implies that the majority of ME is associated with preganglionic axons and terminals, as has been suggested by others (10,26,28,32). Hypoxia reduced MELI in intact SCG, presumably as a result of increased sympathetic activity, but the small residual MELI in decentralized ganglia was unaffected by hypoxia. The hypoxia-induced reductions in neuropeptide levels in intact SCG appear to be a tissue-specific response because the levels of SPLI and MELI in nodose ganglia (SPLI: 580 ± 99 pg/mg protein; MELI: 50 ± 10 pg/ mg protein; mean ± SEM) were not significantly affected by low O_2 exposures in vivo. The possibility that reductions in SPLI were mediated by local afferent fibers that form reflex arcs within the SCG (30) is also unlikely because preliminary experiments in our laboratory have shown that the hypoxic response persists 14 days following resection of the glossopharyngeal nerve (the established source of afferent fibers to the SCG; refs. 2,29), and the results of preliminary experiments suggest that SPLI content is also reduced in ganglia exposed in vitro to low O_2-equilibrated superfusion media.

In a separate series of experiments, we measured the glucose consumption of ganglia that had been decentralized or sham-operated 48 h previously. The data presented in Table 5.2 show that the rate of [³H]2DG uptake in ganglia exposed in vitro to media equilibrated with 20% O_2 (a "hypoxic" stimulus in vitro) was double the rate observed in ganglia similarly exposed to 100% O_2-equilibrated media. Moreover, the response to the low-O_2 media persisted in chronically decentralized ganglia (Table 5.2), suggesting that increased glucose utilization occurs in structures

Table 5.2   Effects of Low O_2 on $^3H[2DG]$ Uptake by Rabbit SCG

	Glucose consumption under:	
	100% O_2 media	20% O_2 media
Normal	2.65 ± 0.13	*5.30 ± 0.33
Decentralized	3.10 ± 0.30	†6.60 ± 0.90

Note: Values (means ± SEM) are given in nmol/g/5min × 10^2.

*$p < .001$, †$p < .005$, for hypoxic versus normoxic conditions (t-test).

other than preganglionic axons and their terminals. In control experiments, we also tested the effects of "hypoxia" on the intermediary metabolism of nodose ganglia, and found that [^3H]2DG uptake in these sensory neurons was unchanged by exposure to the low O_2-equilibrated media (2.19 ± 0.39 × 10^{-2} nmol/g/5min in 100% O_2 media vs. 2.62 ± 0.35 × 10^{-2} nmol/g/5 min in 20% O_2 media; $p > .20$). This result, along with the findings of Ksiezak and Gibson (18), who showed that the ATP content and glucose consumption of brain slices in vitro are not affected by levels of hypoxia similar to those employed in this study, demonstrate that the low O_2-induced increase in glucose consumption observed in isolated SCG is a unique property of this nervous tissue.

DISCUSSION

These results suggest that the SCG contains internal mechanisms that are capable of responding to local chemosensory stimuli independent of preganglionic outflow from the CNS. The large reductions in SPLI observed after short hypoxic episodes in vivo or in vitro suggest that this neuropeptide may be released from its storage site(s) as a consequence of reduced local tissue Po_2. The implicit assumption is that decreases in neuropeptide levels during the relatively short period of exposure to hypoxia are indicative of increased release and subsequent rapid proteolysis. The relatively rapid changes in peptide concentrations that we observed in this study are unlikely to be due to alterations in protein synthesis, because Harmer and Keen (9) have shown that 8 h after complete blockade of protein synthesis, the SP levels in dorsal root ganglia remain unchanged. In the inferior mesenteric sympathetic ganglion, SP acts as an excitatory agent (3,12,17,29); however, an effect of SP on neuronal membrane properties or transmission in the SCG has not been reported. It is known that SP applied to the SCG in vitro modifies the activity of tyrosine hydroxylase (TH) (11,13), the rate-limiting enzyme for catecholamine synthesis. Catecholamines are found in the small, intensely fluorescent (SIF) (20) cells as well as the postganglionic neurons of the SCG; consequently, the release of SP during hypoxia may affect neurotransmission within the SCG, and/or the actions of postganglionic neurons on their peripheral neuroeffector organs.

The functional significance of the hypoxia-induced increase in glucose consumption in the SCG is not readily apparent. The elevated [^{3}H]2DG uptake in normal and decentralized SCG may signal a shift away from oxidative metabolism (i.e., Pasteur effect) in order to maintain neuronal function under conditions of hypoxic stress. However, the fact that levels of hypoxia used in this study failed to affect [^{3}H]2DG uptake by brain or other peripheral nervous tissue (18) suggests that the metabolic changes observed with the SCG might underlie specific chemosensory mechanisms similar to those thought to occur in the chemoreceptor tissue of the carotid body, a well-recognized O_2-sensitive organ. In the carotid body, spectrometric and fluorometric studies have suggested the presence of an unusual cytochrome oxidase with low affinity for oxygen (22), an indication that chemosensory transduction mechanisms in this tissue are linked to its energy metabolism. This suggestion is consistent with a recent report showing that hypoxia and other chemostimulants significantly reduce ATP levels in the carotid body (24), a property that is not shared by other nonchemosensory tissues.

In our experiments with the carotid body, we have observed that low O_2 reduces SP and increases glucose consumption in this tissue in a manner similar to that described here for the SCG (6,25). The chemosensitive apparatus in the carotid body is thought to reside with the type I (glomus) cells, which in many respects are similar to SIF cells of sympathetic ganglia. Both cell types contain neuropeptides and catecholamines, particularly dopamine, and are found in cell groups located adjacent to fenestrated capillaries (2,4,31). In both cases, stimulation of these cells releases dopamine, which acts as a transmitter to the next-order neuron (4,16,20). Whereas SIF cells appear to be interneurons interposed between preganglionic axon terminals and the principal postganglionic neurons (2,31), type I cells of the carotid body are thought to be preneural receptor elements innervated by sensory fibers of the IXth cranial nerve. However, it is noteworthy that type I cells also receive a preganglionic sympathetic innervation (4), and some SIF cells are also innervated by IXth nerve sensory fibers (2). In view of the sensitivity of the SCG to low-O_2 stimuli, the striking similarities between SCG–SIF cells and carotid body type I cells focuses attention on SIF cells as the likely detectors of changes in local tissue P_{O_2} in the SCG. Furthermore, the interneuronal disposition of SIF cells suggests a possible mechanism by which low O_2 might influence impulse traffic through the SCG.

In summary, a study of SCG exposed to brief hypoxic episodes suggests the existence of internal mechanisms that are capable of responding to local chemosensory stimuli. Such responses cannot be attributed to central influences, because the effects could be observed either in vitro or after decentralization in vivo. A recent report may suggest an interesting and important physiological interpretation for our results; it has been shown that postganglionic axons from the SCG are essential for preferentially enhancing the blood flow to cardiac and respiratory control centers in the brainstem during hypoxia (23). Thus, the demonstration that the SCG can respond to local physiological stimuli may have great significance for specific sympathetic ganglion functions under conditions of hypoxic stress. In a broader sense, the results reported here may suggest that neurotransmission through autonomic ganglia, in general, can be subject to local regulatory influences.

REFERENCES

1. Bradford, M. A rapid and sensitive method for the quantitation of micro organism quantities of protein utilizing the principle of protein-dye binding. *Anal. Biochem. 72:* 248–254, 1976.

2. Case, C. P., and M. R. Matthews. A quantitative study of structural features, synapses and nearest-neighbor relationships of small, granule-containing cells in the rat superior cervical sympathetic ganglion at various adult stages. *Neuroscience 15:* 237–282, 1985.

3. Dun, N. J., and A. G. Karczmar. Actions of substance P on sympathetic neurons. *Neuropharmacology 18:* 215–218, 1979.

4. Fidone, S. J., and C. Gonzalez. Initiation and control of chemoreceptor activity in the carotid body. In *Handbook of Physiology,* Sec. 3: *The Respiratory System,* Vol. 2: *Control of Breathing,* ed. N. S. Cherniack and J. G. Widdicombe. Bethesda, MD: Am. Physiol. Soc., 1986, pp. 247–312.

5. Gonzalez, C., and J. Garcia-Sancho. A sensitive assay for ATP. *Anal. Biochem. 114:* 285–287, 1981.

6. Hanson, G. R., L. Jones, and S. Fidone. Physiological chemoreceptor stimulation decreases enkephalin and substance P in the carotid body. *Peptides 7:* 767–769, 1986.

7. Hanson, G., L. Jones, and S. Fidone. Effects of hypoxia on neuropeptide levels in the rabbit superior cervical ganglion. *J. Neurobiol. 17:* 51–54, 1986.

8. Hanson, G., and W. Lovenberg. Elevation of substance P-like immunoreactivity in rat central nervous system by protease inhibition. *J. Neurochem. 35:* 1370–1374, 1980.

9. Harmer, A., and P. Keen. Chemical characterization of substance P-like immunoreactivity in primary afferent neurons. *Brain Res. 220:* 203–207, 1981.

10. Helen, P., P. Panula, H.-Y.T. Yang, A. Hervonen, and S. I. Rapoport. Location of substance P-, bombesin-, gastrin-releasing peptide-, [met⁵]enkephalin- and [met⁵]enkephalin-arg⁶-phe⁷-like immunoreactivities in adult human sympathetic ganglia. *Neuroscience 12:* 907–916, 1984.

11. Ip, N. Y., and R. E. Zigmond. Substance P inhibits the acute stimulation of ganglionic tyrosine hydroxylase activity by a nicotinic agonist. *Neuroscience 13:* 217–220, 1984.

12. Jiang, Z.-G., N. J. Dun, and A. G. Karczmar. Substance P: a putative sensory transmitter in mammalian autonomic ganglia. *Science 217:* 739–741, 1982.

13. Kessler, J. A., J. E. Alder, and I. B. Black. Substance P and somatostatin regulate sympathetic noradrenergic function. *Science 21:* 1059–1061, 1983.

14. Kessler, J. A., J. E. Alder, M. C. Bohn, and I. B. Black. Substance P in principal sympathetic neurons: regulation by impulse activity. *Science 214:* 335–336, 1981.

15. Kessler, J. A., and I. B. Black. Regulation of substance P in adult rat sympathetic ganglia. *Brain Res. 234:* 82–187, 1982.

16. Kobayashi, H. Roles of cyclic nucleotides in the synaptic transmission in sympathetic ganglia of rabbits. *Comp. Biochem. Physiol. 72C:* 197–202, 1982.

17. Konishi, S., and M. Otsuka. Blockade of slow excitatory post-synaptic potential by substance P antagonists in guinea-pig sympathetic ganglia. *J. Physiol. (Lond.) 361:* 115–130, 1985.

18. Ksiezak, H. J., and G. E. Gibson. Oxygen dependence of glucose and acetylcholine metabolism in slices and synaptosomes from rat brain. *J. Neurochem. 37:* 305–314, 1981.

19. Lahiri, S., S. Matsumoto, and A. Mokashi. Responses of ganglioglomerular nerve activity to respiratory stimuli in the cat. *J. Appl. Physiol. 60:* 391–397, 1986.

20. Libet, B., and C. Owman. Concomitant changes in formaldehyde-induced fluorescence of dopamine interneurons and slow inhibitory postsynaptic potentials of the rabbit

superior cervical ganglion induced by stimulation of the preganglionic nerve or by a muscarinic agent. *J. Physiol. (Lond.) 237:* 635–662, 1974.

21. Mata, M., D. J. Fink, H. Gainer, C. B. Smith, L. Davidsen, H. Savaki, W. J. Schwartz, and L. Sokoloff. Activity-dependent energy metabolism in rat posterior pituitary primarily reflects sodium pump activity. *J. Neurochem. 34:* 213–215, 1980.

22. Mills, E., and F. F. Jobsis. Mitochondrial respiratory chain of carotid body and chemoreceptor response to changes in oxygen tension. *J. Neurophysiol. 35:* 405–428, 1972.

23. Neubauer, J. A., and N. H. Edelman. Nonuniform brain blood flow response to hypoxia in unanesthetized cats. *J. Appl. Physiol. 57:* 1803–1808, 1984.

24. Obeso, A., L. Almaraz, and C. Gonzalez. Correlation between adenosine triphosphate levels, dopamine release and electrical activity in the carotid body: support for the metabolic hypothesis of chemoreception. *Brain Res. 348:* 64–68, 1985.

25. Obeso, A., C. Gonzalez, B. Dinger, and S. Fidone. Effects of chemoreceptor stimulation on glucose utilization by the rabbit carotid body in vitro. *Soc. Neurosci. Abstr. 12:* 1357, 1986.

26. Pelto-Huikko, M., A. Hervonen, P. Helen, I. Linnoila, V. M. Pickel, and R. J. Miller. Localization of (met[5])- and (leu[5])-enkephalin in nerve terminals and SIF cells in adult human sympathetic ganglia. *Adv. Biochem. Psychopharmacol. 25:* 379–383, 1980.

27. Robinson, S. E., J. P. Schwartz, and E. Costa. Substance P in the superior cervical ganglion and the submaxillary gland of the rat. *Brain Res. 182:* 11–17, 1980.

28. Schultzberg, M., T. Hokfelt, J. M. Lundberg, C. J. Dalsgaard, and L.-G. Elfvin. Transmitter histochemistry in autonomic ganglia. In: *Autonomic Ganglia,* ed. L.-G. Elfvin. New York: John Wiley, 1983, pp. 205–233.

29. Tsunoo, A., S. Konishi, and M. Otsuka. Substance P as an excitatory transmitter of primary afferent neurons in guinea-pig sympathetic ganglia. *Neuroscience 7:* 2025–2037, 1982.

30. Tuttle, R. S., and M. McCleary. Carotid sinus distension and superior cervical ganglion transmission. *Am. J. Physiol. 240:* H716–H720, 1981.

31. Williams, T., and J. Jew. Monoamine connections in sympathetic ganglia. In: *Autonomic Ganglia,* ed. Lars-Gosta Elfvin. New York: John Wiley, 1983, pp. 235–264.

32. Yoshimasa, T., K. Nakao, H. Ohtsuki, S. Li, and H. Imura. Methionine-enkephalin and leucine-enkephalin in human sympathoadrenal system and pheochromocytoma. *J. Clin. Invest. 69:* 643–650, 1982.

6

Chemoreceptors in Avian Lungs

R. D. TALLMAN, JR.

Carbon dioxide-sensitive pulmonary afferent neurons have been described in several species of Aves (see refs. 4,6,7,22). The exact location of these vagal sensory endings, known as intrapulmonary CO_2 receptors or IPC, has not been histologically verified. However, functional localization studies suggest that their receptive fields are located in the gas exchange areas of the lung (15,23).

The unique anatomy of the avian respiratory system has made it possible to determine unequivocally that airway P_{CO_2} is the adequate stimulus for these receptors. The majority of gas exchange occurs along the parabronchi which are arranged in parallel within the lung parenchyma. Respired gas is propelled through the relatively nonexpanding lungs by thin-walled, compliant air sacs. This anatomical arrangement allows for a technique of artificial ventilation called *unidirectional ventilation*, whereby gas can be directed down the trachea, through the lungs, and out cannulated air sacs in a constant flowing stream. Unidirectional ventilation makes it possible to manipulate independently the distending airway pressure and the gas composition at the pulmonary exchange surfaces. Experiments utilizing this technique have shown that IPC activity is not affected by lung stretch (8), NaCN, or O_2 partial pressure (5,9) and is relatively insensitive to changes in arterial pH (5). IPC discharge is inversely proportional to the partial pressure of CO_2 in the airway gas. The greatest change in discharge frequency occurs between 15 and 25 mmHg, with the average activity of a population of IPC in chickens showing an 80% reduction in maximal discharge when lung P_{CO_2} reaches approximately 28 torr (15,16). IPC will respond to step changes in airway CO_2 within an average of 350 ms, displaying a pronounced overshoot to stepwise decreases in airway CO_2 with little subsequent adaptation (9,17,21). Thus, IPC relay information relating to the rate of change of airway CO_2 as well as the steady-state level.

Because of their location and unique sensitivity to CO_2, it is reasonable to speculate that IPC discharge transmits important information regarding pulmonary CO_2 concentration to the cardiopulmonary control systems. Indeed, changing the P_{CO_2} of the gas during unidirectional ventilation of a vascularly isolated lung in an anesthetized, thoracotomized chicken has a strong influence on respiratory movements. Apnea will result within 460 ms if CO_2 is removed from the ventilating gas, with respiratory movements increasing as CO_2 is increased up to a P_{CO_2} of 50–60 mmHg (9,19). It is therefore clear that under these experimental conditions, IPC discharge is capable of inhibiting breathing.

It has been suggested that IPC are the sensory limb of a control system that allows for regulation of arterial P_{CO_2} (P_aCO_2) in response to changes in the rate of CO_2 delivery to the lung ($\dot{V}_{CO_2}$) (18,21). According to this theory, as lung CO_2 flux increases, IPC discharge is reduced, causing an increase in ventilation proportional to the added CO_2 load. This concept was strengthened by experiments which reported that anesthetized chickens and awake ducks respond to low-level CO_2 inhalation by increasing their ventilation to a level sufficient to maintain a constant P_aCO_2 (18,20).

Several pieces of evidence have since cast doubt on the concept that IPC, responding to changes in lung CO_2 load, stimulate breathing while maintaining P_aCO_2. Cross-perfusion studies stimulating IPC independently from carotid body or central chemoreceptors, demonstrate only small reflex changes in ventilation caused by IPC alone (14). Increasing venous P_{CO_2}, and thus the rate of CO_2 delivery to the lung by venous infusion of CO_2-laden blood (3,24) or gut ventilation with high CO_2 (12), results in a hypercapnic hyperpnea. Awake, spontaneously breathing ducks respond to CO_2 loading via the inspired gas or the venous blood with an increase in both P_aCO_2 and minute ventilation ($\dot{V}_E$), with the slope of the relationship ($\Delta\dot{V}_E/\Delta P_aCO_2$) equal during either route of CO_2 delivery (24). In these experiments, IPC discharge was differentially affected, depending on the route of CO_2 administration. Inspired CO_2 resulted in a significantly lower peak discharge frequency than venous CO_2 loading. On the basis of these findings, it was concluded that a reduction in peak IPC discharge does not represent an added ventilatory drive because minute ventilation was not greater during inspired CO_2 loading at any given P_aCO_2 (25).

Although it appears that IPC do not stimulate breathing when lung CO_2 load is increased, it has been suggested that the greatest influence of IPC on ventilation may be in the hypocapnic range when pulmonary CO_2 is reduced below normal (19). IPC may therefore act to prevent excessive hyperventilation during stressful situations such as exercise, hyperthermia, hypoxia, etc. Indeed the IPC/CO_2 response curve is much steeper at lower airway P_{CO_2}, providing the mechanism for such a nonlinear response to CO_2. Support for this theory comes from experiments which found that venous infusion of blood (over 30 s) containing very little CO_2 greatly reduced ventilation while P_aCO_2 remained unchanged (3). This finding was not confirmed by removal of venous CO_2 using a venovenous bypass circuit containing a membrane lung, although only a small reduction in $\dot{V}_{CO_2}$ (15%) was accomplished (24). The present study was designed to reevaluate this question by lowering lung CO_2 flux over a much larger range, allowing a more complete description of the ventilatory response curve in the steady state, while simultaneously recording from IPC.

METHODS

Eleven adult male Pekin ducks (3.02 kg $\pm$ 0.43) were used in this study. Each was anesthetized with urethan (1 g/kg) and tracheostomized, and the right vagus nerve was exposed midcervically for IPC recording. A silicone rubber catheter (Dow-Corning, 0.76 mm ID, 1.65 mm OD) was advanced through the right ulnar vein past the right ventricle and into the pulmonary artery for taking samples of mixed venous blood. Both brachial arteries were also cannulated for blood pressure monitoring and sampling for blood gas and pH analysis. An extracorporeal venovenous bypass circuit took blood from a jugular vein catheter whose tip was located near the level of the right atrium. The blood was pumped through a silicone membrane blood oxygenator (Sci Med 0800) and heat exchanger, and returned to the animal via the left ulnar vein. A second roller pump was included as part of a shunt circuit in order to recirculate blood through the membrane oxygenator at flow rates independent of the overall bypass flow. This modification made it possible to remove a larger amount of carbon dioxide from the venous blood during the unloading state. The circuit was primed with heparinized blood taken from a donor animal the morning of the experiment. All ventilatory measurements and nerve recordings were made as previously described (25).

Once the animal was attached to the circuit, the first roller pump was slowly turned up to a rate just below the maximum rate possible, and no further adjustments in blood flow were made thereafter. Two experimental states were used in this study. The "control" state was established by not ventilating the oxygenator, thus returning the blood to the duck unaltered. "Venous CO_2 unloading" was accomplished by ventilating the oxygenator with air. The duck was allowed to breathe air spontaneously at all times. The control state was maintained while small slips of the vagus nerve were filamented and placed over bipolar electrodes for recording action potentials. Once an IPC was identified by use of standard techniques (25), a set of control measurements were taken. The membrane lung was then ventilated with air for a minimum of 12 min to establish new steady-state conditions. The physiological measurements made during the unloading state were compared pairwise to the preceding control state. For data from single-breath measurements and analysis of IPC discharge, measurements from four consecutive breaths at each state were used in the analysis.

RESULTS

The activity from 25 IPC was recorded during control and steady-state venous CO_2 unloading. Arterial and mixed venous blood samples were obtained while simultaneously recording from 16 IPC. The rate of extracorporeal bypass flow in these experiments was between 235 and 320 ml/min with an average flow of 284 ml/min. The averages of all of the physiological measurements made during IPC recordings are listed in Table 6.1. CO_2 unloading lowered mixed venous P_{CO_2} from 42.5 to 35 mmHg, reducing $\dot{V}_{CO_2}$ by over 50%, to an average of 16.1 ml/min. Min-

Table 6.1 Steady-State Variables

Variable (units)	Symbol	n	Control	CO_2 unloading
Inspiratory duration (s)	T_I	64	1.89 ± 0.09	*1.95 ± 0.12
Expiratory duration (s)	T_E	64	6.07 ± 0.33	†10.8 ± 35
Respiratory frequency (breaths/min)	f	16	7.9 ± 0.3	†4.6 ± 0.4
Tidal volume (ml)	V_T	64	91.9 ± 4.7	†102.8 ± 9.0
Minute ventilation (ml/min, BTPS)	$\dot{V}_E$	16	723 ± 43	†402 ± 39
Rate of CO_2 production (ml/min, STPD)	$\dot{V}_{CO_2}$	16	34.2 ± 2.0	†16.1 ± 1.1
Arterial blood CO_2 tension (mmHg)	P_aCO_2	16	37.7 ± 3.4	†33.9 ± 2.7
Arterial blood O_2 tension (mmHg)	P_aO_2	16	77.4 ± 3.4	†64.5 ± 2.4
Arterial blood pH	pH_a	16	7.404 ± 0.026	†7.441 ± 0.022
Mixed venous blood CO_2 tension (mmHg)	$P_{\bar{v}}CO_2$	16	42.5 ± 2.8	*35.0 ± 5.0
Mixed venous blood O_2 tension (mmHg)	$P_{\bar{v}}O_2$	16	49.1 ± 5.2	47.0 ± 4.7
Mixed venous blood pH	$pH_{\bar{v}}$	16	7.379 ± 0.011	*7.439 ± 0.032
Impulses/breath	—	64	50.6 ± 5.9	†74.8 ± 9.5
Mean discharge frequency	imp/T_{TOT}	64	6.2 ± 0.71	6.33 ± 0.75

Note: Values are mean $\pm$ SEM.

*$p<.01$, †$p<.002$; significant difference from control, as determined by paired sample t-test.

ute ventilation fell by 44% to 402 ml/min. This fall in ventilation was entirely due to a reduction in breathing frequency since tidal volume actually increased by a small (11%) but significant amount. During venous CO_2 unloading, P_aCO_2 fell a small but significant amount. Figure 6.1 shows the CO_2 response curve; the change in ventilation is plotted as a function of the change in P_aCO_2 from the values measured during the preceding control state. The slope of the CO_2 response during CO_2 unloading was 118.8 ml/mmHg/min, as calculated by means of directional statistics (13).

The average IPC discharge frequency was not affected over this large range of CO_2 flux (see Table 6.1). Although the average frequency was unchanged, the number of impulses per breath was increased. Figure 6.2 shows the average number of impulses per breath over four consecutive breaths during the unloading state, plotted against the control IPC discharge. CO_2 unloading led to a large and significant increase in the number of impulses per breath (Table 6.1) which was seen in nearly all of the fibers studied. This increase was due entirely to an increase in the firing during expiration (mean = 11.9 impulses/breath control vs. 25.8 impulses/breath unloading) since the number of impulses per inspiration was not affected (mean = 38.7 impulses/breath control vs. 36.1 impulses/breath unloading).

DISCUSSION

The results of the present study show that reducing the rate of CO_2 delivery to the lungs of spontaneously breathing ducks results in a significant and progressive fall in P_aCO_2. This hypocapnic response to decreased lung CO_2 load is very similar to the response found in the awake, spontaneously breathing dog (28). On the basis of these findings it seems unlikely that IPC respond to reductions in lung CO_2 load by preventing hyperventilation. This conclusion extends the results from an earlier study that also found a significant hypocapnic response to small amounts of venous CO_2 unloading in the decerebrate duck (24). The slope of the ventilatory response to CO_2 in the hypocapnic range (118 ml/mmHg/min) was less than that previously reported for venous CO_2 loading in decerebrate ducks (308 ml/mmHg/min) (24) but similar to that measured during gut CO_2 loading in the awake duck (137 ml/mmHg/min) (12). Although the reasons for this variability in CO_2 sensitivity are not clear, the use of anesthesia in the present study may have resulted in a somewhat depressed ventilatory response.

The hypothesis has been advanced that IPC discharge provides no significant driving or inhibitory stimulus to ventilation but rather serves as a modulator of breathing pattern much as the slowly adapting pulmonary stretch receptors are thought to act in mammals (14). This is supported by experiments that have shown no difference in the ventilatory CO_2 response despite large reductions in IPC discharge during CO_2 inhalation (24). In these studies, the pattern of breathing was differentially sensitive to the route of CO_2 administration. CO_2 inhalation resulted in a slower, deeper ventilatory pattern than venous CO_2 loading at the same P_aCO_2. This is in contrast to the results described in awake dogs in which the ventilatory pattern was the same (11). Thus, it was concluded that the presence of CO_2 receptors in the avian lung was responsible for these pattern differences.

During spontaneous breathing, all IPC show a modulation in discharge fre-

Fig. 6.1 The steady-state CO_2 response curve measured during IPC recording. Each point is the paired response between unloading and the preceding control. The solid line represents the slope estimated by the maximum likelihood technique of Mardia et al. (13).

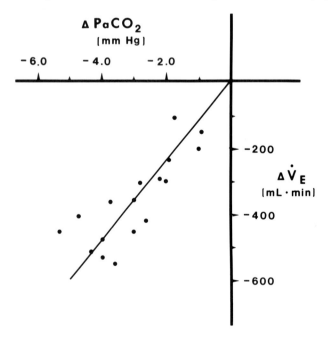

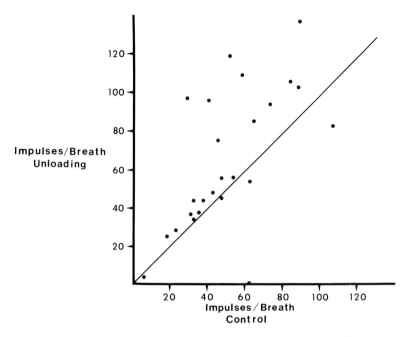

Fig. 6.2 Plot of mean number of IPC impulses/breath measured during venous CO_2 unloading on the ordinate versus the mean of the control discharge on the abscissa. Results from all 25 IPC are plotted, and each point represents the mean from four breaths. The solid line represents the line of identity.

quency that is in phase with breathing, with the average population response exhibiting a peak in discharge near the middle of inspiration (2,10,25). It has been shown that peak IPC discharge frequency was not significantly altered when the rate of CO_2 delivery to the lungs was manipulated over a fivefold range, despite nearly a threefold change in ventilation (25). In these experiments, the switch between inspiration and expiration always occurred when the average IPC discharge had fallen to the same frequency during venous CO_2 loading or unloading, despite a large range of breathing frequencies. A similar finding has been reported in the spontaneously breathing chicken (10). In these experiments, hyperventilation was induced by using almitrine (2 mg/kg, i.v.), a carotid body chemoreceptor stimulant. Despite a fourfold increase in breathing frequency and a doubling of peak IPC discharge, the switch from inspiration to expiration occurred when the discharge frequency had fallen to the same level (10). Indeed, many studies have provided direct and indirect evidence of an important relationship between the IPC discharge profile and inspiratory and expiratory durations (T_I and T_E) (1,26,27). In the present study, the average IPC discharge frequency was not altered by reduction of lung CO_2 delivery by as much as 50% (see Table 6.1). However, the number of impulses per breath was significantly affected by a change in CO_2 delivery to the lung. This increase occurred during expiration where it has been shown that discharge frequency is also increased (25). Previous studies have shown that in eupnea, inspiratory IPC discharge serves to prolong inspiration (1). It is reasonable to suggest that this increased IPC traffic seen during expiration when lung CO_2 flux is decreased serves to prolong expiration. However, the true nature of any possible cause-and-effect relationships between IPC discharge and expiratory duration in the intact, spontaneously breathing bird await further investigation.

REFERENCES

1. Berger, P. J., and R. D. Tallman, Jr. Lengthening of inspiration by intrapulmonary chemoreceptor discharge in ducks. *J. Appl. Physiol. 53:* 1392–1396, 1982.
2. Berger, P. J., R. D. Tallman, Jr., and A. L. Kunz. Discharge of intrapulmonary chemoreceptors and its modulation by rapid F_ICO_2 changes in decerebrate ducks. *Respir. Physiol. 42:* 123–130, 1980.
3. Boon, J. K., W. D. Kuhlmann, and M. R. Fedde. Control of respiration in the chicken: effects of venous CO_2 loading. *Respir. Physiol. 39:* 169–181, 1980.
4. Bouverot, P. Control of breathing in birds compared with mammals. *Physiol. Rev. 58:* 604–655, 1978.
5. Burger, R. E., J. L. Osborne, and R. B. Banzett. Intrapulmonary chemoreceptors in *Gallus domesticus:* adequate stimulus and functional localization. *Respir. Physiol. 22:* 87–97, 1974.
6. Fedde, M. R. Intrapulmonary CO_2 receptors and their role in the control of avian respiration. In: *Advances in Physiological Sciences,* Vol. 10: *Respiration,* ed. I. Hutas, and L. A. Debreczeni. Elmsford, NY: Pergamon Press, 1981, pp. 147–154.
7. Fedde, M. R. Respiration. In: *Avian Physiology* (4th ed.), ed. P. D. Sturkie. Berlin: Springer-Verlag, 1986, pp. 191–220.
8. Fedde, M. R., R. N. Gatz, H. Slama, and P. Scheid. Intrapulmonary CO_2 receptors in the duck: I. Stimulus specificity. *Respir. Physiol. 22:* 99–114, 1974.
9. Fedde, M. R., and D. F. Peterson. Intrapulmonary receptor response to changes in airway-gas composition in *Gallus domesticus. J. Physiol. (Lond.) 209:* 609–625, 1970.
10. Gleeson, M. Changes in intrapulmonary chemoreceptor discharge in response to the adjustment of respiratory pattern during hyperventilation in domestic fowl. *J. Exp. Physiol. 70:* 503–513, 1985.
11. Greco, E. C., Jr., W. E. Fordyce, F. Gonzalez, Jr., P. Reischl, and F. S. Grodins. Respiratory responses to intravenous and intrapulmonary CO_2 in awake dogs. *J. Appl. Physiol. 45:* 109–114, 1978.
12. Jones, D. R., W. K. Milsom, and P. J. Butler. Ventilatory response to venous CO_2 loading by gut ventilation in ducks. *Can. J. Zool. 63:* 1232–1236, 1985.
13. Mardia, K. V., S. Bogle, and R. Edwards. Statistics of response slopes. *J. Appl. Physiol 54:* 309–313, 1983.
14. Milsom, W. K., D. R. Jones, and G.R.J. Gabbott. On chemoreceptor control of ventilatory responses to CO_2 in unanesthetized ducks. *J. Appl. Physiol 50:* 1121–1128, 1981.
15. Nye, P.C.G., and R. E. Burger. Chicken intrapulmonary chemoreceptors: discharge at static levels of intrapulmonary carbon dioxide and their location. *Respir. Physiol. 33:* 299–322, 1978.
16. Osborne, J. L., and R. E. Burger. Intrapulmonary chemoreceptors in *Gallus domesticus. Respir. Physiol. 22:* 77–85, 1974.
17. Osborne, J. L., R. E. Burger, and P. J. Stoll. Dynamic responses of CO_2 sensitive avian intrapulmonary chemoreceptors. *Am. J. Physiol. 233:* R15–R22, 1977.
18. Osborne, J. L., and G. S. Mitchell. Regulation of arterial PCO_2 during inhalation of CO_2 in chickens. *Respir. Physiol. 31:* 357–364, 1977.

19. Osborne, J. L., G. S. Mitchell, and F. Powell. Ventilatory responses to CO_2 in the chicken: intrapulmonary and systemic chemoreceptors. *Respir. Physiol. 30:* 369–382, 1977.

20. Powell, F. L., M. R. Fedde, R. K. Gratz, and P. Scheid. Ventilatory response to CO_2 in birds. I. Measurements in the unanesthetized duck. *Respir. Physiol. 35:* 349–359, 1978.

21. Scheid, P., R. K. Gratz, F. L. Powell, and M. R. Fedde. Ventilatory response to CO_2 in birds. II. Contribution by intrapulmonary CO_2 receptors. *Respir. Physiol 35:* 361–372, 1978.

22. Scheid, P., and J. Piiper. Control of breathing in birds. In: *Handbook of Physiology,* Sec. 3: *Respiration,* Vol. 2: *Control of Breathing,* ed. N. S. Cherniack and J. G. Widdicombe. Bethesda, MD: Am. Physiol. Soc., 1986, pp. 815–832.

23. Scheid, P., H. Slama, R. N. Gatz, and M. R. Fedde. Intrapulmonary CO_2 receptors in the duck: III. Functional localization. *Respir. Physiol. 22:* 123–136, 1974.

24. Tallman, R. D., Jr., and F. S. Grodins. Intrapulmonary CO_2 receptors and ventilatory response to lung CO_2 loading. *J. Appl. Physiol. 52:* 1272–1277, 1982.

25. Tallman, R. D., Jr., and F. S. Grodins. Intrapulmonary CO_2 receptor discharge at different levels of venous P_{CO_2}. *J. Appl. Physiol. 53:* 1386–1391, 1982.

26. Tallman, R. D., Jr., and A. L. Kunz. Changes in breathing pattern mediated by intrapulmonary CO_2 receptors in chickens. *J. Appl. Physiol. 52:* 162–167, 1982.

27. Tallman, R. D., Jr., A. L. Kunz, and D. A. Miller. Effect of timing of $F_I CO_2$ changes on ventilatory period in domestic fowl. *Am. J. Physiol. 237:* R260–R265, 1979.

28. Tallman, R. D., Jr., R. Marcolin, M. Howie, J. S. McDonald, and T. Stafford. Cardiopulmonary response to extracorporeal venous CO_2 removal in awake, spontaneously breathing dogs. *J. Appl. Physiol. 61:* 516–522, 1986.

7

Chemoreflex Control of Bimodal Breathing in Gar *(Lepisosteus)*

N. J. SMATRESK

One of the most significant events in the evolution of vertebrate respiratory systems was the transition from water to air breathing. Air breathing in primitive Sarcopterygian fishes led to the evolution of tetrapod vertebrates, but air breathing has evolved independently in most of the major groups of bony fishes. The obvious advantage of air breathing for these fishes is that it allows them to circumvent the limited availability of O_2 in the aquatic environment. In addition to evolving new structures to breathe air, the nervous system of bimodally breathing animals has to be modified to coordinate the activities of two gas exchangers. In contrast to the relatively rhythmic and regular patterns of gill ventilation seen in most water breathing fish, air breathing in fishes is irregular. This has led to the suggestion that air breathing in most bimodally breathing fishes is not controlled by a centrally generated rhythm, but is instead an on-demand phenomenon, critically regulated by peripheral sensory input (18). The irregular and periodic patterns of gill ventilation seen in many air-breathing fishes further suggest that their central control over gill ventilation is attenuated, and subject to a greater number of modifying influences. Considering the highly variable aquatic O_2 availability, oxygen-sensitive chemoreceptors could be expected to exert dominant control over the balance between aerial and aquatic respiration, but little is known about the specific reflexes they control, their location, or their primary afferent pathways in bimodally breathing fishes.

REFLEX RESPONSES TO HYPOXIA IN AIR-BREATHING FISHES

Most air-breathing fish respond to aquatic hypoxia by increasing the ventilation and perfusion of their air-breathing organ. Some obligate air breathers, like the lungfish and *Electrophorus,* have limited ability for aquatic respiration and respond little to changing water O_2 tensions (7,9,12). The responses of branchial ventilation to hypoxia are quite variable. Air-breathing fish with limited ability to extract O_2 from air, like *Neoceratodus,* may increase branchial ventilation as water O_2 tensions fall (10). Perhaps the most interesting branchial responses are seen in facultative air-breathing fishes that can switch sites for oxygen uptake from gills to their air-breathing organ (ABO). In addition to increasing ventilation and perfusion of their air-breathing organ, many of these fish depress gill ventilation during aquatic hypoxia (e.g. 6,8,17,22). Most of these facultative air-breathing fish have "in-series" circulation of the air-breathing organ and gills. Blood that has been oxygenated in the ABO must pass through the gills before returning to the systemic circulation. When the water Po_2 is lower than the Po_2 in the ventral aorta, oxygen gained by the ABO may diffuse out of the gills down the reversed O_2 gradient. Thus, hypoxic depression of gill ventilation is part of a suite of reflex responses to hypoxia that increase aerial O_2 uptake while minimizing branchial O_2 loss. Some air-breathing fish may also shunt blood flow past the lamellar exchange surfaces to limit O_2 loss during aquatic hypoxia (5).

Recent work in our laboratory has focused on a group of primitive Actinopterygian fish, the gar (*Lepisosteus oculatus* and *L. osseus*), to better understand chemoreflex control of respiration in facultative air-breathing fish. Gar use both gills and a swimbladder, modified as an air-breathing organ, for O_2 uptake and CO_2 excretion. The air-breathing organ is a large, trabecular, and well-vascularized structure invested with both smooth and striated muscle. The gills of gar are greatly reduced when compared to those of similarly sized water-breathing fish (22). In normally aerated water, a 1-kg gar derives about 40% of its O_2 from the air, but in hypoxic water they maintain their metabolic rate exclusively by aerial O_2 uptake (22). As water O_2 tensions (P_wO_2) fall, gar increase ventilation and perfusion of their air-breathing organ, and increase cardiac output and heart rate (19,22). Their branchial response to hypoxia is complex. Branchial ventilation increases as P_wO_2 falls from hyperoxia to about 80 torr, where it is maximal. Below 80 torr, branchial ventilation decreases, and undisturbed gar may ventilate their gills only periodically in severe hypoxia. Because gar have in-series circulation of the gills and ABO, and cannot shunt blood past the lamellar exchange surfaces, this hypoxic depression of gill ventilation is the only means by which they can limit branchial O_2 loss in severely hypoxic water, although the effectiveness of this strategy has been difficult to prove experimentally (22).

RESPONSES TO CHANGING INTERNAL AND EXTERNAL O_2 TENSIONS

The relative contributions of chemoreceptors, which initiate the reflex responses to hypoxia, and of branchial or air-breathing organ mechanoreceptors, which may stimulate secondary reflex responses to hypoxia, are difficult to separate in studies on conscious animals. In an attempt to dissect out the primary and secondary reflex responses to hypoxia, we recently studied the responses of anesthetized, spontaneously ventilating gar to changes in either internal or external O_2 stimulus levels (21). This preparation allowed the P_wO_2 at the gills (external) to be varied while the

P_{O_2} in the ventral aorta ($P_{va}O_2$; internal) was independently regulated by unidirectional ventilation of the ABO with humidified N_2, air, or O_2. ABO volume was held constant during these manipulations, thus eliminating secondary reflex responses to hypoxia due to stimulation of ABO mechanoreceptors. Figure 7.1 illustrates the interactive effects of varying $P_{va}O_2$ and $P_{w}O_2$ tensions on branchial ventilation (P_b) and air-breathing frequency (f_{ab}) in these gar. There was little or no air breathing when the $P_{va}O_2$ was greater than about 40 torr, except during aquatic hypoxia (Fig. 7.1A). Below this level, air breathing was stimulated by reduction of either $P_{w}O_2$ or $P_{va}O_2$ (Fig. 7.1A), with the greatest stimulation seen when the gills were superfused with hypoxic water. These results demonstrate that internal and external O_2 tensions interactively control air-breathing frequency, but whether they do so by stimulating separate internally and externally oriented chemoreceptor loci or by stimulating one set of chemoreceptors located in the diffusion pathway between blood and water cannot be determined from these data.

The chemoreflex control of gill ventilation was quite complex in comparison to the control of air breathing (Fig. 7.1B). When gar were in normally aerated or hyperoxic water, they responded to declining $P_{va}O_2$, tensions by increasing branchial ventilation. At a given $P_{va}O_2$ branchial ventilation also increased when $P_{w}O_2$ was lowered from hyperoxic to normoxic levels. Aquatic hypoxia (Fig. 7.1B, bottom line), on the other hand, depressed branchial ventilation across the observed range of $P_{va}O_2$ tensions, and abolished the correlation between $P_{va}O_2$ and buccal pressure seen in normoxia and hyperoxia.

Gar were also subjected to step changes in $P_{w}O_2$ while branchial ventilation was measured (21). When $P_{w}O_2$ was rapidly increased, from hypoxia to normoxia, buccal pressure amplitude increased simultaneously with the change of P_{O_2} measured at the gills, suggesting the presence of water-facing chemoreceptors. Stimulation of these receptors during aquatic hypoxia reflexively inhibits gill ventilation regardless of internal O_2 tension.

These studies also provided some insight into the extent of chemoreflex control over the cardiovascular system. Air breathing in gar and other bimodally breathing fish is generally accompanied by tachycardia (5,9,11,22). The anesthetized, spontaneously ventilating gar showed little or no cardiac response to internal or external hypoxia or air-breathing attempts, suggesting that tachycardia following air breathing in conscious gar results from stimulation of ABO mechanoreceptors. The effects of hypoxia on blood flow distribution were not directly measured in these studies, but it was noted that aquatic hypoxia significantly altered $P_{va}O_2$, increasing it when the ABO was being ventilated with air or O_2, and decreasing it when the ABO was ventilated with N_2. This apparent increase in the O_2 transfer factor across the ABO suggests that stimulation of externally oriented chemoreceptors may have also reflexly increased ABO blood flow.

These studies suggest that gar use two sets of chemoreceptor loci, one set monitoring the $P_{w}O_2$, the other set monitoring the mixed systemic venous and pulmonary venous blood. The different reflex responses to stimulation of internal and external chemoreceptor loci may help to explain the irregular patterns of gill and ABO ventilation and the responses to increased metabolic demands in gar. After an air breath, ABO P_{O_2}, hence $P_{va}O_2$, falls slowly. Progressive stimulation of internally oriented chemoreceptors could then account for the gradual increase in gill

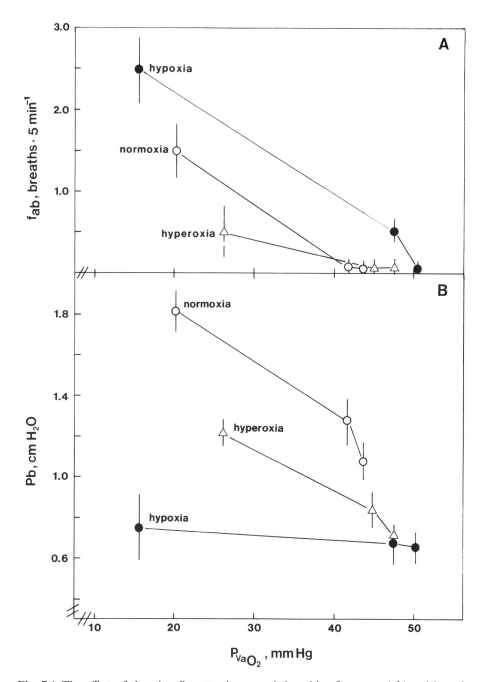

Fig. 7.1 The effect of changing $P_{va}O_2$ tensions on air-breathing frequency (f_{ab}) and buccal pressure amplitude (P_b) in anesthetized spontaneously ventilating *L. osseus* during superfusion of the gills with hyperoxic (△), normoxic (○), or hypoxic (●) water. $P_{va}O_2$ changes were made by ventilation of the lung with humidified N_2 air, or O_2. [Reproduced by permission from Smatresk et al., 1986 (21).]

ventilation normally observed during the interbreath interval, and may also terminate the breath-hold period by stimulating the next air breath. Stimulation of internally oriented chemoreceptors may also account for increased gill ventilation and air breathing when metabolic demands are increased, during exercise or as temperature rises (23,24). When gar are in well-aerated water, the low level of stimulation of external chemoreceptor loci favors branchial ventilation over air breathing. As P_wO_2 falls, stimulation of these receptors shifts the balance of respiration from water to air breathing by inhibiting branchial ventilation and increasing ABO ventilation and possibly ABO perfusion.

LOCALIZATION OF CHEMORECEPTORS

The observation that the exclusively stimulatory effect of internal hypoxia on gill ventilation could be abolished by aquatic hypoxia argues strongly for anatomically distinct internal and external chemoreceptor loci. The reflex responses to internally or externally administered cyanide helped to confirm this conclusion and further localize putative internal and external loci (19,21). Cyanide put into the inspired water flow (0.5 mg diluted into approx. 8 liters of water) to conscious unrestrained gar promptly depressed gill ventilation and vigorously stimulated air breathing, but stimulated both gill ventilation and air breathing when injected into the dorsal aorta. The reflex responses stimulated by giving internal or external cyanide were thus consistent with the responses to changing P_wO_2 or $P_{va}O_2$ levels. In anesthetized gar, cyanide injected upsteram from the gills (20 μg in 0.3 ml saline) into the conus arteriosus or ventral aorta stimulated air breathing and gill ventilation with a 5- to 10-s latency, but had about a 60-s latency when injected into the dorsal aorta (downstream from the gills). The short response latency to cyanide injections upstream from the gills indicates that the internal chemoreceptors probably lie in or near the vascular pathway between the ventral aorta and dorsal aorta, most probably in the gills. Interestingly, cyanide injected into the ventral aorta first stimulated and then slightly depressed gill ventilation. It seems likely that cyanide given as a concentrated bolus immediately upstream from the gills may diffuse through the gills and stimulate external chemoreceptor loci, thereby depressing gill ventilation.

External PO_2 tensions could be effectively monitored by water-facing chemoreceptors; alternatively, the PO_2 of the efferent (arterialized) circulation of the gills or head could be monitored. If the water-sensing chemoreceptor loci were in the efferent branchial circulation, however, internal cyanide should have depressed gill ventilation regardless of where it was injected. Because dorsal aorta and conus cyanide injections stimulated only gill ventilation, it seemed most likely that the externally oriented chemoreceptors lay close to the water flow, perhaps in superficial epithelial layers of the gills. Dunel-Erb et al. (4) recently described glomuslike cells in the primary epithelium, facing the water flow, in teleost gills, which could potentially respond to changing P_wO_2 tensions. There is some evidence that lungfish may have both internal and external chemoreceptor loci. Johansen and Lenfant (9) used internal and external injections of nicotinamide as a chemoreceptor probe, and found that it stimulated gill ventilation and air breathing in African lungfish. Lahiri et al. (14) also found that cyanide injected into the gill arch circulation of *Protopterus* stimulated air breathing.

Unimodal water-breathing fish may have a similar arrangement of chemoreceptor loci. External hypoxia or cyanide injections elicited reflex bradycardia and stimulated gill ventilation in trout and catfish (1,2,25), but intravascular cyanide had no effect on heart rate, and stimulated only gill ventilation in catfish (1). Bilateral section of the innervation to the first gill arch (branches of cranial nerves IX and X) in salmonids, or the first two gill arches of catfish (IX, + branches 1–3 of X), abolished the reflex bradycardia, but not the ventilatory responses to hypoxia (1,25). Complete branchial deafferentation was needed to abolish all chemoreflex responses to hypoxia in catfish (1). Branchial chemoreceptor loci have been unequivocally demonstrated by Milsom and Brill (15), who recently characterized chemoreceptor activity from the first gill arch of tuna.

From these studies, it seemed likely that the branchial branches of cranial nerves IX and X form the afferent limb of the chemoreflex responses to hypoxia in gar. We tested this hypothesis by observing the effects of bilateral section of all branchial branches of the vagus (X), thus interrupting sensory activity to the brain from gill arches 2 through 4, in anesthetized, spontaneously ventilating *L. oculatus*. Figure 7.2 illustrates the changes in branchial ventilation and air breathing during normoxia and hypoxia, before and after nerve section. Prior to nerve section, hypoxia severely depressed gill ventilation, and stimulated air breathing in sham-operated gar. Following nerve section, aquatic hypoxia had no noticeable effect on branchial ventilation, and attenuated the air-breathing response in three out of four of the gar tested (Smatresk, unpublished data). These studies clearly demonstrate that the external chemoreceptors lie in the gills, and that their stimulation by aquatic hypoxia reflexly inhibits gill ventilation. The attenuation of air breathing suggests that gill arches 2–4 may also have internal chemoreceptors, but the remaining, albeit attenuated, air breathing during hypoxia further suggests that the pseudobranch or first gill arch (innervated by IX) contains the remaining chemoreceptor loci. The role of these remaining chemoreceptors remains to be determined however, because sectioning the glossopharyngeal was difficult in this preparation.

CONCLUSIONS

Oxygen-sensitive chemoreceptors exert dominant control over the respiratory mode and complex patterns of branchial and aerial ventilation in gar. Other peripheral sensory receptors, including ABO mechanoreceptors or branchial defense receptors, may help to coordinate the activities of the gills and ABO, but their contribution appears to be secondary to the ventilatory priorities set by the internal and external chemoreceptor loci (3,13,16,18,20). Stimulation of internally oriented receptors, which appear to monitor the Po_2 of the branchial afferent circulation, increases the overall level of both gill ventilation and air breathing (i.e., hypoxic drive). Stimulation of external branchial chemoreceptors, which monitor the P_wO_2,

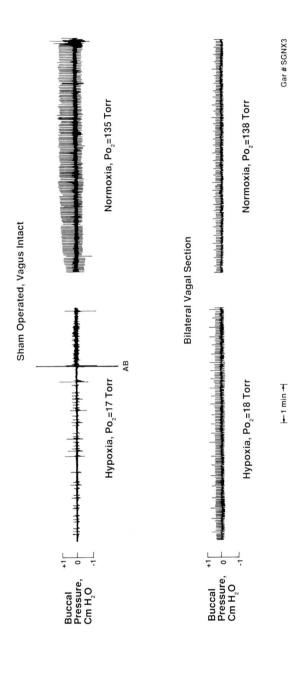

Fig. 7.2 Recording of the steady-state responses of gill ventilation (measured by buccal pressure, P_b) to aquatic hypoxia from an anesthetized, spontaneously ventilating gar (*L. oculatus*), before and after sectioning of the branchial branches of the vagus. Hypoxia depressed ventilation in sham-operated animals, but after nerve section hypoxia had little or no effect on branchial ventilation.

shifts the ventilatory emphasis from water to air breathing by inhibiting gill ventilation and by increasing ABO ventilation and perfusion. The precise anatomical location of these receptors, their responses to varying water or arterial O_2 stimulus levels, and their central integration remain to be determined. Similar studies on the role of chemoreceptors in other unimodally or bimodally breathing fishes suggest that the internal/external arrangement may be relatively common; thus the different branchial responses to hypoxia in bimodally breathing fishes may result from different central integration of peripheral chemoreceptor activity.

ACKNOWLEDGMENTS

This research was supported by National Science Foundation Grant DCB-8317914. I would like to thank B. Shipman for helpful comments on the manuscript, and also S. Lahiri and the University of Pennsylvania for their help and support, which led to my participation in the Julius H. Comroe Memorial Symposium.

REFERENCES

1. Burleson, M. L., and N. J. Smatresk. Effects of sectioning cranial nerves IX and X on the reflex response to hypoxia in catfish [Abstract]. *Am. Zool. 26:* 51, 1986.
2. Daxboeck, C., and G. F. Holeton. Oxygen receptors in the rainbow trout, *Salmo gairdneri. Can. J. Zool. 56:* 1254–1259, 1978.
3. DeLaney, R. G., P. Laurent, R. Galante, A. Pack, and A. P. Fishman. Pulmonary mechanoreceptors in the dipnoi lungfish *Protopterus* and *Lepidosiren. Am. J. Physiol. 244:* R418–R428, 1983.
4. Dunel-Erb, S., Y. Bailly, and P. Laurent. Neuroepithelial cells in fish gill primary lamellae. *J. Appl. Physiol. 53:* 1342–1353, 1982.
5. Farrell, A. P. Cardiovascular events associated with air breathing in two teleosts, *Hoplerythrinus unitaeniatus* and *Arapima gigas. Can. J. Zool. 56:* 953–958, 1978.
6. Hughes, G. M., and B. Singh. Gas exchange with air and water in an air-breathing catfish, *Saccobranchus (Heteropneustes) fossilis. J. Exp. Biol. 53:* 281–298, 1971.
7. Johansen, K. Air breathing in the teleost *Symbranchus marmoratus. Comp. Biochem. Physiol. 18:* 383–395, 1966.
8. Johansen, K., D. Hanson, and C. Lenfant. Respiration in the primitive air breather, *Amia calva. Respir. Physiol. 9:* 162–174, 1970.
9. Johansen, K., and C. Lenfant. Respiration in the African lungfish *Protopterus aethiopicus.* II. Control of breathing. *J. Exp. Biol. 49:* 453–468, 1968.
10. Johansen, K., C. Lenfant, and G. Grigg. Respiratory control in the lungfish, *Neoceratodus forsteri* (Krefft). *Comp. Biochem. Physiol. 20:* 835–854, 1967.
11. Johansen, K., C. Lenfant, and D. Hanson. Cardiovascular dynamics in the lungfishes. *Z. Vergl. Physiol. 59:* 157–186, 1968.
12. Johansen, K., C. Lenfant, K. Schmidt-Nielsen, and J. Petersen. Gas exchange and control of breathing in the electric eel, *Electrophorus electricus. Z. Vergl. Physiol. 61:* 137–163, 1968.
13. Jones, D. R., and W. K. Milsom. Peripheral receptors affecting breathing and cardiovascular function in non-mammalian vertebrates. *J. Exp. Biol. 100:* 59–91, 1982.
14. Lahiri, S., J. Szidon, and A. P. Fishman. Potential respiratory and circulatory adjustments to hypoxia in the African lungfish. *Fed. Proc. 29:* 1141–1148, 1970.
15. Milsom, W. K., and R. W. Brill. Oxygen sensitive afferent information arising from the first gill arch of yellowfin tuna. *Respir. Physiol. 66:* 193–203, 1986.

16. Milsom, W. K., and D. R. Jones. Characteristics of mechanoreceptors in the air-breathing organ of the holostean fish, *Amia calva. J. Exp. Biol. 117:* 389–399, 1985.
17. Pettit, M. J., and T. Beitinger. Oxygen acquisition of the reedfish, *Erpetoichthys calabaracus. J. Exp. Biol. 114:* 289–306, 1985.
18. Shelton, G., D. R. Jones, and W. K. Milsom. Control of breathing in ectothermic vertebrates. In: *Handbook of Physiology,* Sec. 3: *The Respiratory System,* Vol. 2: *Control of Breathing,* ed. N. S. Cherniack and J. G. Widdicombe. Bethesda: Am. Physiol. Soc. 1986, Part 2, pp. 857–909.
19. Smatresk, N. J. Ventilatory and cardiovascular responses to hypoxia and NaCN in *Lepisosteus osseus,* an air-breathing fish. *Physiol. Zool. 59:* 385–397, 1986.
20. Smatresk, N. J., and S. Q. Azizi. Characteristics of pulmonary mechanoreceptors in the air-breathing fish, *Lepisosteus oculatus. Am. J. Physiol. 252:* R1066–R1072, 1987.
21. Smatresk, N. J., M. L. Burleson, and S. Q. Azizi. Chemoreflexive responses to hypoxia and NaCN in longnose gar: evidence for two chemoreceptor loci. *Am. J. Physiol. 251:* R116–R125, 1986.
22. Smatresk, N. J., and J. N. Cameron. Respiration and acid–base physiology of the spotted gar, a bimodal breather. I. Normal values and the response to severe hypoxia. *J. Exp. Biol. 96:* 263–280, 1982.
23. Smatresk, N. J., and J. N. Cameron. Respiration and acid–base physiology of the spotted gar, a bimodal breather. II. Responses to temperature change and hypercapnia. *J. Exp. Biol. 96:* 281–293, 1982.
24. Smatresk, N. J., and J. N. Cameron. Respiration and acid–base physiology of the spotted gar, a bimodal breather. III. Response to a transfer from fresh water to 50% sea water, and control of ventilation. *J. Exp. Biol. 96:* 295–306, 1982.
25. Smith, F., and D. R. Jones. Localization of receptors causing hypoxic bradycardia in trout *(Salmo gairdneri). Can J. Zool. 56:* 1260–1265, 1978.

Part II
CAROTID BODY: SENSORY MECHANISMS

Introduction

N. S. CHERNIACK

The eight chapters in this section focus on the mechanisms responsible for the conversion of changes in P_{CO_2} and P_{CO_2}/H^+ to nerve impulses by the carotid body. It is hoped that information on the operation of the carotid body will be useful in elucidating more general principles of operation of other respiratory chemoreceptors. The central chemoreceptors are yet to be definitely located; likewise little is known or established regarding peripheral "metaboreceptors" that have been suggested by some investigators to be involved in the ventilatory response to exercise.

In Chapter 8, Eyzaguirre reviews the membrane responses of the carotid body to a variety of stimulating and inhibiting agents and concludes that the effects of CO_2 and hypoxia on glomus cell membrane potential and resistance are not the same. His studies suggest that the pattern of membrane changes produced depends on the intensity of glomus cell stimulation. Inhibitory stimuli hyperpolarize the cell and increase membrane resistance, as do agents that greatly increase carotid body discharge (i.e., by more than six fold). However, stimuli that moderately excite the glomus cell depolarize and reduce membrane resistance.

It is known that the same fibers in the carotid sinus nerve respond to hypoxia and hypercapnia, but evidence is accumulating that the mechanisms that produce carotid body stimulation by hypercapnia and hypoxia are different. For example, in Chapter 9, Fitzgerald et al. suggest that ionic pumps are involved in the excitation of the carotid body by CO_2, but not by hypoxia. Their experiments also show that there may be an antiport that allows Na^+-H^+ exchange to occur and modifies the response to increased CO_2 levels.

The studies by Fidone et al. (Chap. 10) demonstrate that there are interactions among the different neuroactive substances found in the glomus cell—acetylcholine, dopamine, met-enkephalin, and substance P. Cholinergic agents affect the release of dopamine produced in hypoxia. Met-enkephalin and substance P levels in the rabbit carotid body decrease with hypoxia and increase when the carotid sinus nerve is sectioned. Dopamine release can be modulated by both of these neuropeptides.

The amines and polypeptides that may act as neurotransmitters or neuromodulators in the carotid body are discussed in three chapters in this section. In Chapter 11, Prabhakar and Cherniack focus on the possible importance of tachykinins such as substance P and neurokinin A in mediating the hypoxic response in both cats and rabbits. Their study also provides evidence that these tachykinins influence both carotid and aortic body function, and supports the idea that CO_2 and hypoxia act in different ways on the carotid body.

Why the carotid body is so sensitive to changes in Po_2 remains unclear. In Chapter 13, Acker et al. suggest that the sensing of hypoxia by the carotid body may depend on chromophores and O_2-sensitive enzymes. Activation of these sensing mechanisms may change cytosolic calcium levels, releasing neurotransmitters.

In Chapter 15, Sirahata reports on the effects of exogenous substance P on the chemosensory responses to natural stimuli and the effects of anti-SP infusion on the chemoreceptor responses to O_2 and CO_2. Results suggest that SP is probably the principal neurotransmitter for hypoxic stimulation of carotid body chemoreceptors.

Taken together, this group of chapters suggests that hypoxia and hypercapnia release a mixture of inhibitory and excitatory agents. The neural response of the carotid body may depend on relatively small changes in the proportions of these constituents. Moreover, there seem to be several sites at which carotid body excitation can be triggered. More studies at the cellular level will be needed to elucidate the pathways involved.

In Chapter 14, O'Donnell et al. demonstrate the application of patch-clamp methods to isolated carotid body cells. The authors believe that this method will prove useful in investigating the ionic mechanisms underlying the response of the carotid body to hypoxia and hypercapnia.

In Chapter 12, Hansen et al. report that the brain can appreciably modify the effects of hypoxia on breathing in the fetus and newborn. Their studies make several interesting points. First, ventilatory responses to hypoxia do not adequately reflect carotid body responses, since ventilatory depressions by hypoxia in the newborn and fetus can occur despite carotid body excitation. Second, in the newborn there are hypoxia-sensitive structures in the brain that depress the ventilatory response. It is possible that similar structures exist in the adult.

8

Membrane Properties of Glomus Cells During Stimulation and Inhibition of Carotid Nerve Discharges

C. EYZAGUIRRE

The carotid body glomus (type I) cells are innervated by fibers of the carotid nerve; the nerve terminals and cells form chemoreceptor synapses. Morphologically, these junctions have been described as afferent, efferent, or reciprocal and are enveloped by processes of the sustentacular (type II) cells (12).

From a neurophysiological point of view, it is tempting to assume that the glomus cell is the presynaptic structure and the nerve ending is the postsynaptic element. In this view, the glomus cells would be the primary site for chemoreception, transmitting this information to the nerve endings. However, the morphology suggests a more complex relationship, and there is no consensus that, functionally, this is the case. In fact, the glomus cell, the enveloping type II cells, and the nerve terminals have been assigned the role of primary transducer elements (3,8,9). Further, it is well established that the glomus cell is a secreting structure and that the products of secretion—acetylcholine (ACh), catecholamines (especially dopamine), and the neuropeptides (enkephalins and substance P)—influence the nerve discharge when exogenously applied (3,8,9). Therefore, secretions could affect not only the nerve terminals but also the glomus cells if the latter have autoreceptors for the released chemicals. Another complication is that chemoreceptor stimuli and the released substances could also affect the behavior of the sustentacular cells which, in turn, might modify the chemoreception process. Thus, for proper understanding of the mechanisms of chemoreception, it is essential to obtain direct evidence on the physiological behavior of the three elements of the chemoreceptor junction.

It should be stated at the outset that we have no information on the properties of sustentacular cells. This is not surprising since, physiologically, they are difficult to identify and intracellular recordings from them are extremely difficult to perform, at least in mammalian preparations. We know, however, that they appear to be similar to glial cells in the central nervous system and to capsule cells of peripheral automatic ganglia (11). There is information about some properties of the carotid nerve terminals in that they give rise to small and slow depolarizing potentials, similar to those recorded from postsynaptic elements in other junctions. During receptor stimulation, their frequency increases and they fuse, forming larger and slower depolarizations (6). However, intracellular penetrations for voltage recordings have been difficult, and crucial experiments to determine if they are pre- or postsynaptic have not been performed. It has been easier to obtain physiological and pharmacological information by intracellular recordings from glomus cells (1,2,5,6,10). However, the relationship between changes in their membrane properties and variations in the sensory discharge frequency has not been established.

The purpose of this chapter is to present a brief overview of what is known about the membrane of glomus cells and some recent findings from this laboratory regarding their resting properties and changes during excitation and depression of the sensory discharge.

METHODS

The membrane of glomus cells can be studied during intracellular penetrations with microelectrodes used to record the resting potential (E_m), input resistance (R_0), and voltage noise (E_{rms}). These studies have been conducted in vitro; in vivo experiments have not been reported, possibly because it is difficult to maintain good and long-lasting microelectrode penetrations owing to respiratory movements and arterial pulsations which tend to dislodge an impaling microelectrode. Intracellular recordings from glomus cells in vitro are relatively simple to accomplish since the preparations survive for many hours in modified Tyrode's solution equilibrated with either pure oxygen or 50% O_2 in N_2, pH 7.43. They can be tested by using natural (low Po_2, high Pco_2, acidity, high temperature, and osmolarity) and chemical (NaCN, and cholinomimetic and catecholaminergic) agents. Discharge depressants such as alkalinity and cooling have also been tried. It is possible to record simultaneously the sensory discharge from the carotid nerve and membrane changes from the glomus cells in intact carotid body–nerve preparations, as shown in the upper part of Fig. 8.1. In other experiments, cultured glomus cells and carotid body slices have been used (1,5). These preparations permit intracellular recordings under visual observation with Nomarski or phase contrast optics. Slices and cultured glomus cells have the advantage that one is certain about the location of the microelectrode without resorting to staining of the recorded element, but they have the disadvantage that one cannot record the sensory discharges simultaneously.

RESULTS

Resting Membrane Potential (E_m)

The values reported for the membrane potential of glomus cells are generally low if one compares them with the norm for excitable tissues. Different authors have

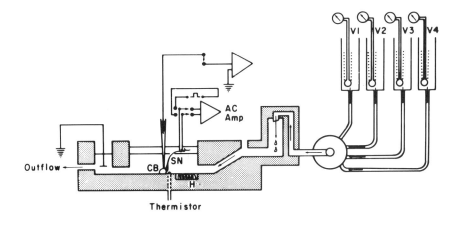

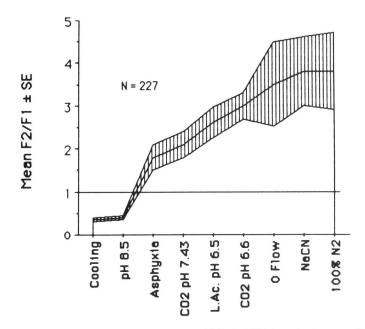

Fig. 8.1 (Top) The experimental setup. The carotid body (CB) is at the bottom of the chamber, and its sinus nerve (SN) is lifted into oil covering the flowing modified Tyrode's solution. The nerve is placed on platinum–iridium recording electrodes connected to an AC amplifier for recording of sensory discharges. A microelectrode is lowered into the bath for intracellular recordings of the glomus cells. The temperature is controlled by a thermistor operating in conjunction with an insulated nichrome wire heater. Solutions flow under the oil from vessels (V1 to V4), where they are equilibrated with different gas mixtures. The preparation is transilluminated and visualized with a dissecting microscope at 10–40X. (Courtesy of Dr. Y. Hayashida.) **(Bottom)** The effects of different agents (abscissa) on the carotid sinus nerve (SN) sensory discharge. The ordinate represents the frequency ratio (test frequency/control frequency, F_2/F_1) $\pm$ SE (shaded area). N, total number of observations. The horizontal line at $F_2/F_1 = 1.0$ is the level at which no changes in frequency are observed. Ratio values higher than 1 result in an increase in frequency; values lower than 1 discharge depression. The values were plotted and the charts were drawn by computer in this and the following illustrations. L. Ac., lactic acid.

reported different values, and there has been a general concern that low values may be due to injury induced by the microelectrode's penetration of these small (about $10 \mu m$) cells. However, even if some injury has occurred, there is the real possibility that glomus cells may never be in a "resting" state. A muscle fiber that is not stimulated may be at rest. However, carotid body chemoreceptors may always have some basal activity even when one thinks that the preparation is at rest. In fact, these receptors respond to such variety of stimuli that even basal conditions such as temperature ($37°C$), pH 7.43, proper oxygenation, and low CO_2 may induce some receptor activation. If, under these conditions, one records the sensory discharge from the carotid nerve, there are some discharges. Therefore, glomus cells could behave similarly, and "resting" conditions may indicate only that one is not doing something obvious to the preparation.

At "rest," the membrane potentials recorded by different authors have varied between 10 and 100 mV, the most frequent values being between 20 and 50 mV. As a comparison, one should note that resting potential of autonomic ganglion cells varies between 50 and 70 mV.

Input Resistance (R_0)

This parameter has been measured by passing current pulses (0.1 and 1.0 nA) through the recording microelectrode via a bridge circuit. The resistance has been calculated as the amplitude of the recorded pulse (V) divided by the injected current (I). Values for R_0 have also varied greatly (10 to >100 megohm, $M\Omega$) with an approximate mean of 40–60 $M\Omega$. These values are low as compared with those recorded in excitable cells, when one considers the size of glomus cells. Again, injury induced by the electrode could account for these low values, but the cells may always have some basal activity.

Voltage Noise (E_{rms})

This interesting phenomenon was first reported by Hayashida and Eyzaguirre (10). Careful observation of the oscilloscope screen during an intracellular penetration reveals small fluctuations of the baseline which are of irregular amplitude, duration, and polarity. Their amplitude can be measured by use of high-AC amplification, and an rms voltage meter. Their mean amplitude is about 2 mV, which is large when compared to noise recorded in other systems. Its origin is still obscure because noise may be produced by channel activity of the membrane surface or by coupling between two or more cells. In fact, gap junctions between cells have been described (12), and coupling can be a noise generator. Another possibility is that secretory channels may contribute to the total voltage noise. However, this possibility is remote because, if secretion is produced by exocytosis, this phenomenon is electroneutral and unlikely to generate noise. An alternative would be secretion via electroactive channels. However, when a medium containing no calcium and an excess of Mg was used, there was no change in noise amplitude (unpublished). Furthermore, secretion is known to be either absent or markedly decreased under these conditions. Thus, surface channel activity and coupling between cells are the most likely candidates for its generation.

Effects of Some Stimulants and Inhibitors of the Sensory Discharge on the Glomus Cell Membrane

The lower part of Fig. 8.1 illustrates the effects of several agents on the sensory discharge of the cat carotid nerve. The most powerful stimuli were pure nitrogen (anoxic anoxia), boluses of 1–25 μg sodium cyanide (histotoxic anoxia), and interruption of flow of the bathing saline. These effects were followed in intensity by 6% CO_2 at an external pH (pH_o) of 6.6, lactic acid (pH 6.5), 6% CO_2 at pH 7.43, and asphyxia. The latter was provoked by superfusing a solution equilibrated with 100% CO_2 for 30 s, followed by long periods of rest. Cooling (from 36°C to 32°C) and alkalinity (pH 8.5) depressed the sensory discharge. The following description covers the effects of these agents on the glomus cell membrane.

Effects of Zero Saline Flow, and Anoxic and Histotoxic Anoxia

Flow interruption elicited cell depolarization, reduced input resistance, and decreased membrane noise. The other two powerful enhancers of the sensory discharge induced either cell depolarization (reduction) or hyperpolarization (increase) of the resting potential. For simplicity, the effects of these three agents were pooled. Figure 8.2 (top left) shows the effects of these agents on the resting potential (ΔE_m) of glomus cells. The changes in voltage noise (ΔE_{rms}) and input resistance (ΔR_0) varied from increase to decrease as depicted in Fig. 8.2 (middle and bottom left). These variations, which became evident after a few experiments, have been reported in previous communications (8). Therefore, to determine if there were statistically significant correlations between these parameters, it was necessary to sample a large population. Changes in resistance (ΔR_0) were used as the independent or explanatory variable, under the assumption that conductance ($1/R_0$) changes could be responsible for ΔE_m and E_{rms}. Results of these analyses are presented in Fig. 8.2 (right). The upper panel shows that as resistance fell (increased conductance) the cells became depolarized, whereas when resistance increased there was a tendency toward an increased (more negative) membrane potential. The lower panel illustrates a significant and positive correlation between ΔR_0 and changes in voltage noise (ΔE_{rms}). As resistance increased (decreased conductance), the noise also increased, and vice versa. Thus, changes in resistance had opposite effects on the membrane potential and voltage noise.

It is unknown why the cells reacted differently to these stimuli. In the case of NaCN there was no correlation between doses (1–25 μg) and changes in membrane potential or noise. We do not know if this is exclusively an effect of CN or if the same phenomenon occurs with the other stimuli. The negative correlation between changes in resistance and membrane potential is conventional. As resistance decreased (increased conductance), the membrane potential was reduced. This effect could be produced by opening of ionic channels, leading to cell depolarization, and channel closing, leading to a larger membrane potential. It is more difficult to explain why increased conductance reduced membrane voltage noise. If the latter represents opening of ionic channels, one would expect the opposite—that is, augmented noise. Yet this did not occur. The noise reduction was probably due to

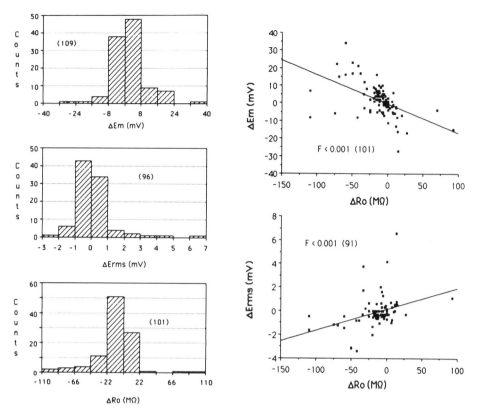

Fig. 8.2 The effects of zero saline flow, anoxia (100% N_2), and NaCN boluses on glomus cell membrane. **(Left panels)** Histograms depicting distribution of changes in membrane properties during application of these stimuli. The upper record depicts changes in membrane potential (ΔE_m) in millivolts (mV), where negative values indicate membrane hyperpolarization, and positive ones, depolarization. The middle record shows changes in membrane noise (ΔE_{rms}) in millivolts (mV), which either increased or decreased. The lower record illustrates changes in input resistance (ΔR_0) in megohms (MΩ), which also either decreased or increased. The number of observations is shown in parentheses. **(Right panels)** The upper record shows a regression analysis plotting changes in resistance against changes in membrane potential; the lower record, the same analysis plotting changes in resistance against changes in membrane voltage noise. $F <$, statistical probability of F. The number of observations is shown in parentheses. Notice the statistically significant correlations in the upper and lower regressions.

the small amplitude of voltage noise and the relatively large changes in resistance, in accordance with Ohm's law. When changes in resistance were plotted against the estimated membrane *current* noise, there was a significant and negative correlation between these parameters. As resistance decreased, there was a tendency toward larger current noise. However, this is only an indirect estimate of the measured values, and a definite conclusion will have to wait until current and conductance measurements are made in voltage-clamp experiments.

Effects of Hypercapnia and pH$_o$ on the Glomus Cell Membrane

As shown in Fig. 8.1, hypercapnia (6% CO_2 in 44% O_2) at pH 7.43, 6% CO_2 at pH 6.6, and lactic acid at pH 6.5 induced a carotid nerve sensory discharge increase which was less marked than that elicited by the previously described (anoxic and histotoxic anoxia and zero flow) stimuli. Asphyxia (100% CO_2) at pH 5.5 was even less effective. Alkalinity (pH$_o$ 8.5) depressed the sensory discharge.

Figure 8.3A illustrates the changes in sensory discharge frequency elicited by these agents. As pH decreased from 8.5, there was considerable increase in sensory discharge frequency. However, the increase in discharge was much less marked when pH$_o$ fell to 5.5 during asphyxia. The latter observation is not unusual since there is a limit to the tolerance of these receptors to acid (and other) stimulation as shown earlier (4,7).

With regard to the effects of these agents on the glomus cell membrane, Fig. 8.3B shows that as extracellular pH fell there was a tendency toward cell depolarization, represented by the regression line with a significant negative slope. This illustration also shows that there was ample variation in the results obtained during application of different solutions to the bath. In fact, at a given pH$_o$ some cells underwent depolarization, whereas others were hyperpolarized. Nevertheless, the trend was clear and significant. Figure 8.3C depicts something similar with regard to voltage noise. As pH$_o$ fell, the tendency was toward increased noise in spite of the variations of the data obtained during applications of a given agent. Likewise, Fig. 8.3D shows that the input resistance tended to increase with lower pH$_o$.

These results suggested that the major effect of increased external acidity was an increase in resistance and that, perhaps, R_0 changes led to cell depolarization and increased noise. This assumption seemed correct because regression analyses showed a significant and *positive* correlation between changes in resistance versus changes in membrane potential and voltage noise (not illustrated). This correlation is not unusual since acidity and CO_2 are considered to be membrane "stabilizers" (14).

It should be noted that the positive and significant correlation between changes in resistance and in voltage noise was similar to that reported for the more potent chemoreceptor stimuli. However, the correlation between ΔR_0 and ΔE_m was opposite to that recorded for the other stimuli. One possible explanation for this difference is that the glomus cell membrane may be permeable not only to CO_2 (or HCO_3), but also to other organic (such as lactic) acids. Internal acidification would deposit an excess of H^+ ions on the inside of the membrane, contributing to cell depolarization if the cell resting potential is dependent on this ion. This could be the case if there is Na^+-H^+ exchange across the membrane as previously suggested (2). However, there is no experimental proof that this exchange occurs. Cell hyperpolarization during alkalinity could have been produced by acid extrusion which would deposit H^+ ions on the outside of the membrane. Likewise, the increased resting potential seen during acid stimulation of some cells could be accounted for by acid extrusion if these cells became too acid. In fact, cell depolarization followed by hyperpolarization was seen in a few instances when pH$_o$ was lowered (not illustrated). Nevertheless, a possible permeability to organic acids has to be reconciled with an increased resistance.

pH Effects on Discharge and Glomus Cells

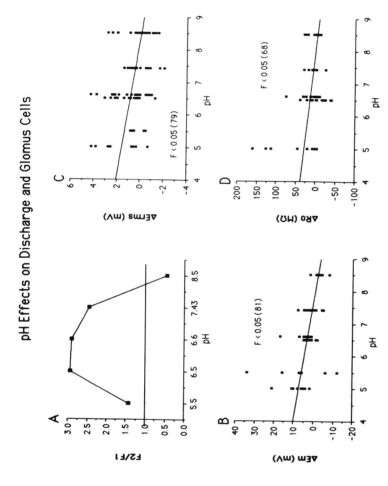

Fig. 8.3 Effects of pH$_o$ on carotid nerve sensory discharge (**a**) and on glomus cell membrane parameters (**B-D**). (**A**) At pH 8.5, the sensory discharge is depressed. As pH decreases to 6.5, there is a progressive increase in discharge frequency. This increase is less marked when pH reaches 5.5. (**B**) There is a tendency toward cell depolarization with a lower pH. (**C**) There is a tendency toward an increase in membrane noise as acidity increases. (**D**) Resistance tends to increase as pH falls. Abscissae, pH$_o$ units. Ordinates, as in Figs. 8.1 and 8.2. $F <$, probability of F. The number of observations is shown in parentheses.

Effects of Rapid Cooling on the Glomus Cell Membrane

We have reported that rapid cooling (36–37°C to 31–32°C) of in vitro preparations depresses the sensory discharge (also shown in Fig. 8.1). This effect was accompanied by marked cell depolarization and decreased input resistance (2).

We repeated those observations in 22 cells, adding measurements of voltage noise. Cooling produced the effects previously described but failed to change voltage noise. Thus, cooling elicited changes in resting potential and input resistance similar to those obtained during zero flow, but the effects of these two agents on voltage noise were quite different. What is noteworthy is that cooling is a powerful depressant of the sensory discharge, whereas flow interruption is one of the more potent ones (7,8). At this point, trying to discuss this puzzle would lead only to speculation.

Correlation Between Glomus Cell Membrane Changes and Sensory Discharge Frequency

One of the most frustrating experiences in recording intracellularly from glomus cells has been the variability of results obtained during applications of stimulants or depressants of the carotid nerve discharge, as indicated before and elsewhere (3,8,9). This variability of the glomus cell response occurred concomitantly with consistent effects on the nerve. Until recently, it appeared that there was no correlation between these events. However, a more recent analysis using a large number of observations has shown that glomus cell and nerve activity are not entirely independent.

Experiments were designed to record simultaneously discharges from the whole nerve and intracellularly from a glomus cell. Once a successful penetration was made, the "resting" values for membrane potential, input resistance, and membrane noise were recorded, as was the frequency of the carotid nerve discharges. During the action of a chemoreceptor stimulant or depressant, changes in membrane parameters and the new frequency of the sensory discharge were again recorded. Differences (test minus control) in membrane parameters (ΔE_m, ΔR_0, and ΔE_{rms}) and the ratio between test and control frequency (F_2/F_1) were used as variables for regression analyses. Ratios are more accurate that ΔF's because recordings were made from multifiber preparations and it was important to normalize the results.

In 98 trials, simultaneous recordings from the nerve and from glomus cells were analyzed; results are presented in Fig. 8.4. The linear regression was constructed by plotting changes in membrane potential (ΔE_m) against F_2/F_1 during the effects of all stimulants and depressants of the sensory discharge. This analysis shows a direct and positive regression between the membrane potential changes and the sensory discharge. The correlation was highly significant ($F < .013$), in spite of the fact that cooling depressed the discharge and induced cell depolarization. However, for this observation to be valid without question, one needs further analyses to avoid biases due to an uneven number of categories. Nevertheless, the present data suggest that an increased sensory discharge elicited by any agent is more likely to occur when the cell membrane potential is reduced. No significant

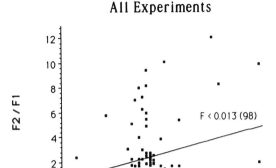

Fig. 8.4 Linear regression illustrating the correlation between the effects of different agents on the glomus cell membrane and the sensory discharge frequency in all experiments. Abscissa, changes in membrane potential (ΔE_m in millivolts, mV). Positive numbers indicate membrane depolarization; negative ones, hyperpolarization. Ordinate, ratio of frequency changes (F_2/F_1) as in Fig. 8.1. $F <$, significance of F. The number of observations is in parentheses. The horizontal line through 1.0 in the ordinate is as defined in Figs. 8.1 and 8.3A.

correlations between changes in resistance or membrane noise and F_2/F_1 have been found.

For the moment, these empirical analyses do not establish a cause–effect relationship between changes in glomus cell properties and the sensory discharge. However, they illustrate that events in the glomus cell and the nerve discharge are not totally independent.

DISCUSSION

It appears that interruption of flow and anoxia (both anoxic and histotoxic) affect the glomus cell membrane, but the mechanisms are different from those acting during either hypercapnia (at neutral or acid pH) or external acidity. Different mechanisms for the effects of hypoxia and hypercapnia on the sensory discharge have been reported by Mulligan and Lahiri (13). It is possible, therefore, that this difference may be produced by different behavior of the glomus cells reacting under these stimuli. It is too early to be definite about this point, but further exploration of this possibility is worthwhile.

As to the effects of hypercapnia and external acidity, it is interesting to note that a lowering of pH_o affected the glomus cell membrane when carbonic and lactic acids were used. No effects were obtained when the external pH was lowered by use of HCl, which may indicate that inorganic acids do not penetrate into the glomus cell. Further, it shows that a high external concentration of H^+ ions per se does not affect the membrane. It seems that acids have to penetrate or leave the cell to be effective. It may be that during this exchange there is also an exchange of other (e.g., Na^+) ions which may be important in regulating the membrane potential of these cells, as suggested in a previous publication (2; see also Fitzgerald et al., Chap. 9, this volume). However, we still do not have evidence about the activities of intracellular H^+ and Na^+ ions in these cells.

The lack of effect of HCl on the glomus cells is interesting in view of previous observations in which the lowering of pH_o by manipulations of the Tris-HCl buffer increased the carotid nerve sensory discharge (4,7). This author is not aware of studies comparing the effects of organic versus inorganic acids on the sensory discharge. This point ought to be studied since it may give an indication of a possible role of the glomus cell in these processes. Also, if the acidic hypothesis of chemosensory excitation (15) is correct, external acidification of the carotid nerve terminals may suffice, whether it is achieved by organic or inorganic acids. However, as expressed elsewhere (8), one problem with this hypothesis is that H^+ ions are membrane stabilizers (14). Therefore, it is difficult to conceive how a high H^+ concentration could destabilize (depolarize) the membrane of the nerve terminals unless they have some special properties or are indirectly activated by acid-induced chemical release from the glomus cells.

As to discharge depressants, cooling and alkalinity appeared to act on the glomus cell membrane by very different mechanisms even when the end product, discharge depression, was about the same. Again, we do not have precise information about the effects of these depressants on the intracellular activities of different ions. And, as stated previously, it is puzzling that cooling and interruption of flow acted almost identically on the membrane potential and resistance whereas their action on the sensory discharge was exactly the opposite. The only recorded difference was that whereas zero flow affected membrane noise, cooling did not. However, we need more information about the physiological meaning of membrane noise to understand this phenomenon.

In conclusion, we are still far from understanding the role of glomus cells in chemosensory transduction. We know that usual carotid body stimulants induce release of endogenous substances from the glomus cells and that these agents, when exogenously applied, change the frequency of the carotid nerve sensory discharges (3,8,9). Thus, there may be complex feedback mechanisms (from cell to nerve and vice versa) in addition to communication between glomus cells. These interactions, probably involving electrical and chemical messages, have prevented us from assigning unequivocal roles to the main elements of the chemosensory synapse, namely, the glomus cells and nerve terminals.

ACKNOWLEDGMENTS

The original experimental material used for this presentation was obtained in collaboration with Drs. Margarita Brown, L. Monti-Bloch, and Y. Hayashida. The technical assistance of Messrs. P. Lenoir, J. Fisher, and B. Evans is gratefully acknowledged. This work was supported by NIH grants NS-05666 and NS-07938 and American Heart Association Grant 860662.

REFERENCES

1. Acker, H., and F. Pietruschka. Meaning of the type I cell for the chemoreceptive process—an electrophysiological study on cultured type I cells of the carotid body. In:

Chemoreception in the Carotid Body, ed. H. Acker, S. Fidone, D. Pallot, C. Eyzaguirre, D. W. Lubbers, and R. W. Torrance. New York: Springer-Verlag, 1977, pp. 92–96.

2. Baron, M., and C. Eyzaguirre. Effects of temperature on some membrane characteristics of carotid body cells. *Am J. Physiol. 233 (Cell Physiol. 2):* C35–C36, 1977.

3. Eyzaguirre, C., R. S. Fitzgerald, S. Lahiri, and P. Zapata. Arterial chemoreceptors. In: *Handbook of Physiology,* Sec. 2: *The Cardiovascular System,* Vol. 3: *Peripheral Circulation and Organ Blood Flow,* ed. J. T. Shepherd and F. M. Abboud. Bethesda: Am. Physiol Soc., 1983, pp. 557–621.

4. Eyzaguirre, C., and H. Koyano. Effects of hypoxia, hypercapnia and pH on the chemoreceptor activity of the carotid body in vitro. *J. Physiol. (Lond.) 178:* 385–409, 1965.

5. Eyzaguirre, C., and L. Monti-Bloch. Nicotinic and muscarinic reactive sites in mammalian glomus cells. *Brain Res. 252:* 181–184, 1982.

6. Eyzaguirre, C., L. Monti-Bloch, Y. Hayashida, and M. Baron. Biophysics of the carotid body receptor complex. In: *Physiology of the Peripheral Arterial Chemoreceptors,* ed. H. Acker and R. G. O'Regan. New York: Elsevier, 1983, pp. 59–87.

7. Eyzaguirre, C., and P. Zapata. Pharmacology of pH effects on carotid body chemoreceptors in vitro. *J. Physiol (Lond.) 195:* 557–588, 1968.

8. Eyzaguirre, C., and P. Zapata. Perspectives in carotid body research. *J. Appl. Physiol. 57:* 931–957, 1984.

9. Fidone, S. J., and C. Gonzalez. Initiation and control of chemoreceptor activity in the carotid body. In: *Handbook of Physiology, Sec. 3: The Respiratory System,* Vol. 2: *Control of Breathing,* ed. N. S. Cherniack and J. G. Widdicombe. Bethesda, MD: Am. Physiol. Soc., 1986, pp. 247–312.

10. Hayashida, Y., and C. Eyzaguirre. Voltage noise of carotid body type I cells. *Brain Res. 167:* 189–194, 1979.

11. Kondo, H., T. Iwanaga, and T. Nakajima. Immunocytochemical study on the localization of neuron-specific enolase and S-100 protein in the carotid body of rats. *Cell Tissue Res. 227:* 291–295, 1982.

12. McDonald, D. M., and R. A. Mitchell. The innervation of glomus cells, ganglion cells and blood vessels in the rat carotid body: a quantitative ultrastructural analysis. *J. Neurocytol. 4:* 177–230, 1975.

13. Mulligan, E., and S. Lahiri. Separation of carotid body chemoreceptor responses to O_2 and CO_2 by oligomycin and by antimycin A. *Am. J. Physiol. 242:* C200–C206, 1982.

14. Shanes, A. M. Electrochemical aspects of physiological and pharmacological actions in excitable cells. *Pharmacol. Rev. 10:* 59–273, 1958.

15. Torrance, R. W. A comparison of central and peripheral chemoreceptors. In: *Acid Base Homeostasis of the Brain Extracellular Fluid and the Respiratory Control System,* ed. H. H. Loeschcke. Stuttgart: Thieme, 1976, pp. 95–103.

9

Testing for Ionic Pumps in the Carotid Body

R. S. FITZGERALD, M. SHIRAHATA, AND S. LAHIRI

The carotid bodies in the cat play a key role in several of the cardiopulmonary responses to hypoxia; they increase ventilation, functional residual capacity, cardiac output, and ventricular contractility, thereby offsetting the precipitous fall in total peripheral resistance in the systemically hypoxic animal. The carotid bodies also are responsible for changes in airway resistance and airway secretions generated by hypoxia. They participate as well in the hydroxycorticosteroid response to hypoxia.

The carotid bodies also increase their neural output in response to hypercapnia and to metabolic acidosis. Indeed, the resting ventilation in the carotid body-resected animal is lower and the resting P_aCO_2 is higher, very probably due more to CO_2 drive than to O_2 drive at the carotid bodies. There is evidence that the mechanisms involved in the chemotransduction of arterial hypoxia differ at least in part from those responsible for the chemotransduction of arterial hypercapnia into neural activity.

However, the mechanisms involved in the chemotransduction of hypoxia and hypercapnia into increased neural activity are not well understood. Not long ago, Hanson, Nye, and Torrance (5) proposed that nerve endings in the carotid body responded to changes in the pH of an extracellular compartment surrounding the nerve fiber. Hypercapnia increased neural activity by the carbonic anhydrase-assisted generation of H^+. Hypoxia increased neural activity by shutting down an O_2-dependent HCO_3^- pump which regulated the $[H^+]$ of the compartment. However, some experiments using acetazolamide and benzolamide produced data not consistent with their hypothesis. They suggested that the pH change might be intracellular, either in the nerve endings or in the type I cell.

This group then tried several drugs that poison a cell's ability to manipulate its intracellular pH. One such drug was amiloride. Given in 1 mM concentration, this drug is known to poison a Na^+–H^+ antiporter which operates in many tissues. The Na^+–H^+ antiporter or exchanger has several functions, but the most common is the regulation of intracellular pH. [One of us has recently used amiloride in studies of the rat diaphragm's response to hypercapnia. In the in vitro rat diaphragm exposed to hypercapnia, the pH_i decreased significantly more when the superfusate contained 0.6–0.8 mM amiloride than when it did not (4).]

Hanson et al. evaluated their results, treating the carotid body with amiloride as negative (5). However, there seemed to be only one animal in their study; moreover, the concentration of the drug at the carotid body was not specified, nor was it clear how long after the administration of the drug the hypercapnic or hypoxic challenges were given.

We hypothesized that if the chemosensitive structure responsive to hypercapnia was in a compartment where the pH was regulated by a $Na^+–H^+$ antiporter, then the output from the structure would be greater in response to hypercapnia after the antiporter was blocked with amiloride than with no amiloride block. We further hypothesized that the response to hypoxia would not be altered by amiloride, the chemoreceptive response to hypoxia involving, perhaps, the energy status of the carotid body (7) and not necessarily H^+ concentration.

METHODS

Cats ($n = 6$) were anesthetized with sodium pentobarbital (32 mg/kg), paralyzed, and artificially ventilated. All of the arterial branches around the carotid sinus were ligated except the occipital artery supplying the carotid body and the external carotid artery. The latter was prepared so that a clip could be placed on the artery, thus diverting flow through the carotid body only.

A loop containing a three-way stopcock was then inserted into the common carotid artery. The stopcock was arranged so that for the most part the cat perfused its own carotid body and external carotid artery with its own arterial blood. When the protocol required selective perfusion of the carotid body with a solution, the common carotid artery was clamped, the external carotid artery was clamped, the stopcock was turned, and a peristaltic pump delivered at a comparable mean pressure a pulsatile flow of the solution through water-jacketed catheters from flasks in a water bath at constant temperature (37–38°C). These solutions were gassed with 95% O_2/5% CO_2.

The carotid sinus nerve was prepared for recording neural activity from single- or few-fiber chemoreceptor axons. Femoral arterial and venous catheters allowed for the measurement of arterial blood gas values (P_aO_2, P_aCO_2, pH_a; Radiometer BMS 3Mk2 Blood Micro System, Copenhagen) and blood pressure, and for the renewal of anesthetic and administration of sodium bicarbonate when necessary.

The overall plan of our selective carotid body perfusion technique was to make the cat hypercapnic (or hypoxic), allowing arterial blood to perfuse the carotid body. Then the carotid body was selectively perfused with a Krebs–Ringer bicarbonate solution after which hypercapnic (or hypoxic) arterial blood again perfused the carotid body for 4 min. Then the amiloride-containing solution selectively per-

Table 9.1 Experimental Protocol

Step	Carotid body area perfused with:	Cat ventilated on:	Duration (min)
1.	Common carotid arterial blood	Room air	20
2.	Common carotid arterial blood	7.5% CO_2, 21% O_2; balance, N_2	5
3.	Krebs–Ringer bicarbonate solution	7.5% CO_2, 21% O_2; balance, N_2	2.5
4.	Common carotid arterial blood (hypercapnic)	7.5% CO_2, 21% O_2; balance, N_2	4
5.	Krebs–Ringer Bicarbonate + *amiloride* (0.6–0.8 mM) solution	7.5% CO_2, 21% O_2; balance, N_2	2.5
6.	Common carotid arterial blood (hypercapnic)	7.5% CO_2, 21% O_2; balance, N_2	4
7.	Rest; cf. step 1		
8–12.	Repetition of steps 2–6	Then 8% O_2, 92% N_2	

fused the carotid body, after which the hypercapnic (or hypoxic) blood was allowed to perfuse the carotid body again for 4 min.

Impulses per second were counted for 4 min after the blood flow was reestablished in each case. This value was normalized by dividing by the P_aCO_2 (or P_aO_2). The details of the protocol are shown in Table 9.1.

RESULTS

Figure 9.1 presents the carotid body response to hypercapnic blood after 12 paired infusions in six animals. The open histograms represent the neural response to hypercapnic blood following control infusions (normal Krebs–Ringer bicarbonate solution); solid histograms represent the carotid body response to hypercapnic blood following amiloride-containing infusions. As demonstrated by analysis of variance and Duncan's new multiple range tests, the only significant difference between the two sets occurred in the first 25 s. In other words, there appears to be no sustained significant difference between the neural responses to hypercapnic blood after selective perfusion of the carotid body with ordinary Krebs–Ringer bicarbonate solution and the response after perfusion with the amiloride-containing solution.

We then determined the response to hypoxic blood after the control and amiloride-containing infusions. We had hypothesized that there would be no effect due to amiloride. On the other hand, if as Torrance had proposed, an O_2-dependent HCO_3^- pump failed, one might reasonably expect in our preparation a larger increase in output in response to hypoxic blood after amiloride than after control, at least transiently. This would occur because amiloride presumably had poisoned a Na^+–H^+ antiporter somewhere in the chemoreceptive process. The result would be to allow a larger accumulation of H^+ for a given level of CO_2 because the influx of the HCO_3^- buffer would be reduced.

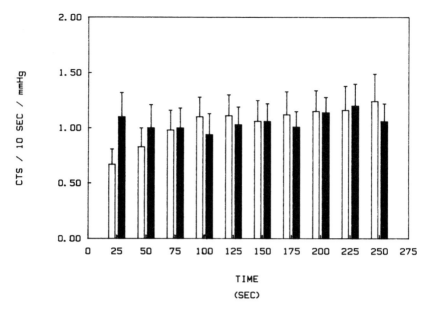

Fig. 9.1 Carotid body response to hypercapnic arterial blood after a 150-s perfusion. Mean values ($\pm$ SE) of impulses per 10 s in response to hypercapnic arterial blood perfusing the carotid body after an extracorporeal infusion of standard Krebs–Ringer bicarbonate solution (open histograms) or a Krebs–Ringer bicarbonate solution containing 0.6–0.8 mM amiloride (solid histograms). There were 12 infusions of each kind in six animals. The responses have been normalized by dividing the responses by the arterial partial pressure of CO_2 (P_aCO_2 = 48–64 mmHg). Only the histograms at 25 s are significantly different from each other.

Figure 9.2 presents the results of 10 paired infusions in six animals. Open histograms represent the neural response to hypoxia after a control infusion; and the solid histograms, the carotid body response after an amiloride-containing infusion. Using analysis of variance and Duncan's test, we found the response to hypoxia after the amiloride infusions to be significantly less than the corresponding response to hypoxia after the control infusions.

The Na^+–H^+ antiporter is also blocked by an extracellular fluid containing a decreased concentration of sodium. We reduced Na concentration from 140 mM to 24 mM (only that contained in the $NaHCO_3^-$), and to make up for the decreased chloride ion, we substituted 120 mM choline chloride. This solution was infused in place of the amiloride-containing solution during hypercapnia. Figure 9.3 compares, in that animal, the effect of the control and low-sodium infusions on the carotid body response to subsequent hypercapnic blood. The response seems remarkably similar to the carotid body response to hypercapnia after amiloride.

We then made the animal hypoxic and perfused with, first, control solution and, then, the low sodium solution. The carotid body responses to hypoxic blood after each of these two infusions are shown in Fig. 9.4. Clearly the carotid body response to hypoxic blood is very similar to the response after amiloride.

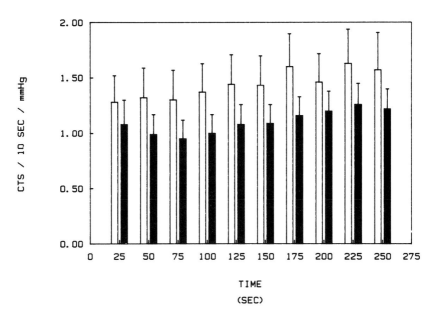

Fig. 9.2 Carotid body response to hypoxic arterial blood after a 150-s perfusion. The symbols are defined as in Fig. 9.1. In this case the impulses per 10 s have been normalized by dividing by the arterial oxygen tension (P_aO_2 = 35–45 mmHg). The hypoxic response of the carotid body after a control infusion of Krebs–Ringer bicarbonate solution (open histograms) is significantly greater than the corresponding hypoxic response points after the amiloride-containing perfusion (solid histograms).

Fig. 9.3 Carotid body response to hypercapnic arterial blood after a 150-s infusion of low-sodium Krebs–Ringer bicarbonate solution. Instead of 140 mM Na, the perfusate contained 24 mM Na and 120 mM choline chloride. The plot resembles Fig. 9.1, suggesting that sodium exchange is not important for the chemoreception of hypercapnia.

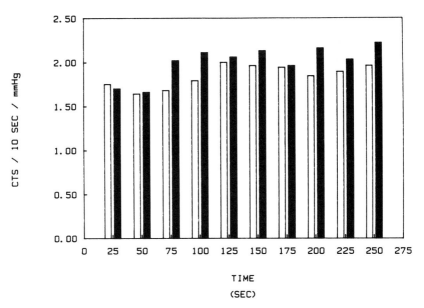

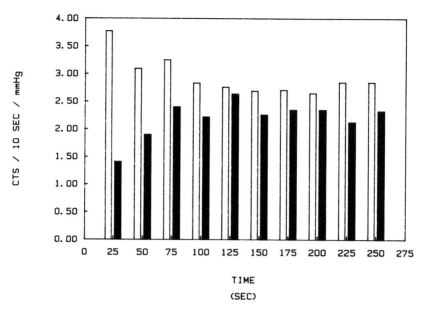

Fig. 9.4 Carotid body response to hypoxic arterial blood after a 150-s infusion of low-sodium Krebs–Ringer bicarbonate solution. The details are as in Fig. 9.3. The plot resembles Fig. 9.2, suggesting that sodium exchange is important for the chemoreception of hypoxia.

DISCUSSION

In summary, our data show that the response of the carotid body to hypercapnic blood after being perfused with either an amiloride-containing solution or a solution of low sodium concentration does not seem to differ significantly from the responses to hypercapnic blood after the infusion of control solutions, whereas the response to hypoxic blood after these infusions is significantly lower than the responses after the appropriate control infusions. The data are absolutely contrary to our initial hypothesis. But they do provide evidence of two receptor mechanisms, one for hypoxia, attenuatable by amiloride or low sodium, and one for hypercapnia, unaffected by these agents.

We are aware of the potential problems of using amiloride. Because amiloride and Na compete for access to the external transport site of the Na^+–H^+ exchanger and because the K_m for Na is quite low, amiloride is not an effective inhibitor of Na^+ in the presence of physiological Na concentrations (140–150 mM) unless 10^{-4} or 10^{-3} M amiloride concentrations are used. At these concentrations other effects may occur, including the interruption of protein synthesis, the inhibition of paracellular cation permeability in epithelia, the inhibition of Na^+,K^+-ATPase, and, as amiloride is a weak base, the nonspecific alteration of transmembrane pH gradients (6). In spite of these possible constraints, amiloride has been used in many studies in 10^{-4}–10^{-3} M concentrations (1). We feel that the low sodium experiment corroborates the action of amiloride in inhibiting a Na^+–H^+ antiporter in the carotid body.

The Na^+–H^+ antiporter or exchanger has been found in ova, sperm, erythrocytes, lymphocytes, skeletal and cardiac muscle, Purkinje fibers, neurons, capillary endothelia, fibroblasts, renal tubular cells, intestinal and gall bladder epithelia, and a variety of cells in culture (2). We are unaware of any study reporting its presence in the carotid body. The presence of a Na^+–H^+ exchanger in the carotid body needs further supporting evidence, and also needs characterization. The data do not support our first hypothesis. We propose, then, the following model incorporating the antiporter to explain the data presented:

1. The chemoreception of hypercapnia involves the release of ACh from the type I cell, but it is postulated that although ACh contributes to the increased neural activity in the chemoreceptive fibers during hypercapnia, it is not necessary for it to occur.
2. The increase in neural activity during hypoxia is essentially dependent on the release of ACh in the presence of an appropriate pH.
3. The Na^+–H^+ antiporter is located on the type I cell.
4. We postulate that the choline uptake system, which is reported to be Na-sensitive (3), is compromised by amiloride's inhibition of the Na^+–H^+ exchanger or by the low sodium perfusate. The uptake of extracellular Na falls. The synthesis and release of ACh is decreased and the response to hypoxic blood is reduced.

In conclusion, there may be other antiporters operating in carotid body chemoreception, for example, the Cl^-–HCO_3^- exchanger. The important point to be learned from these results, regardless of whether the model we present is accurate, is that the chemoreception of hypoxia by the carotid body depends either directly or indirectly on that structure's ability to pump Na across some compartment's boundary (cell wall?), whereas the chemoreception of hypercapnia is not dependent on this process.

ACKNOWLEDGMENTS

This work was supported in part by NHL BI Grants HL-19737, HL-10342 and HL-30021. We thank Mr. A. Mokashi for technical assistance.

REFERENCES

1. Aickin, C., and R. Thomas. An investigation of the ionic mechanisms of intracellular pH regulation in mouse soleus muscle fibers. *J. Physiol. (Lond.), 273:* 295–316, 1977.
2. Aronson, P. S. Kinetic properties of the plasma membrane Na^+–H^+ exchanger. *Annu. Rev. Physiol. 47:* 545–560, 1985.
3. Fidone, S., S. Weintraub, W. Stavinoha, C. Stirling, and L. Jones. Endogenous acetylcholine levels in cat carotid body and autoradiographic localization of a high affinity component of choline uptake. In: *Chemoreception in the Carotid Body,* ed. H. Acker, S. Fidone, D. Pallot, C. Eyzaguirre, D. W. Lubbers, and R. W. Torrance. Berlin: Springer-Verlag, 1977, pp. 106–113.
4. Fitzgerald, R., M. Pike, D. Westcott, S. Howell, and W. Jacobus. ^{31}P NMR determination of intracellular pH control in the in vitro resting rat diaphragm during an acid challenge. *Am. Rev. Respir. Dis. 135:* A333, 1987.

5. Hanson, M., P. Nye, and R. Torrance. The exodus of an extracellular bicarbonate theory of chemoreception and the genesis of an intracellular one. In: *Arterial Chemoreceptors, Proc. Sixth Int. Meeting,* ed. by C. Belmonte, D. Pallot, H. Acker, and S. Fidone. Leicester, UK: Leicester University Press, 1981, pp. 362–372.

6. Mahnensmith, R., and P. Aronson. The plasma membrane sodium-hydrogen exchanger and its role in physiological and pathophysiological processes. *Circ. Res. 56:* 773–788, 1985.

7. Mulligan, E., and S. Lahiri. Separation of carotid body chemoreceptor responses to O_2 and CO_2 by oligomycin and by antimycin A. *Am. J. Physiol. 242 (Cell Physiol. 11):* C 200–C206, 1982.

10

Transmitter Interactions in Peripheral Arterial Chemoreceptors

S. FIDONE, C. GONZALEZ, B. DINGER, A. OBESO,
L. ALMARAZ, K. YOSHIZAKI, R. RIGUAL, AND G. HANSON

The arterial chemosensory tissue of the mammalian carotid body contains morphologically distinct parenchymal cells in synaptic association with afferent terminals of the carotid sinus nerve (CSN). These type I (glomus) parenchymal cells store multiple neuroactive substances, including biogenic amines (dopamine, DA: norepinephrine, NE; acetylcholine, ACh) and neuropeptides (substance P, enkephalins). An important problem in chemoreception is to understand the interactions among these putative transmitters in initiating and/or modulating the chemosensory activity on the CSN.

NEUROACTIVE SUBSTANCES IN CAROTID BODY CHEMORECEPTION

Catecholamines

In recent years, attention has been focused on the role of type I cell catecholamines, notably DA, in the chemoreception process. However, the results of these studies have often been inconclusive and controversial (for a review, see ref. 9). For example, neurochemical studies disagree in regard to the effects of chemoreceptor stimulation on the catecholamine content of the carotid body (see refs. 8, 10). Likewise, studies aimed at characterizing the pharmacological actions of exogenously applied DA and its agonists and antagonists have produced confounding results. A common finding has been that DA may behave as either an excitatory or an inhibitory agent in the carotid body, depending upon dose (35), animal species (26), and whether the organ is studied in vivo or in vitro (e.g., compare ref. 5 vs. 26 and ref. 6 vs. 28). At present, the role of catecholamines in carotid body chemoreception remains unclear.

Acetylcholine

It is well known that cholinergic agonists and antagonists profoundly alter chemoreceptor discharge. Neurochemical investigations seem to indicate that the metabolic machinery necessary for ACh synthesis, storage, and inactivation is associated with the type I cells (13,14,20,22), and that CSN afferent fibers are virtually devoid of cholinergic activity (13,15). It has also been shown that an ACh-like substance is released upon stimulation of the organ in vitro (7). Although these data suggest that ACh may play a role in carotid body chemoreception, its actions in the sensory process have been elusive, particularly with respect to its putative role as mediator or transmitter of chemosensory information between type I cells and CSN afferent fibers. Disagreement about the function of ACh stems from the observations that (a) anticholinergic agents completely block the effects of exogenously applied ACh, but not the response to natural stimuli (31; but see also ref. 9); and (b) exogenous ACh enhances chemosensory discharge in the cat (7,12) whereas similar doses in the rabbit produce inhibition of discharge (5,26). A fundamental problem regarding the actions of ACh in the carotid body has been the uncertainty about the locus of its specific effects on type I cells versus afferent nerve terminals. Thus, previous attempts to demonstrate pharmacologically the chemosensory involvement of ACh have not been convincing, because neither the sites of action of the applied drugs, nor the nicotinic versus muscarinic nature of the cholinergic receptors were clearly defined.

Neuropeptides

The neuropeptides met- and leu-enkephalin (ME, LE) have been localized to the type I cells with immunohistochemical techniques (23,33), whereas substance P (SP)-like immunoreactivity (SPLI) has been reportedly found in both nerve fibers (21) and 20% of the type I cells (1). Little is known regarding the role of these substances in carotid body function, but recent pharmacological studies suggest that administration of exogenous neuropeptides is able to modify chemoreceptor activity of both in vivo and in vitro carotid body preparations (24,25,29). Consequently, these substances are now thought to play a role in the genesis of the normal chemoresponse.

In studying the role of biogenic amines and neuropeptides in the carotid body, an important step is to determine the response of these putative transmitters to natural stimuli which are known to alter the physiological activities of this organ. In our laboratory, we have investigated the synthesis and release of, and the receptor sites of action for these substances as they relate to carotid body chemoreception.

METHODS

Synthesis of Catecholamines In Vitro

These methods are described in detail in our previous publications (8–11). Briefly, carotid bodies are removed from anesthetized animals, cleaned of surrounding connective tissue in a chamber containing 100% O_2-equilibrated Tyrode's solution at 0–4°C, and then transferred to scintillation vials containing 1.5 ml of Tyrode's (100% O_2) and 40 μM [³H]tyrosine ([2,6-³H]tyrosine, 2 Ci/mM), 1 mM ascorbic acid (as antioxidant and dopamine β-hydroxylase [DβH] cofactor), and 100 μM 6-tetrahydromercaptopurine (6-MPH$_4$) (i.e., tyrosine hydroxylase [TH] cofactor). After incubation for 2–3 h in a waterbath shaker at 37°C, each carotid body is weighed in the humidified chamber of a Cahn electrobalance (sensitivity, 50 ng). This basic protocol is utilized to label catecholamine stores, whether the experiments deal with synthesis or release of labeled catecholamines. (In release experiments, however, the specific activity of [³H]tyrosine is 20–40 Ci/mmol, and experiments utilize a superfusion chamber that permits simultaneous recording of chemoreceptor discharge; see ref. 11.)

Measurement of Catecholamine Release

The superfusates are collected in vials containing a carrier solution consisting of 0.3 N acetic acid, 1 mM ascorbic acid, and 100 μM unlabeled DA, at a final pH = 3.6. The solutions are processed with the alumina adsorption method for recovery of [³H]catecholamines (11). In experiments without monoamine oxidase (MAO) inhibitors, after elution of [³H]DA with 0.3 N acetic acid (recovery, 65 ± 5%), further elution with 1 N HCl permits the recovery of dihydroxyphenyl acetic acid (DOPAC), the principal DA catabolite in the carotid body (17). The eluate of 0.3 N acetic acid is further analyzed by means of high-voltage paper electrophoresis; the eluate containing [³H]DOPAC is directly counted in a liquid scintillation spectrometer. Recovery of preformed [³H]DA and [³H]NE after electrophoresis is approximately 95%. After electrophoresis, the channels are led through a radiochromatogram scanner, and the peaks for DA and NE are cut out and combusted in a sample oxidizer to yield tritiated water in an aqueous counting cocktail.

General Methods for Receptor Binding Studies

After weighing, tissue samples are transferred to glass scintillation vials containing 1 ml of modified Tyrode's solution in a waterbath-shaker and preincubated in the presence or absence of competing drugs. A subsequent incubation period begins with the addition of 100 μl of media containing the radiolabeled ligand. After incubation, the carotid bodies are washed, and tissue samples containing tritium are combusted in a sample oxidizer and counter in a liquid scintillation spectrometer. Samples containing ¹²⁵I are solubilized in 40 μl NCS II (Amersham) plus 200 μl of water at 60°C for 12–24 h. Prior to the addition of scintillation fluor for counting, the samples are neutralized with 750 μl of 1.3% acetic acid.

Radioimmunoassay (RIA) of Carotid Body Neuropeptides

Tissue samples are homogenized in 0.01 N HCl, and aliquot is removed for protein determination, and the remainder is heated in boiling water (10 min) to denature proteases. The samples are centrifuged (5000 × g, 20 min), and the resulting supernatant is removed and lyophilized for storage at −80°C until assayed. The lyophilized samples are reconstituted in phosphate-buffered saline with gelatin (0.1 M monobasic sodium phosphate, 0.9% sodium chloride, and 0.1% gelatin; pH 7.4) and centrifuged to remove insoluble material. The supernatant is then assayed for SP-like immunoreactivity (SPLI) and ME-like immunoreactivity (MELI). The investigators have their own supply of SP-specific antiserum and use commercially prepared antisera for ME (Immunonuclear). The SP antiserum can reliably detect 10 pg of synthetic bovine hypothalamic SP at a 1:200,000 dilution and displays less than 2% cross-reactivity with eledoisin and physalaemin, two peptides structurally similar to substance P. The antiserum for ME can reliably detect 10 pg at a 1:2000 dilution and displays insignificant cross-reactivity with leu-enkephalin (less than 3%), SP (less than 0.002%) β-endorphin (less than 0.002%), and porcine dynorphin[1-13] (less than 0.002%). The assays are carried out by preincubating one of the antisera with the samples for 2 h at room temperature. The radiolabeled SP or ME (New England Nuclear) are added to their respective incubation mixtures (5000–8000 dpm/tube) and allowed to incubate for an additional 24 h at either room temperature (SPLI) or 4°C (MELI). Antibody-bound and free ^{125}I-labeled peptides are separated by mixing the reactant with a dextran-coated charcoal slurry. The SPLI and MELI are determined by comparing the ratio of bound to free radiolabeled peptide for each sample with a standard curve.

RESULTS

Catecholamines

We have examined the purported species differences for catecholamine actions in the carotid body of the rabbit versus the cat, with emphasis on a comparison of the effects of natural stimuli on synthesis and release. The release of catecholamines has been correlated with stimulus intensity and the resultant CSN chemoreceptor discharge.

Effects of Natural Stimuli on [³H]Catecholamine Synthesis

In these experiments (10,30), unanesthetized animals were exposed either to 10% O_2 in N_2 (hypoxia) or to room air (normoxia) for 3 h in a chamber. The carotid bodies were quickly removed and incubated, either for 3 h in 40 μM [³H]tyrosine or for 2 h in 10 μM [³H]dopa. Carotid bodies from both hypoxic rabbits and cats, incubated with [³H]tyrosine, exhibited significant increases in the rate of [³H]DA synthesis, but no change in [³H]NE synthesis (Fig. 10.1A). This increase in [³H]DA synthesis was the likely result of increased release of endogenous DA during the hypoxic episode and subsequent removal of feedback inhibition exerted by DA at the level of tyrosine hydroxylase (TH), the rate-limiting step in catecholamine synthesis. Consistent with this interpretation, our results showed that when the TH step was obviated by incubation of the tissue with [³H]dopa instead of [³H]tyrosine (Fig. 10.1B), the hypoxic episode failed to produce any change in the rate of [³H]DA synthesis in either rabbit or cat carotid bodies, which agrees with findings in other tissues after physiologic stimulation (see ref. 9).

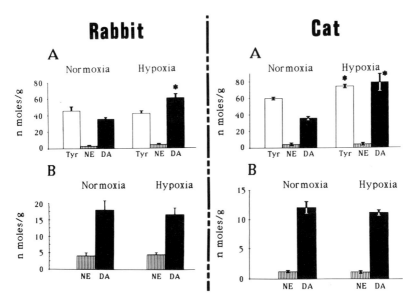

Fig. 10.1 Effects of in vivo hypoxia (3 h; 10% O_2 in N_2) on the rate of [³H]catecholamine synthesis in rabbit and cat carotid bodies using **(A)** [³H]tyrosine (40 μM) or **(B)** [³H]dopa (10 μM) as precursors. Control carotid bodies were obtained from animals similarly exposed to air. Note the specific increase in [³H]DA synthesis ($p < .01$) from [³H]tyrosine; no change was observed with [³H]dopa. Data are means ± SEM for 6–8 carotid bodies.

Effects of Natural Stimuli on [³H]Catecholamine Release

In release experiments, CSN chemoreceptor discharge was monitored along with the release of [³H]DA. In the absence of MAO inhibitors in the superfusate, the time course of resting release of [³H]DA had two phases: an initial rapid decline lasting 2 h, and a subsequent slower phase which could be followed for up to 8 h. Release of [³H]DA, efflux of [³H]DOPAC (the principal catabolite of DA in the carotid body), and chemoreceptor discharge from the CSN were monitored simultaneously. The total stimulus-related [³H]DA release was taken as the sum of the increased [³H]DA and [³H]DOPAC recoverable in the superfusates (neglecting reuptake). In the rabbit, there was a close relationship between chemoreceptor activity and [³H]DA release throughout the entire range of low O_2 stimulation (11), whereas in the cat the release of [³H]DA increased more rapidly than did the chemoreceptor discharge (30). The correlation between release of [³H]DA and CSN activity in the cat was better for low pH stimuli, as well as for low pH + high CO_2, CN^-, 2,4-dinitrophenol (DNP), 2-deoxy-D-glucose, and nicotine. The release of [³H]DA by all the above stimuli in both species was found to be dependent on the presence of extracellular Ca^{2+}.

In summary, these studies characterized the relationship between catecholamine synthesis, release, and chemoreceptor discharge, and also established that natural stimuli cause the release of DA from carotid bodies of both rabbit and cat. Our findings with a variety of natural and pharmacological stimuli suggest that DA plays an identical role in chemoreception in these animals. However, it remains to be established precisely what this role is in relation to the other putative neuro-transmitters present in the organ.

Acetylcholine

In earlier studies, we characterized and localized putative nicotinic receptors in the cat carotid body with ^{125}I-labeled α-bungarotoxin ([^{125}I]α-BGT) and muscarinic receptors in the rabbit carotid body with [^{3}H]quinuclydinylbenzilate ([^{3}H]QNB). These biochemical and autoradiographic studies showed that nicotinic sites in the cat and muscarinic sites in the rabbit are localized within lobules of type I and type II parenchymal cells (3,4). Selective denervation experiments indicated that cholinergic sites were absent from CSN afferent terminals. More recently, we have examined muscarinic binding sites in the cat and nicotinic binding sites in the rabbit, in an effort to test the correspondence between the pharmacological effects of cholinergic drugs in each of these species and the number of nicotinic versus muscarinic receptors and their location within the carotid body cell lobules.

Table 10.1 summarizes our earlier data for [^{125}I]α-BGT binding in the cat carotid body and [^{3}H]QNB binding in the rabbit carotid body. In normal, unoperated animals (Table 10.1), the per gram content (B_{max}) of nicotinic sites in the cat and muscarinic sites in the rabbit are nearly identical. The equilibrium dissociation constants (K_D) for the respective binding sites are in close agreement with similar parameters for specific muscarinic and nicotinic receptors detected in other tissues with these ligands (27,34). We found that chronic CSN denervation did not change the number of [^{125}I]α-BGT binding sites in the cat (3) or [^{3}H]QNB binding sites in the rabbit (4), but degeneration of the sympathetic fibers from the superior cervical ganglion reduced the specific [^{125}I]α-BGT binding in the cat and [^{3}H]QNB binding in the rabbit by approximately 50%. These latter results may reflect the presence of presynaptic cholinergic receptors associated with sympathetic terminals, because in other sympathetically innervated tissues, muscarinic and nicotinic drugs can modulate the evoked release of catecholamines (32).

Table 10.2 compares the relative numbers of [^{125}I]α-BGT and [^{3}H]QNB binding sites in cat versus rabbit carotid body. Binding was assayed at a single concentration of radioligand (either 11.00 nM [^{125}I]α-BGT or 350 pM [^{3}H]QNB), chosen in accordance with our earlier studies to provide near saturation of the nicotinic or muscarinic sites, with minimal nonspecific binding. In Table 10.2, the nonspecific binding of [^{125}I]α-BGT is identical ($p > .10$) in cat and rabbit chemosensory tissue, suggesting that the toxin is equally accessible to the carotid bodies in both species. The portion of the total binding displaceable by 10^{-3} M ACh (specific binding) is

Table 10.1   Binding Parameters[a] of Nicotinic ([^{125}I]α-BGT) and Muscarinic ([^{3}H]QNB) Sites in Cat and Rabbit Carotid Body

	K_D	B_{max} (pmol/g)	Displacing drugs
[^{125}I]α-BGT (cat)	5.56 nM	9.21	10^{-3} M curare; 10^{-3} M ACh
[^{3}H]QNB (rabbit)	71.46 pM	9.23	10^{-7} M QNB; 10^{-6} M atropine

[a]Based on Scatchard analysis of equilibrium data.

Table 10.2 Comparative Binding Data (Relative Number of $[^{125}I]\alpha$-BGT and $[^3H]$QNB Sites) in Cat vs. Rabbit Carotid Body

	$[^{125}I]\alpha$-BGT binding[a]		$[^3H]$QNB binding[b]	
	Rabbit	Cat	Rabbit	Cat
Total	2.41 ± 0.30 (11)[c]	7.78 ± 0.45 (4)	7.25 ± 1.30 (4)	4.35 ± 0.45 (7)
Nonspecific	1.87 ± 0.08 (17)	1.58 ± 0.23 (4)	0.45 ± 0.10 (4)	0.60 ± 0.50 (7)
Specific	*0.54 ± 0.16	‡6.20 ± 0.33	†6.80 ± 0.75	†3.75 ± 0.35

[a]$[^{125}I]\alpha$-BGT = 11.0 nM; nonspecific binding was determined in the presence of ACh (10^{-3} M) plus eserine (10^{-5} M).
[b]$[^3H]$QNB = 350 pM; nonspecific binding was measured in the presence of 1.0 μM atropine.
[c]Values are expressed in pmol/g of tissue; n values are given in parentheses.
*$p < .025$, †$p < .005$, ‡$p < .001$, for comparison of total vs. nonspecific binding.

6.25 pmol/g of tissue in the cat carotid body, which is similar to that found in our earlier studies (3). In contrast, specific $[^{125}I]\alpha$-BGT binding in the rabbit carotid body amounts to only 0.54 pmol/g, or 8.6% of cat specific binding.

The data in Table 10.2 also compare the binding of $[^3H]$QNB (350 pM) in normal rabbit and cat carotid body. Again, nonspecific binding in the presence of 10^{-6} M atropine was comparable in the two species, indicating equal access of the ligand. The specific binding of $[^3H]$QNB in rabbit carotid body amounted to 6.78 ± 0.72 pmol/g of tissue, whereas under identical binding conditions, 3.77 ± 0.47 pmol/g was specifically bound in cat carotid body. Thus, assuming identical dissociation constants (K_D) for $[^3H]$QNB in the cat and rabbit, the data indicate a 55.6% relative abundance of specific binding sites in the cat as compared to the rabbit chemosensory tissue. In the rabbit, muscarinic sites account for over 90% of the total cholinergic receptor population. Conversely, nicotinic receptors dominate cat carotid bodies by approximately 2 to 1 over muscarinic sites.

Cholinergic Receptor Coupling to Catecholamine Release and Chemoreceptor Discharge

Because specific α-BGT and QNB binding sites are localized primarily within glomerular lobules in the carotid body but are absent from the sensory terminals of the CSN, it follows that the type I cells are the most likely site for these receptors. We have therefore investigated whether the dominant receptor subtype in each animal—that is, nicotinic receptors in the cat and muscarinic receptors in the rabbit—are able to modulate both the release of DA from the type I cells and CSN chemoreceptor discharge. We found that in cat carotid body, α-BGT (50 nM) depressed the increase in chemosensory discharge and the release of DA elicited by nicotine (10^{-5} M) as well as low O_2 (Fig. 10.2). In contrast to this dominant excitatory effect of nicotinic agents on discharge and release in the cat, our preliminary data with muscarinic agents in the rabbit carotid body suggest a very different effect on chemoreceptor discharge and $[^3H]$DA release. In 100% O_2-equilibrated superfusion media, basal release was unaffected by the muscarinic agonist, bethanechol (100 μM), but during normal hypoxia, bethanechol severely reduced the evoked release, and this effect could be reversed by atropine (0.5 μM; Fig. 10.3). These data suggest that muscarinic receptors in this species primarily inhibit DA release.

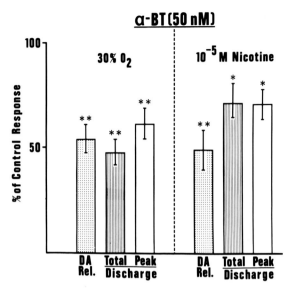

Fig. 10.2 Effects of α-BGT on [³H]DA release, and total and peak CSN discharge evoked by hypoxia (30% O₂ equilibrated media) or 10^{-5} M nicotine. Data are expressed as percentages of control responses determined prior to the introduction of 50 nM α-BGT. *$p < .01$ and **$p < .005$ levels of significance.

Neuropeptides

Effects of Hypoxia on Neuropeptide Stores in the Carotid Body

In a study of the effects of hypoxia on carotid body peptides, rabbits were placed singly into a clear Lucite chamber which was continuously flushed (4 1/min) with either room air or 5% O₂ in N₂ for two 30-min periods, with a 20-min interim. The animals were then anesthetized with pentobarbital sodium and respired with the given gas mixture during surgical removal of the carotid bodies (and in some experiments, the nodose ganglion and the striatum, which served as control tissues for nonspecific effects of hypoxia on peptide stores). The tissues were then processed by RIA as described in Methods.

Animals exposed to hypoxia had significantly reduced levels (approx. 40% decrease; for details see ref. 18) of both SPLI and MELI in their carotid bodies, compared to animals exposed only to room air in the chamber. The SPLI and

⟶

Fig. 10.3 Effects of muscarinic agents on the low-O₂-induced release of [³H]catecholamines and CSN discharge frequency in the rabbit carotid body. In **(A)**, 10^{-4} M bethanechol completely blocked [³H]catecholamine release and markedly reduced the CSN discharge evoked by superfusion media equilibrated with 20% O₂ (a potent chemoreceptor stimulus in vitro). In **(B)** (same preparation), the response to low O₂ has recovered after a 45-min washout period. The subsequent application of 10^{-4} M bethanechol in the presence of 0.5 μM atropine did not significantly affect [³H]catecholamine release or CSN discharge. Apparent delay in release of recoverable [³H]catecholamines is due to the use of a conventional flow-type (not drop-type) chamber which has a significantly greater dead space on the outflow side of the preparation.

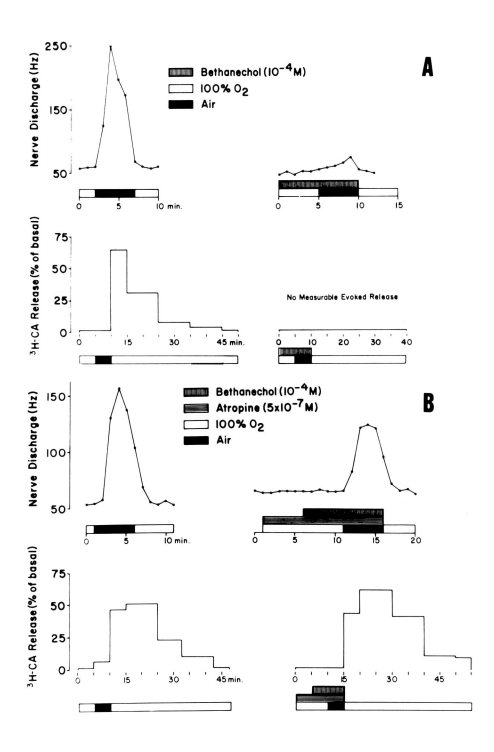

MELI levels in the nodose ganglion and in the striatum were unchanged after exposure to hypoxia. We also investigated the effects of chronic CSN section on peptide levels in the carotid body, because our previous studies had shown that this nerve exerts long-term trophic effects on biosynthetic enzyme levels and transmitter release by the carotid body (16). Twelve to 15 days following section of the CSN, the basal (unstimulated) level of SPLI was significantly increased (52%) in spite of the loss of CSN SPLI, whereas the level of MELI was reduced (24%).

Localization of Peptidergic Receptors in the Carotid Body

Pharmacological studies by other investigators (24,25,29) have demonstrated that SP and ME alter chemoreceptor discharge from the carotid body. In addition, these peptides modify responses to natural stimuli and to certain pharmacologically active agents (e.g., ACh and nicotine). The results from these experiments have been difficult to interpret, however, because each peptide has been shown to have both excitatory and inhibitory actions. Moreover, the data for the effects of SP obtained from in situ verus in vitro preparations are conflicting, suggesting that this peptide may have indirect effects on chemoreceptor activity via the carotid body vasculature.

In an effort to resolve this uncertainty regarding the sites of peptide action in this organ, we have initiated ligand binding studies using radiolabeled SP and various opiate ligands to localize peptide receptors. [^{3}H]Etorphine binds to mu (μ) and delta (δ) opiate receptors with approximately equal affinity, and in preliminary experiments we found that high concentrations of the unlabeled μ and δ agonist, levorphanol, reduced total binding of [^{3}H]etorphine by 34% in the carotid body. In other experiments, we also examined [^{125}I]SP binding in the carotid body, and found that 42% of total labeled SP binding was displaced by unlabeled SP. These data confirm the presence of receptors for these peptides in the carotid body.

We have also begun experiments aimed at clarifying the role of these peptides in modulating the actions of biogenic amines in the carotid body. Our preliminary data already demonstrate that SP and ME are able to modify the nicotine-evoked release of labeled catecholamines from the cat carotid body, but that the release evoked by high-K^{+} is unaffected by these peptides. Although we have no data at the present time to indicate a direct action of the peptides on the type I cells, studies with isolated adrenal chromaffin cells have shown that both SP and ME (or morphine) cause similar reductions in the nicotine-evoked release of catecholamines, and also leave unaffected the release evoked by high K^{+}. These findings suggest that the effects of these peptides in the cat carotid body may be specific for the nicotine-evoked release by the type I cells.

DISCUSSION

Catecholamines

An important feature of neurotransmiter metabolism is the capacity to adjust synthetic rates to meet altered transmitter demand. We have compared the effects of hypoxia on [³H]catecholamine synthesis from [³H]dopa and [³H]tyrosine in rabbit and cat carotid bodies. No alterations in synthesis were observed when [³H]dopa was used as precursor, and this finding is in agreement with that found for other catecholaminergic systems (see ref. 10). In contrast, use of the natural precursor, tyrosine, resulted in a significant increase in [³H]DA synthesis in both species. Our results therefore suggest that in the carotid body, as in other catecholaminergic structures, the short-term regulation of catecholamine levels by natural stimuli is mediated through end-product inhibition of this rate-limiting step in the biosynthetic pathway. This increased synthesis of carotid body DA with hypoxia is a markedly different effect from the actions of low O_2 on catecholamine synthesis in other structures. In brain, *decreased* synthesis of catecholamines has been shown to accompany low O_2 exposures, even at the moderate levels of hypoxia employed in this study (10% O_2 in N_2; see ref. 10). It would thus appear that the increase in DA synthesis in the carotid body may be a specific response to the hypoxic stimulus.

In experiments where [³H]DA and [³H]DOPAC in the superfusate were monitored as total [³H]DA release, we found in both rabbit and cat carotid bodies that over a wide range of stimulus intensities there was a definite relationship between stimulus-induced [³H]DA release and peak chemosensory discharge. Average discharge frequency increased more slowly than total [³H]DA release throughout the entire range of stimulus intensities. This relationship between the intensity of the low-O_2 stimulus, on the one hand, and [³H]DA release and chemosensory activity on the other, suggests a role of DA in the mechanisms of chemoreception. Although our data do not provide incontrovertible evidence for a *causal* relationship between DA release and chemosensory activity, the correspondence between these two phenomena in normal Tyrode's medium suggests that DA participates in an important way in the overall genesis of the chemoresponse. Furthermore, DA receptors (D_2) are known to be located on the sensory neural elements in the carotid body (as well as the type I cells; see ref. 9). However, it must also be considered that some agent in addition to DA, perhaps one of the neuropeptides present in this organ, may be released to excite the sensory nerve endings. Other possible roles of DA in the mammalian carotid body should also be considered. DA may act as a "modulator" of the chemoresponse, its presence in the carotid body being required for optimal chemosensitivity. This might be achieved through modifications of ionic permeabilities in the sensory nerve membrane, which could change the threshold to natural stimuli.

In conclusion, our data demonstrate that the synthesis and release of DA in the carotid body respond to natural stimuli in a manner very similar to that seen in other tissues where catecholamines act as neurotransmitters. We conclude that DA actively participates in the immediate reactions that comprise the chemoresponse and ultimately lead to the initiation of chemosensory activity on the CSN. Further, a comparison of the synthesis and release of [³H]catecholamines in rabbit and cat carotid body has shown that the basic neurochemical aspects of [³H]DA metabolism in this organ are similar in both species. These findings help resolve the controversy regarding the effects of hypoxia on the release of DA in the cat versus the rabbit, and suggest that the apparent species differences observed in pharmacological experiments do not accurately reflect the physiological function of this amine. It is likely, therefore, that this putative neurotransmitter may play analogously important roles in chemoreception in both species.

Acetylcholine

Our study comparing the amounts of specific [^{3}H]QNB and [^{125}I]α-BGT binding sites in rabbit and cat carotid bodies indicates that rabbit carotid bodies are dominated by inhibitory muscarinic receptors to an extent that correlates with the ability of ACh to depress the CSN discharge. Cat carotid bodies, in contrast, contain mostly nicotinic cholinergic sites which mediate a large excitatory response to nicotinic drugs. A substantial population of [^{3}H]QNB binding sites in cat chemosensory tissue is not associated with the sympathetic or sensory innervation, and the function and localization of these muscarinic sites remain obscure.

An antagonistic effect on catecholamine release by nicotinic and muscarinic receptors has been described for isolated bovine adrenal chromaffin cells (2). In that system, muscarinic inhibition paralleled increased cyclic GMP levels, and phosphodiesterase inhibitors also inhibited catecholamine secretion. However, in other species, adrenal chromaffin cell secretion has been shown to be stimulated by both nicotinic and muscarinic agents. At the present time, the physiological significance of these species differences in regards to cholinergic coupling to catecholamine secretion remains unclear for both the adrenal medulla and the carotid body. Nonetheless, it is noteworthy that for the carotid body the increase in [^{3}H]DA release produced by nicotinic receptors in the cat, and the antagonistic effects of muscarinic agents on release in the rabbit, correspond to the actions of nicotinic and muscarinic agents on CSN impulse activity in these two species.

Neuropeptides

Our results suggest that SP and ME are released from the carotid body by natural stimuli and therefore may play a role in the regulation and/or mediation of carotid body chemoreception (see Prabhakar and Cherniack, Chap. 11, this volume). The implicit assumption is that decreases in neuropeptide levels during the relatively short period of exposure to hypoxia are indicative of increased release and subsequent rapid proteolysis. Such an assumption may not be unreasonable, since the relatively rapid changes in peptide concentrations that we observed in this study are unlikely to be due to alterations in protein synthesis; thus, it has been shown that 8 h after complete blockade of protein synthesis, SP levels in dorsal root ganglia remain unchanged (19). Although our experiments do not rule out possible nonspecific effects of hypoxia on the carotid body, such as those unrelated to direct changes in chemoreception (e.g., local tissue hypoxia, blood pressure changes, hormonal and temperature effects, etc.), the lack of effect of hypoxia on neuropeptides in nodose ganglia and corpus striatum suggests that tissue peptide stores may be resistant to such sequelae, and that changes observed in carotid body peptide levels reflect a true physiological response dependent on altered chemoreceptor drive. In sum, our data suggest that the SP and ME systems in the carotid body are responsive to natural stimuli that affect the physiological activity of this chemoreceptor organ.

REFERENCES

1. Cuello, A. C., and D. S. McQueen. Substance P: a carotid body peptide. *Neurosci. Lett.* *17:* 215–219, 1980.
2. Derome, G., R. Tseng, P. Mercier, I. Lemarre, and S. Lemarre. Possible muscarinic regulation of catecholamine secretion mediated by cyclic GMP in isolated bovine adrenal chromaffin cells. *Biochem. Pharmacol. 30:* 855–860, 1981.
3. Dinger, B., C. Gonzalez, K. Yoshizaki, and S. Fidone. Localization and function of cat carotid body nicotinic receptors. *Brain Res. 339:* 295–304, 1985.
4. Dinger, B. G., T. Hirano, and S. J. Fidone. Autoradiographic localization of muscarinic receptors in rabbit carotid body. *Brain Res. 367:* 328–331, 1986.
5. Docherty, R. J., and D. S. McQueen. The effects of acetylcholine and dopamine on carotid chemosensory activity in the rabbit. *J. Physiol. (Lond.) 288:* 411–423, 1979.
6. Donnelly, D. F., E. J. Smith, and R. E. Dutton. Neural response of carotid chemoreceptors following dopamine blockade. *J. Appl. Physiol. 50:* 172–177, 1981.
7. Eyzaguirre, C., and P. Zapata. The release of acetylcholine from carotid body tissues. Further study on the effects of acetylcholine and cholinergic blocking agents on the chemosensory discharge. *J. Physiol. (Lond.) 195:* 589–607, 1968.
8. Fidone, S. J., and C. Gonzalez. Catecholamine synthesis in rabbit carotid body in vitro. *J. Physiol. (Lond.) 333:* 69–79, 1982.
9. Fidone, S. J., and C. Gonzalez. Initiation and control of chemoreceptor activity in the carotid body. In: *Handbook of Physiology, Sec.* 3: *The Respiratory System,* Vol. 2: *Control of Breathing,* ed. N. S. Cherniack, and J. G. Widdicombe. Bethesda: Am. Physiol. Soc., 1986, pp. 247–312.
10. Fidone, S. J., C. Gonzalez, and K. Yoshizaki. Effects of hypoxia on catecholamine synthesis in rabbit carotid body in vitro. *J. Physiol. (Lond.) 333:* 79–93, 1982.
11. Fidone, S. J., C. Gonzalez, and K. Yoshizaki. Effects of low oxygen on the release of dopamine from the rabbit carotid body in vitro. *J. Physiol. (Lond.) 333:* 93–110, 1982.
12. Fidone, S. J., A. Sato, and C. Eyzaguirre. Acetylcholine activation of carotid body chemoreceptor A fibers. *Brain Res. 9:* 374–376, 1968.
13. Fidone, S. J., S. Weintraub, and W. B. Stavinoha. Acetylcholine content of normal and denervated cat carotid bodies measured by pyrolysis gas chromatography/mass fragmentometry. *J. Neurochem. 26:* 1047–1049, 1976.
14. Fidone, S. J., S. Weintraub, W. B. Stavinoha, C. Sterline, and L. Jones. Endogenous acetylcholine levels in the cat carotid body and the autoradiographic localization of a high affinity component of choline uptake. In: *Chemoreception in the Carotid Body,* ed. H. Acker, S. Fidone, D. Pallot, C. Eyzaguirre, D. W. Lubbers, and R. W. Torrance. Berlin: Springer, 1977, pp. 106–113.
15. Goldberg, A. M., A. P. Lentz, and R. S. Fitzgerald. Neurotransmitter mechanism in the carotid body: absence of ACh in the carotid sinus nerve. *Brain Res. 140:* 374–377, 1978.
16. Gonzalez, C., Y. Kwok, J. W. Gibb, and S. J. Fidone. Reciprocal modulation of tyrosine hydroxylase activity in rat carotid body. *Brain Res. 172:* 572–576, 1979.
17. Hanbauer, I., and S. Hellstrom. The regulation of dopamine and noradrenaline in the rat carotid body and its modification by denervation and by hypoxia. *J. Physiol. (Lond.) 282:* 21–34, 1978.
18. Hanson, G. R., L. F. Jones, and S. Fidone. Physiological chemoreceptor stimulation decreases enkephalin and substance P in the carotid body. *Peptides 7:* 767–769, 1986.
19. Harmer, A., and P. Keen. Chemical characterization of substance P-like immunoreactivity in primary afferent neurons. *Brain Res. 220:* 203–207, 1981.

20. Hellstrom, S. Putative neurotransmitters in the carotid body. Mass fragmentographic studies. *Adv. Biochem. Psychopharmacol. 16:* 257–263, 1977.
21. Jacobowitz, D. M., and C. J. Helke. Localization of substance P immunoreactive nerves in the carotid body. *Brain Res. Bull. 5:* 195–197, 1980.
22. Jones, J. V. Localization and quantitation of carotid body enzymes: their relevance to the cholinergic transmitter hypothesis. In: *The Peripheral Arterial Chemoreceptors,* ed. M. J. Purves. Cambridge: Cambridge University Press, 1975, pp. 143–162.
23. Lundberg, J. M., T. Hokfelt, J. Fahrenkrug, G. Nilsson, and L. Terenius. Peptides in the cat carotid body *(glomus caroticum):* VIP-, enkephalin- and substance P-like immunoreactivity. *Acta Physiol. Scand. 107:* 279–281, 1979.
24. McQueen, D. S. Pharmacological aspects of putative transmitters in the carotid body. In: *Physiology of the Peripheral Arterial Chemoreceptors,* ed. H. Acker and R. G. O'Regan. Amsterdam: Elsevier, 1984, pp. 149–195.
25. Monti-Bloch, L., and C. Eyzaguirre. Effects of methionine–enkephalin and substance P on the chemosensory discharge of the cat carotid body. *Brain Res. 338:* 297–307, 1985.
26. Monti-Bloch, L., and C. Eyzaguirre. A comparative physiological and pharmacological study of cat and rabbit carotid body chemoreceptors. *Brain Res. 193:* 449–470, 1980.
27. Moore, W. M., and R. N. Brady. Studies of nicotinic acetylcholine receptor protein from rat brain. *Biochim. Biophysica Acta 444:* 252–260, 1976.
28. Nolan, W. F., D. F. Donnelly, E. J. Smith, and R. E. Dutton. Inhibition of carotid chemoreception by haloperidol in vitro. *Fed. Proc. 43:* 813, 1984.
29. Prabhakar, N. R., M. Runold, Y. Yamamoto, M. Langercrantz, and C. von Euler. Effects of substance P antagonist on the hypoxia-induced carotid chemoreceptor activity. *Acta Physiol. Scand. 121:* 301–303, 1984.
30. Rigual, R., E. Gonzalez, C. Gonzalez, and S. Fidone. Synthesis and release of catecholamines by the cat carotid body in vitro: effects of hypoxic stimulation. *Brain Res. 374:* 101–109, 1986.
31. Sampson, S. R. Effects of mecamylamine on responses of carotid body chemoreceptors in vivo to physiological and pharmacological stimuli. *J. Physiol. (Lond). 212:* 655–666, 1971.
32. Westfall, T. C. Local regulation of adrenergic neurotransmission. *Physiol. Rev. 57:* 659–728, 1977.
33. Wharton, J., J. M. Polak, A.G.E. Pearse, G. P. McGegor, M. G. Bryant, S. R. Bloom, P. C. Emson, G. E. Bisgard, and J. A. Will. Enkephalin-, VIP-, and substance P-like immunoreactivity in the carotid body. *Nature 284:* 269–271, 1980.
34. Yamamura, H. I., and S. H. Snyder. Muscarinic cholinergic binding in rat brain. *Proc. Natl. Acad. Sci. U.S.A. 71:* 1725–1729, 1974.
35. Zapata, P. Effects of dopamine on carotid chemo- and baroreceptors in vitro. *J. Physiol. (Lond.) 244:* 235–251, 1975.

11

Importance of Tachykinin Peptides in Hypoxic Ventilatory Drive

N. R. PRABHAKAR AND N. S. CHERNIACK

Substance P (SP) is an undecapeptide first isolated from the extracts of brain and intestine by Euler and Gaddum (4) and subsequently characterized and synthesized by Leeman and her colleagues in 1971 (1). Now it is recognized that SP belongs to a group of structurally related peptides called *tachykinins* (2). Although the precise physiological roles of tachykinins are uncertain, currently it is believed that SP-like peptides may function as neurotransmitters or modulators in certain peripheral and central nervous structures (10,22). The recent development of antagonists for substance P has helped to elucidate further the potential importance of tachykinins in various physiological systems (30).

Respiratory augmenting effects of SP were reported by Euler and Pernow 30 years ago (5). SP has been shown to be present at a number of different sites in the respiratory system. For example, immunocytochemical studies have demonstrated SP-like peptides in vagal sensory fibers innervating bronchopulmonary regions (see refs. 10,22, for review). Furthermore, the nucleus tractus solitarii, which receives various respiratory afferents, has also been shown to contain substantial amounts of tachykinins (16). Since the early 1980s, our research has centered on assessing the physiological significance of tachykinins in regulation of breathing, particularly on chemical control. This review summarizes recent evidence concerning the possible role of tachykinins in the expression of the hypoxic ventilatory response.

ARTERIAL CHEMORECEPTOR RESPONSES TO EXOGENOUS SUBSTANCE P

Close carotid body injections of SP increase respiration (5), which is prevented by section of carotid sinus nerves (25). McQueen (17) was the first to report that increasing doses of SP results in progressive increases in carotid body activity. We

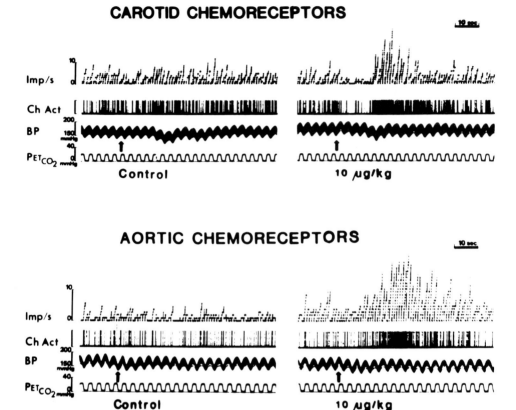

Fig. 11.1 Examples of experiments illustrating the effect of exogenous SP on carotid and aortic chemoreceptor activity (Ch. Act.) from two separate cats. In the case of carotid chemoreceptors, the superior cervical ganglion was removed surgically. Both chemoreceptors, the superior cervical ganglion was removed surgically. Both chemoreceptors responded with an augmented discharge to substance P injections, but showed no response to control saline administration (left panel). $P_{ET}CO_2$, end-tidal PCO_2; BP, arterial blood pressure.

compared the responses to SP of single fibers in the carotid and aortic chemoreceptors in anesthetized cats that were paralyzed and artificially ventilated with room air. All experiments on the carotid chemoreceptors were performed after surgical removal of the superior cervical ganglia to eliminate the influence of sympathetic innervation on blood flow to the carotid body. SP increased the activity of both aortic and carotid chemoreceptors (Fig. 11.1). Increasing the concentrations of SP to 1, 3, and 10 μg/kg augmented carotid body activity by 330 ± 39%, 609 ± 81%, and 780 ± 75% (mean ± SE), respectively. The corresponding percent increases in aortic body activity were 309 ± 48%, 550 ± 52%, and 826 ± 43%, respectively. Occasionally, a transient depression of the discharge was observed preceding these increases. However, unlike the augmentation, neither the magnitude of the depression nor the frequency of its appearance was dose dependent. With 10 μg/kg of SP

(Fig. 11.1), the increased activity reached its peak within 9 s in the carotid body and 18 s in the aortic body.

After SP injection arterial pressure decreased. However, it is unlikely that the chemosensory augmentation was secondary to cardiovascular changes. Unlike the rise in chemosensory activity, the size of the hypotensive response was not dose dependent. Furthermore, with repeated injections of SP, the magnitude of the chemosensory discharge remained the same, but the hypotensive response became smaller or even disappeared. It has also been shown that SP increases the activity of the carotid body in vitro, suggesting a direct effect of the peptide on chemosensory elements (19).

Cats and rabbits are most commonly used in chemoreceptor research. Although systemic hypoxia increases chemosensory activity in both species, the effects of chemical substances such as acetylcholine and dopamine on the carotid body have been reported to differ qualitatively. It is not known whether there is a similar species difference with respect to the effects of SP. Therefore, in another series of experiments we assessed the carotid body responses to SP in anesthetized and paralyzed rabbits ventilated with room air. As in the cat, exogenous SP augmented carotid body activity in a dose-dependent manner (Fig. 11.2). The peak activity was reached within 2–3 s—faster than in cats. A notable difference from the results obtained in cats was that extremely low concentrations of SP stimulated rabbit chemoreceptors. Thus even 0.2 ng/kg of SP increased chemosensory activity by 310%, even though there were no noticeable changes in arterial blood pressure.

Thus, these studies establish that both aortic and carotid chemoreceptors of cats are stimulated by exogenous SP, and that rabbits require lower concentrations of SP than cats. By contrast, baroreceptor activity recorded from carotid sinus nerve seems to be unaffected by exogenous SP (Prabhakar et al., unpublished observations).

SUBSTANCE P AND HYPOXIC STIMULUS

A number of observations seem to support the idea that SP is involved in the response of the peripheral chemoreceptor to hypoxia. In the course of the experiments with exogenous SP, it was observed that SP caused almost negligible chemoreceptor stimulation under hyperoxic conditions ($P_aO_2 > 300$ mmHg), but the same fiber could be excited by SP by lowering arterial PO_2 to normoxic values (Fig. 11.3). These observations suggested that the magnitude of SP-induced excitation might be related to arterial PO_2. In cats, SP (3 μg/kg) increased carotid body activity at levels of arterial PO_2 ranging from 444 ± 17 mmHg to 25 ± 1.5 mmHg. However, the magnitude of stimulation at the lowest arterial PO_2 was greater than that at the highest P_aO_2 ($+11.8 \pm 1.8$ imp/s vs. $+3 \pm 1.3$ imp/s). Although it could be argued that the chemoreceptor activity, which is already elevated during hypoxia, alone contributes to the greater SP response, this is not likely since 5-HT-induced augmentation was the same at all levels of P_aO_2 (unpublished observations).

SP enhanced the hypoxic responses of both the carotid and aortic bodies. For example, before the administration of SP, aortic chemoreceptors responded to hypoxia (P_aO_2 = 42 ± 2.4 mmHg) by increasing the discharge rate by 5 ± 0.9 imp/s; after SP, the same hypoxic challenge increased the activity of the same fibers by 11 ± 1.2 imp/s. Monti-Bloch and Eyzaguirre (19) reported that SP diminished the excitation caused by hypoxia in an isolated in vitro carotid body preparation. One reason for the discrepancy could be differences in the preparation used (i.e., in vitro vs. in vivo). Second, the hypoxic stimulus used by the in vitro study may have been

Fig. 11.2 Example illustrating the effect of substance P on carotid chemoreceptor activity (C.A) of a rabbit. Intralingual arterial administration of saline (control; top panel) did not affect the chemoreceptor activity, whereas SP increased chemoreceptor activity in a dose-dependent manner. Note that nanogram concentrations of SP were needed, as compared to microgram concentrations in cats (Fig. 11.1).

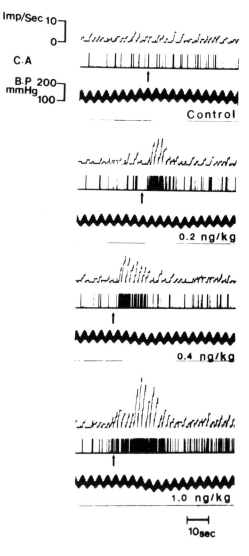

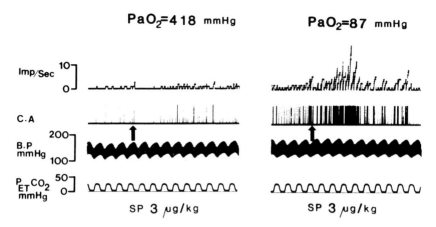

Fig. 11.3 Effect of intraaortic administration of SP at two levels of arterial P_{O_2} on an aortic chemoreceptor discharge. Note that at high P_aO_2, SP caused a negligible increase in discharge, whereas at low P_{O_2}, the same concentration substantially increased activity.

too severe. In our study, P_{O_2} (50 mmHg) during hypoxia was probably much greater than that in vitro because the superfusing solution was equilibrated with 100% N_2. Severe hypoxia can have depressive effects on carotid body activity (6), and so also may SP.

SP enhances not only chemoreceptor responses to systemic hypoxia but also the responses to histotoxic hypoxia caused by sodium cyanide. Others have also noticed the potentiating effects of SP on the chemoreceptor response to sodium cyanide (17,19). Like Mulligan and Lahiri (20), we noted that during hyperoxia sodium cyanide was unable to excite chemoreceptors. However, after SP, cyanide markedly stimulated chemoreceptor activity despite continued hyperoxia.

Mulligan and Lahiri (21) showed that the carotid body responses to hypoxia but not to hypercapnia can be blocked by oligomycin and antimycin A, a finding which suggested to them that the hypoxic response depends on the phosphate potential. We assessed the chemoreceptor responses to SP, hypoxia, hypercapnia, and lobeline before and after administration of oligomycin (60–80 $\mu g/kg$) (25). After oligomycin, chemoreceptor augmentation caused by SP (3–10 $\mu g/kg$), like the response to hypoxia, was markedly attenuated ($p < .01$), whereas the magnitude of excitation caused by hypercapnia and lobeline (10 $\mu g/kg$) was unaffected ($p > .05$). In two experiments, we examined the effect of antimycin A; the results were found to be qualitatively the same as with oligomycin. The fact that inhibitors of oxidative processes inside the cell also blocked the SP responses further supports the notion that the mechanisms for SP and hypoxic excitation are interrelated. The possibility that oligomycin might have blocked the SP receptor binding sites, however, remains open.

Further evidence that an SP-like peptide is involved in the chemoreceptor stimulation caused by hypoxia comes from experiments with SP antagonists. We have shown that hypoxic excitation of the carotid body in the cat can be attenuated after administration of "Spantide"—[D-Arg^1-D-Pro^2-D-Trp^{7,9}-Leu^{11}]-SP—an Sp antagonist (24–26). In recent studies using [D-Pro^2-D-Trp^{7,9}]-SP, another SP antagonist, we could effectively block hypoxic excitation not only of the cat carotid body but also the cat aortic body and the rabbit carotid body (24,25,28). Blockade of hypoxic stimulation in the rabbit carotid body required as little as 0.2 μg/kg of SP antagonist as opposed to 10–15 μg/kg needed in cats. Also, SP antagonists were able to prevent the stimulatory effects of sodium cyanide. By contrast, excitatory effects of nicotine were not affected by antagonists, indicating the specificity of the SP antagonist. These important results require independent confirmation (see Shirahata, Chap. 15, this volume).

EFFECT OF SP ON CO$_2$-INDUCED STIMULATION
OF THE CHEMORECEPTORS

The increase in chemoreceptor activity caused by hypercapnia occurs even after the administration of SP antagonists. This suggests that the effects of hypoxia and hypercapnia on the carotid body may not be mediated by a common mechanism. Carotid body stimulation by CO$_2$ was also not blocked by doses of oligomycin which eliminated responses to hypoxia.

Several investigators have shown that hypoxic hypercapnia has a multiplicative (positive interaction) effect on the discharge of single nerve fibers from the carotid body (11). In recent studies we have tested the possibility that antagonists to SP might affect this interaction of hypoxia and CO$_2$ on carotid body activity (24). Before SP antagonist, hypoxic hypercapnia (P_aO_2 = 42.0 $\pm$ 2 mmHg; P_aCO_2 = 57 $\pm$ 1 mmHg) increased carotid body activity from 2.7 $\pm$ 0.5 to 22 $\pm$ 4.7 imp/s, and the slope of the response ($\Delta imp/\Delta P_aCO_2$) was 0.90 $\pm$ 0.2. After SP antagonist, the hypoxic CO$_2$ response of the same fibers was significantly attenuated ($p < .01$), and the response slope was decreased to 0.36 $\pm$ 0.06. These studies support the idea that endogenous SP may play an important role in carotid body responses to hypoxia but not to CO$_2$.

If two separate mechanisms are responsible for carotid body excitation by hypoxia and hypercapnia, how do they interact to produce greater than additive effects? Different neuroactive substances might be released independently by hypoxia and hypercapnia, which by temporal summation produce greater than additive effects at the afferent nerve endings. The chemical substance for hypoxic expression might be a tachykinin, perhaps SP. Relevant to this idea is the observation that close carotid body injection of SP potentiated the carotid body response to hyperoxic CO$_2$, much as did hypoxia (24).

BIOCHEMICAL IDENTIFICATION OF TACHYKININS
IN THE CAROTID BODY

Although immunocytochemical studies indicate the presence of SP-like peptides in the carotid body, information regarding their chemical identity is lacking. We analyzed the characteristics of tachykinins in carotid body extracts using high-pressure liquid chromatography (HPLC) (23). Carotid bodies were surgically removed from anesthetized, artificially ventilated cats and were placed in 1.0 M formic acid (1 ml) containing dithiothreitol (DTT, 10^{-4} M) and a proteolytic enzyme inhibitor, phenylmethyl-sulfonyl fluoride (PMSF), and constantly mixed for 24 h at 4°C. The supernatants were collected after centrifugation. After separation of the proteins with acetone precipitation, the supernatant was lyophilized and subjected to analysis using a reverse-phase HPLC (C-18 Synchropak, Dupont). The eluates were monitored at 220 nM for peptide absorption. The carotid body extracts, as expected, showed elution profiles corresponding to synthetic substance P (SP) and neurokinin A (NKA) (Fig. 11.4). In addition, distinct peak corresponding to C-terminal fragment of substance P were observed. Two more elution profiles corresponding to physalaemin and eledoisin, peptides structurally related to SP were also noticed. The occurrence of these latter two peptides was unexpected because they are believed to be present only in nonmammalian tissues (22). Recent studies, however, indicate that tachykinins other than SP and NKA may be found in higher animals (2).

The presence of SP and NKA in the carotid body was further confirmed with radioimmunoassay technique (RIA) using specific antisera. Owing to its high sensitivity, this assay also offered an advantage to measure changes in peptide content under controlled arterial Po_2 conditions. Thus under room air conditions (P_aO_2 = 110 ± 2.4 mmHg), average SP and NKA values of the carotid bodies were 56.5 ± 7.8 and 85 ± 14 fmol/mg (wet weight), respectively. To date, there are two reports on SP content of the carotid bodies, one in cats (34), and the other in rabbits (8). The values of SP content in our experiments are close to those reported in cats (34). On the other hand, the SP content of rabbit carotid body was found to be 2.97 ng/mg of protein or 10 pmol/mg of protein. This value is approximately four times higher than that found in cats. Thus there appears to be substantial species variation in carotid body SP content.

Whether or not alterations in arterial oxygenation affect the tachykinin content of the carotid body was tested in experiments in anesthetized cats. After artificial ventilation for 1 h with 100% O_2, the carotid body on one side was removed. Thereafter, the animals were exposed for 1 h to an hypoxic challenge (6% O_2 + N_2) and the remaining carotid body was removed. The SP content of the hypoxic carotid bodies was 83% (43 ± 15 to 68 ± 19 fmol/mg) and the NKA content 44% (52 ± 12 to 73 ± 11 fmol/mg) higher than in the hyperoxic controls. In contrast, Hansen et al. (8) reported a decrease in SP content of rabbit carotid bodies with intermittent hypoxia (5% O_2 in N_2). The variations in the results may have been caused by species differences or by differences in the experimental protocol. Hansen et al. exposed unanesthetized rabbits to an hypoxic challenge and then, after anesthetizing them, removed the carotid bodies. It is also possible that cats might require more prolonged hypoxia than rabbits before there is a detectable decrease in tachykinin content (see Fidone et al., Chap. 10, this volume).

Various factors such as rates of synthesis, formation from precursor molecule, and degradation all contribute to the tissue content of a substance. For example, carotid body levels of dopamine can be best shown to be reduced by hypoxia after blockade of tyrosine hydroxylase, a rate-limiting enzyme in catecholamine biosynthesis (7). Increases in tachykinin content could have occurred despite increased

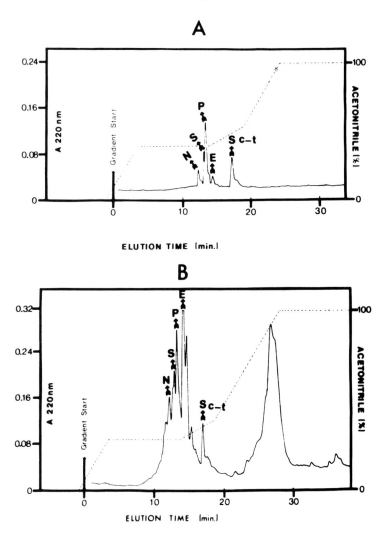

Fig. 11.4 High-pressure liquid chromatographic analysis (HPLC) of carotid body extracts. **(A)** Elution profiles with synthetic substance P (S), neurokinin A (N), physalaemin (P), eledoisin (E), and substance P C-terminal fragment (S_{C-t}). **(B)** Elution profiles generated by cat carotid body extracts.

release during hypoxia if hypoxemia enhanced SP and NKA synthesis even more. Unfortunately, detailed information concerning the enzymes involved in synthesis and degradation of tachykinins is not well understood. Nonetheless, the present results, like the study of Hansen et al. (8), do indicate that changes in arterial P_{O_2} affect the carotid body tachykinin content.

The presence of NKA in the carotid body raises the question of whether it affects chemosensory activity. Experiments were performed on anesthetized cats, paralyzed and artificially ventilated with room air ($P_aO_2 = 115 \pm 6.8$; and $P_aCO_2 = 32 \pm 3.3$ mmHg). Close carotid body injection of SP (50 nM) increased sensory discharge by 4.7 ± 0.9 imp/s (from 2.9 ± 0.7 to 7.6 ± 1.5 imp/s, $n = 6$), whereas an equimolar dose of NKA augmented activity by 4.8 ± 0.8 imp/s (from 3 ± 1.2 to 7.7 ± 1.8 imp/s)—nearly the same amount.

LOCALIZATION OF SP-LIKE TACHYKININS IN THE CAROTID BODY

Until recently, SP was regarded as the only tachykinin occurring in mammalian neural and nonneural tissues. Because our biochemical studies indicate that NKA, a structurally related peptide, is also present in the carotid body, we reexamined the immunoreactivity of tachykinins in cat carotid bodies with respect to localization of SP and NKA (12). Immunoreactivity to NKA and SP was localized in many type I cells (Fig. 11.5). In addition, both fine and coarse nerve fibers also displayed SP- and NKA-like immunoreactivity (SPLI and NKLI).

The source of tachykinins in the carotid bodies is not known. In the somatosensory system, for example, SP is synthesized in the cells of the dorsal root ganglion and is transported axonally to the afferent terminals (see ref. 10). By analogy, the sensory cell bodies in the petrosal ganglion may synthesize tachykinins and transport them to the carotid body via the sensory axons. Alternatively, SP and NKA may originate in either the superior cervical or the nodose ganglion and are transported via the sympathetic and parasympathetic axons innervating the carotid body. To test these possibilities, we examined the tachykinin immunoreactivity after chronic denervation of the carotid sinus, sympathetic, and parasympathetic nerves to the carotid bodies (12). Sectioning of the carotid sinus nerve (CSN) two weeks prior to assay did not affect NKLI and SPLI in type I cells but eliminated all the fine nerve fibers, leaving a sparse plexus of coarse axons. Removal of the superior cervical and nodose ganglion had no effect on SPLI and NKLI in type I cells or on fine terminal plexus, but eliminated the coarse plexus. These studies provide indirect evidence that tachykinins are formed in the carotid body, presumably in type I cells.

In addition to tachykinins, cat carotid body also contains a variety of other peptides (e.g., calcitonin-gene related peptide [CGRP]). Of all these peptides, interestingly enough, only two peptides are localized in type I cells, namely the tachykinins (SP and NKA) and enkephalins. The depressant effects of enkephalins on chemosensory activity are well known (18), which leaves the SP and NKA as the only excitatory peptides present in glomus cells, the putative receptive element of the carotid body.

EFFECTS OF SP ON RESPIRATION VIA PULMONARY RECEPTORS

Recent studies on anesthetized, spontaneous breathing rabbits (29) showed that right atrial injections of SP (25–100 ng/kg) increased respiratory rate and peak phrenic activity. In addition, SP elicited augmented breaths in 67% of the trials. By contrast, intraaortic injections of SP (also 25–100 ng/kg) did not provoke aug-

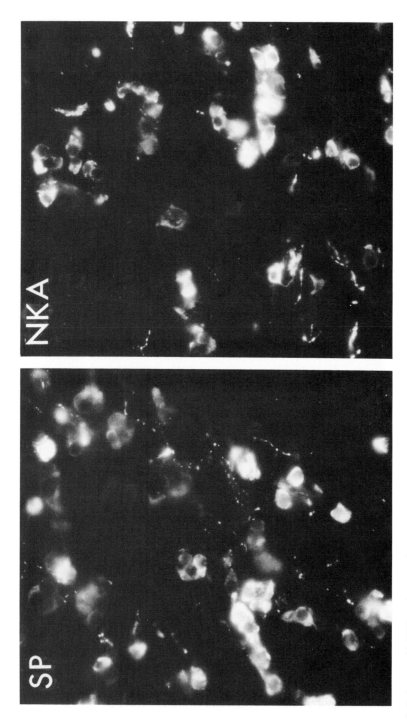

Fig. 11.5 Substance P (SP) and neurokinin A (NKA) immunofluorescence of cat carotid body. Magnification, ×500. Note that SP- and NKA-like immunoreactivity (SPLI and NKLI, respectively) is present in cells. SPLI axons are more abundant than NKLI axons.

mented breaths and caused no increase in respiratory rate. Tidal phrenic activity rose with intraaortic injection, but the change was substantially less than that observed with right atrial injections. Because both routes of administration decreased the arterial blood pressure to the same extent, these respiratory responses likely were not secondary to cardiovascular changes. After administration of an SP antagonist ([D-Arg^1-D-Pro^2-D-Trp^{7,9}-Leu^{11}]-SP), but not antihistamine, respiratory responses to right atrial injections of SP were significantly attenuated. Interestingly, the rate of occurrence of augmented breaths elicited by releasing tracheal occlusions was also reduced (control 95%, vs. 14% after SP antagonist). Bilateral vagotomy abolished the tachypneic response and reduced the magnitude of the phrenic nerve increases caused by right atrial injections of SP, indicating the reflex nature of the response. Recording from single fibers indicated that two types of vagal fibers (both involved in pulmonary nociception) could be stimulated by SP: (a) sensory fibers, whose discharge coincided with peak inspiration and showed adaptation to main-tained inflation, which were probably supplied by rapidly adapting mechanorecep-tors ("irritant" receptors); and (b) the sensory fibers, which were sensitive to phen-ylbiguanide and normally have low resting activity, presumably the "C" fibers (3). The activity of high-threshold pulmonary stretch receptors was unaffected by sub-stance P (29), but the low-threshold pulmonary stretch receptors responded with an increase in activity, especially when the lungs were not being inflated (unpub-lished observations).

Neuroepithelial bodies in the lungs of rabbits have been shown to have pep-tides and also respond to hypoxic stimulus (13). It is tempting to speculate that SP may be involved in hypoxic excitation of neuroepithelial bodies.

EFFECTS OF SUBSTANCE P ON CENTRAL RESPIRATORY NEURONS

Injections of crude extracts containing SP into the lateral ventricles of adult cats and rabbits increased respiratory rate and tidal volume (5). SP caused similar respi-ratory effects in rabbit pups after application to the dorsal medullary surface (33). Prompted by the finding that SP may be involved in the hypoxic ventilatory response (24,26,28), Yamamoto and Lagercrantz (32) studied the hypoxic ventila-tory response in rabbit pups before and after administration of an SP antagonist ([D-Arg^1-D-Pro^2-D-Trp^{7,9}-Leu^{11}]-SP) near the vicinity of the respiratory neural com-plex on the dorsal medullary surface. According to these authors, the SP antagonist blocked the ventilatory response to SP and hypoxia but not to elevated CO_2. Sub-sequently, with the use of a microdialysis technique, increased release of SP was measured in the nucleus tractus solitarii of adult cats during an hypoxic challenge (14).

Localized areas near the ventral medullary surface appear to be involved in central chemoreceptive functions (15). Substance P-like immunoreactivity was localized in the nerve fibers and cell bodies of this region and was thought to be involved in cardiovascular regulation (9). It is also possible that the SP-containing neural elements may also be important in chemical control of breathing. Therefore, the respiratory effects of topical ventral surface applications of SP were assessed in anesthetized, paralyzed, vagotomized, and peripherally chemodenervated cats. In response to SP applications, efferent phrenic, hypoglossal, and recurrent laryngeal nerve activities increased within 5–10 s after application (27). Furthermore, after the animals were ventilated to "apnea," phasic phrenic activity could be provoked with application of SP to the ventral medullary surface. Control applications of artificial cerebrospinal fluid (CSF) elicited no response. During eucapnic breathing, topical application of SP antagonist ([D-Pro^2-D-Trp^{7,9}]-SP) did not affect the phrenic activity; however, it did depress the ventilatory response to elevated CO_2. These observations indicate that SP-like peptides in the ventral surface can potentially modulate the CO_2 response in the same way that it enhances the hypoxic–hypercapnic interaction of peripheral chemoreceptors. In this context, it is well worth noting that this region of the ventrolateral medulla has been implicated in influencing cerebral blood vessel dilation by hypoxia (31).

These observations suggest that SP is involved centrally, as well as peripherally, in the expression of hypoxic ventilatory response.

ACKNOWLEDGMENTS

We are grateful to Professor C. von Euler for his encouragement and in whose laboratory the initial experiments were performed. We also gratefully acknowledge the help of Professor Susan Leeman in the radioimmunoassay measurements. We greatly appreciate the collaboration of Drs. Story Landis, Ganesh Kumar, Michael Runold, and Jyoti Mitra. This research was supported in part by NIH Grant HL-25830.

REFERENCES

1. Chang, M. M., and S. E. Leeman. Isolation of a sialogigic peptide from bovine hypothalamic tissue and its characterization as substance P. *J. Biol. Chem. 245:* 4784–4790, 1970.
2. Erspamer, V. Tachykinin peptide family. *Trends Neurosci. 4:* 267–269, 1981.
3. Euler, C. von. The contribution of sensory inputs to the pattern generation of breathing. *Can J. Physiol. Pharmacol. 59:* 700–706, 1981.
4. Euler, U. S. von, and J. H. Gaddum. An unidentified depressor substance in certain tissue extracts. *J. Physiol (Lond.) 72:* 76–87, 1931.
5. Euler, U. S. von, and B. Pernow. Neurotropic effects of substance P. *Acta Physiol. Scand. 36:* 265–274, 1956.
6. Fidone, S. J., and C. Gonzalez. Initiation and control of chemoreceptor activity in the carotid body. In: *Handbook of Physiology, Sec. 3: The Respiratory System,* Vol. 2: *Control of Breathing,* ed. N. S. Cherniack and J. G. Widdicombe. Bethesda: Am. Physiol. Soc., 1986, pp. 267–312.
7. Fitzgerald, R. S., P. Garger, M. C. Hauer, H. Raff, and L. Fechter. Effect of hypoxia and hypercapnia on catecholamine content in cat carotid body. *J. Appl. Physiol. 54:* 1408–1413, 1983.
8. Hansen, G., L. Jones, and S. Fidone. Physiological chemoreceptor stimulation decreases enkephalin and substance P in the carotid body. *Peptides 7:* 767–769, 1986.
9. Helke, C. J. Neuroanatomical localization of substance P: implications for central cardiovascular control. *Peptides 3:* 479–483, 1982.
10. Jessell, R. M. Substance P in the nervous system. In: *Handbook of Psychopharmacology,* Vol. 16, ed. L. Iverson, S. D. Iverson, and S. H. Snyder. New York: Plenum, 1983, pp. 1–105.

11. Lahiri, S., and R. G. DeLaney. Stimulus interaction in the response of carotid body chemoreceptor single afferent fibers. *Respir. Physiol. 24:* 249–266, 1975.

12. Landis, S. C., N. R. Prabhakar, J. Mitra, and N. S. Cherniack. Localization of substance P and CGRP immunoreactivity in cat carotid body. *Fed. Proc., 46:* 824, 1987.

13. Lauweryns, J. M., and M. Cockelaere. Intrapulmonary neuro-epithelial bodies: hypoxia-sensitive neuro(chemo-)receptors. *Experimentia 29:* 1384–1386, 1973.

14. Lindefors, N., Y. Yamamoto, T. Pantaleo, H. Lagercrantz, E. Brodin, and U. Ungerstedt. In vivo release of substance P in the nucleus tractus solitarii increases during hypoxia. *Neurosci. Lett. 69:* 94–97, 1986.

15. Loeschcke, H. H. Central chemosensitivity and the reaction theory. *J. Physiol. (Lond.) 332:* 1–24, 1982.

16. Maley, B., and R. Elde. Immunohistochemical localization of putative neurotransmitters within the feline nucleus tractus solitarii. *Neuroscience 7:* 2469–2490, 1982.

17. McQueen, D. S. Effect of substance P on the carotid chemoreceptor activity in the cat. *J. Physiol. (Lond.) 302:* 31–47, 1980.

18. McQueen, D. S., and J. A. Ribeiro. Inhibitory actions of methionine–enkephalin and morphine on cat carotid chemoreceptors. *Br. J. Pharmacol. 71:* 297–305, 1980.

19. Monti-Bloch, L., and C. Eyzaguirre. Effects of methionine–enkephalin and substance P on the chemosensory discharge of the cat carotid body. *Brain Res. 338:* 297–307, 1985.

20. Mulligan, E., and S. Lahiri . Dependence of carotid chemoreceptor stimulation by metabolic agents on P_aO_2 and P_aCO_2. *J. Appl. Physiol. 50:* 884–891, 1981.

21. Mulligan, E., and S. Lahiri. Separation of carotid body chemoreceptor responses to O_2 and CO_2 by oligomycin and by antimycin A. *Am. J. Physiol. 242:* C200–C206, 1982.

22. Pernow, B. Substance P. *Pharmacol. Rev. 35:* 85–141, 1983.

23. Prabhakar, N. R., G. K. Kumar, J. Mitra, C. von Euler, and N. S. Cherniack. A comparison of presence and chemoreceptive function of different tachykinins in the carotid body. *Soc. Neurosci. Abstr. 12:* 494, 1986.

24. Prabhakar, N. R., J. Mitra, N. S. Cherniack. Role of substance P in hypercapnic excitation of carotid chemoreceptors. *J. Appl. Physiol., 63:* 2418–2425, 1988.

25. Prabhakar, N. R., J. Mitra, H. Lagercrantz, C. von Euler, and N. S. Cherniack. Substance P and hypoxic excitation of the carotid body. In: *Substance P and Neurokinins,* ed. J. L. Henry. New York: Springer-Verlag, 1988, pp. 263–265.

26. Prabhakar, N. R., M. Runold, J. Mitra, H. Lagercrantz, and N. S. Cherniack. Role of substance P in the transduction process of carotid chemoreceptors. In: *Neurobiology of the Control of Breathing,* ed. C. von Euler and H. Lagercrantz. New York: Raven Press, 1986, pp. 101–107.

27. Prabhakar, N. R., M. Runold, Y. Yamamoto, C. von Euler, J. Mitra, and N. S. Cherniack. Substance P induced excitation of tracheopulmonary receptors and central chemosensitive structures. *Soc. Neurosci. Abstr. 10:* 1124, 1984.

28. Prabhakar, N. R., M. Runold, Y. Yamamoto, H. Lagercrantz, and C. von Euler. Effect of substance P antagonist on the hypoxia induced carotid chemoreceptor activity. *Acta Physiol. Scand. 121:* 301–303, 1984.

29. Prabhakar, N. R., M. Runold, Y. Yamamoto, H. Lagercrantz, N. S. Cherniack, and C. von Euler. Role of the vagal afferents in substance P induced respiratory responses in anaesthetized rabbits. *Acta Physiol. Scand. 131:* 63–71, 1987.

30. Rosell, S., and K. Folkers. Substance P antagonists: a new type of pharmacological tool. *Trends Neurosci. 211* (May): 212, 1982.

31. Underwood, M. D., C. Iadecola, and D. J. Reis. Brainstem mechanisms mediating the cerebrovascular vasodilation to hypoxia: role of C_1 area of rostral ventrolateral medulla. *Fed. Proc., 46:* 1244, 1987.

32. Yamamoto, Y., and H. Lagercrantz. Some effects of substance P on central respiratory control in rabbit pups. *Acta Physiol. Scand. 124:* 449–455, 1985.

33. Yamamoto, Y., H. Lagercrantz, and C. von Euler. Effects of substance P and TRH on ventilation and pattern of breathing in newborn rabbits. *Acta Physiol. Scand. 113:* 541–543, 1981.
34. Wharton, J., Polak, J. M., Pearse, A.G.E., McGregor, G. P., Bryant, M. G., Bloom, S. R., Emson, P. C., Bisgard, G. E., and Will, J. A. Enkephalin-, VIP-, and substance P-like immunoreactivity in the carotid body. *Nature 284:* 269–271, 1980.

12

Peripheral Chemoreceptors and Other Oxygen Sensors in the Fetus and Newborn

M. A. HANSON, G. J. EDEN, J. G. NIJHUIS, AND P. J. MOORE

Fetal breathing movements (FBM) in the sheep differ in several respects from postnatal breathing movements (see ref. 6 for review): (a) They are episodic, occurring mainly during periods of low-voltage electrocortical activity (LV ECoG) associated with rapid eye movements (REM); (b) they are abolished, apart from occasional, isolated movements, by a reduction in arterial P_{O_2} (P_aO_2) to approximately 15 mmHg, even though the carotid chemoreceptors increase their discharge over this P_aO_2 range (2); (c) they are stimulated by a rise in arterial P_{CO_2} (P_aCO_2), although this response is weaker than that of the neonate; and finally, (d) they serve no purpose in gas exchange, and in fact necessitate a substantial expenditure of energy. Although fetal breathing in humans has been known for many years (1; see ref. 19 for review), and is also episodic, its relation to the ECoG is unknown; recent studies (18) suggest that although it is more common in REM sleep, it occurs also in non-REM sleep.

This chapter is concerned in part with the effects of hypoxia on breathing movements in the fetal lamb. In the fetus, the effects have been suggested to involve a descending inhibition arising from some structure above the pons (7) and not involving the cerebrum (13). In this respect, the site of the inhibition appears to differ from that reported to arise from the frontal lobes in the adult cat (17). Recently, Gluckman and Johnston (11) reported that lesions in the region of the trigeminal nuclei in the rostrolateral pons in the fetal lamb abolished the effects of hypoxia on fetal breathing. Whether such lesions destroyed a specific hypoxia-sensitive (i.e., chemoreceptive) structure, or whether they affected axons passing through the area as part of more complex neural circuitry, is not known. Nor is it known unequivocally whether or not the effects of hypoxia on FBM requires intact peripheral arterial chemoreceptors: Dawes et al. (7) reported that the effect of hypoxia on FBM was unaffected by section of the carotid sinus nerves, although the technique that they used (i.e., stripping the carotid bifurcation region) might also have destroyed other structures. Also, they did not section the vagi, and thus aortic chemoreceptor afferents would have remained intact. We reasoned that if the cessation of FBM does indeed represent descending inhibition, rather than hypoxic depression, of the medullary respiratory neurons, then it should be possible to stimulate FBM pharmacologically even in hypoxia. Moreover, such a stimulation of FBM should not require the presence of carotid chemoreceptor afferents. We reinvestigated the question and report the results in this chapter.

The inhibitory effect of hypoxia on breathing movements does not disappear immediately at birth (3). It has been suggested to play a role in the secondary fall in ventilation ($\dot{V}_E$) which occurs after an initial stimulation when neonatal animals or babies are exposed to actue hypoxia (12). In the rat, the "adult" respiratory response to hypoxia (i.e., a sustained increase in $\dot{V}_E$) matures gradually over the first two postnatal weeks; the age at which a "biphasic" $\dot{V}_E$ response is detectable depends on the intensity of the hypoxia to which the animal is exposed (9). Exposing rat pups from birth to chronic hypoxia delays the maturation of the adult $\dot{V}_E$ reponse, whereas exposure to chronic hyperoxia accelerates its maturation (8,10). We proposed two possible explanations for these observations: (a) The P_aO_2 achieved postnatally determined the rate of disappearance of the fetal suprapontine inhibitory mechanism; or (b) the P_aO_2 achieved altered the rate of postnatal resetting of the carotid chemoreceptors. Either explanation would account for the "blunted" response of chronically hypoxic neonates to superimposed episodes of acute hypoxia. We decided to test these ideas by exposing kittens from birth to hypoxia or hyperoxia. This species is large enough to permit us to make recordings from carotid chemoreceptor afferents in the neonate. We could thus define the extent to which alterations in chemoreceptor hypoxic sensitivity were responsible for the different $\dot{V}_E$ responses to acute hypoxia.

METHODS

Fetal Lambs

Nine mule cross-bred sheep at 115–120 days' gestation were anesthetized (thiopentone, 1.5 g i.v. for induction; halothane, 2% in O_2 for maintenance). Using sterile techniques, we exteriorized the fetus and chronically instrumented it according to the procedure of Boddy et al. (4). Briefly, catheters were placed in a jugular vein, a carotid artery, the trachea, and the amniotic cavity. Bipolar electrodes were placed in the diaphragm, and also on the parietal dura for measurement of ECoG activity. In three fetuses, we identified the carotid sinus nerves under a dissecting microscope at the junction with the glossopharyngeal nerves. Two ligatures were placed around the carotid sinus nerves which we then sectioned in between. The vagus nerves were also ligated and cut in the midcervical region. These fetuses were deemed to be chemodenervated. In the remaining (sham-operated) fetuses, the dissections of the carotid sinus and vagus nerves were similar, but the nerves were not cut. The fetuses were returned to the uterus and the incisions were closed. Catheters and electrode cables were led out through the flank of the ewe. Ewe and fetus were given antibiotics postoperatively, and measurements were not made until at least 5 days after surgery.

Initially, over a period of 4 h, control measurements were made, after which 2 mg pilocarpine was injected i.v. When the full effects of the drug had been produced (in about 4 min), 2 mg atropine sulfate was given i.v. On a subsequent day, we subjected the fetus to isocapnic hypoxia by giving the ewe 10% O_2 in N_2 to breathe. When FBM had been abolished, 2 mg of pilocarpine was injected i.v. Again 2 mg of atropine sulfate was then given i.v. after about 4 min. This protocol was repeated on successive days. At about 138 days' gestation, the ewe and fetus were killed and the fetus was delivered. In the chemodenervated group, the anatomical completeness of the denervation was then confirmed.

Newborn Kittens

Pregnant cats were placed individually in a normobaric environmental chamber (10) through which air was passed at about 15 l/min. A few days before they were expected to litter, the inspired O_2 fraction (F_1O_2) in the chamber was reduced to 0.13–0.15 by blending N_2 with the inflowing air (chronic hypoxia) or was increased to 0.30 by blending O_2 with the air (chronic hyperoxia). The chamber was housed in a constant temperature room with a 12-h light/12-h dark cycle. The F_1O_2 and the temperature in the chamber were measured automatically every 15 min and their values recorded on a data logger; humidity and the P_{CO_2} in the chamber were checked daily. Normoxic cats and their litters were kept in standard cages in the same room as the environmental chamber and breathed room air.

When the kittens were 12–13 days old, we measured their respiratory responses to an acute reduction in F_1O_2. To this purpose, they were placed in a plethysmograph to which a pneumotachometer was connected to measure breathing continuously (16). The plethysmograph was placed in a nylon hood through which gas was passed of the same F_1O_2 as the kitten had been exposed to from birth. When the kitten was asleep (judged visually, or in some experiments by the ECoG), the F_1O_2 was reduced abruptly to 0.08 for 6 min. In order to validate comparison of their responses with those of the chronically hypoxic kittens, the normoxic kittens were exposed to an F_1O_2 of 0.13–0.15 for 15 min before the F_1O_2 was reduced to 0.08. Similarly, for comparison with the chronically hyperoxic kittens, they were exposed to an F_1O_2 of 0.30 for 15 min before the acute hypoxic challenge.

At postnatal age 12–23 days, the kittens were anesthetized (pentobarbitone, 30 mg/kg, i.p.), paralyzed, and artificially ventilated. Single- or few-fiber chemoreceptor afferent preparations were dissected from the cut left carotid sinus nerve and their steady-state responses to graded levels of isocapnic hypoxia were measured.

RESULTS

Fetal Lambs

In all fetuses, pilocarpine produced a vigorous stimulation of FBM which lasted up to an hour and could not be mistaken for normal FBM. On a subsequent day, reducing P_aO_2 to about 11 mmHg produced a cessation of spontaneous FBM. When pilocarpine was administered intravenously, a vigorous stimulation of breathing again occurred (Fig. 12.1). The ECoG switched to a low-voltage pattern which per-

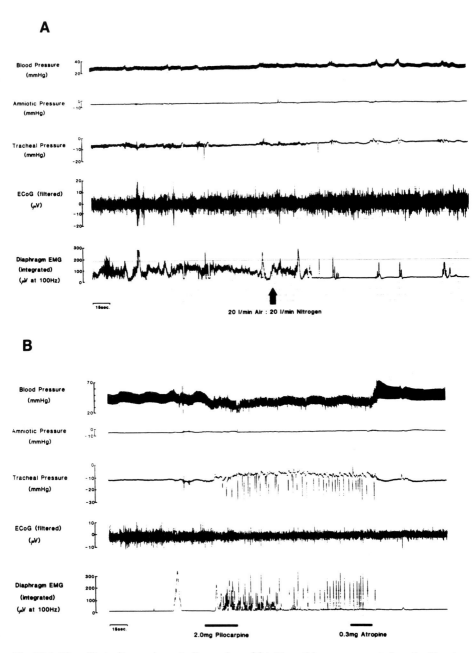

Fig. 12.1 The effect of hypoxia and pilocarpine of fetal breathing movements in a fetal lamb at 126 days' gestation. In **A,** fetal hypoxia induced by giving the ewe 10% O$_2$ to breathe caused a cessation of spontaneous breathing movements. Then in **B,** pilocarpine induced a large stimulation of breathing, which was blocked by atropine.

sisted for the duration of the stimulation of FBM. Administration of atropine rapidly abolished the stimulation of FBM and the ECoG returned to a high-voltage pattern. These effects were similar in both the chemodenervated and the sham-operated fetuses.

Newborn Kittens

On postnatal day 12/13, the normoxic kittens showed a sustained increase in ventilation ($\dot{V}_E$) during the acute exposure to an F_IO_2 of 0.08 (Fig. 12.2). This was true whether they had been exposed to an F_IO_2 of 0.13–0.15 (7 kittens) or of 0.30 (6 kittens) for 15 min before the exposure to F_IO_2 of 0.08. In contrast, both the chronically hypoxic ($n = 6$) and the chronically hyperoxic ($n = 5$) kittens showed a poor respiratory response to the acute hypoxia. This was particularly true of the hypoxic animals, which showed a progressive decline in $\dot{V}_E$ (Fig. 12.2).

We also observed striking differences in the steady-state response curves of the carotid chemoreceptors to isocapnic hypoxia (see Fig. 12.3). The curves were flatter for the chronically hypoxic kittens (10 chemoreceptor preparations from 6 kittens) and hyperoxic kittens (8 preparations from 4 kittens) than for the normoxic kittens (9 preparations from 5 kittens).

DISCUSSION

The observation that pilocarpine can stimulate FBM even during hypoxia, when FBM are normally absent, provides further evidence that the effects of hypoxia occur via a descending inhibitory mechanism acting upon the respiratory neurons, rather than via a direct depression of neuronal activity. Further work is needed to establish the site of origin of this inhibition and the means by which it detects hypoxia.

At present, we do not know where pilocarpine exerts its effects; unlike Brown et al. (5), we did not find any evidence for its action via the peripheral chemoreceptors. It might act (a) through the pathways by which ECoG state modulates FBM, as suggested by its effect in producing a switch to low-voltage ECoG; (b) at the suprapontine hypoxic sensor; or (c) through some completely independent cholinergic system impinging upon the respiratory neurons. If (b) or (c) is true, pilocarpine must, in addition, have independent effects on the ECoG.

Our experiments with kittens confirm those of Eden and Hanson (10) in rats, in showing that chronic hypoxia from birth reduces the $\dot{V}_E$ response to acute hypoxia, as if it delays the maturation of the "adult" response. In the rat, however, there was no evidence for a reduced peripheral chemoreceptor response to hypoxia. The studies in the rat had, of necessity, to be performed by recording the activity of the whole carotid sinus nerve, a method that gives an indication of the relative increase in discharge in hypoxia in any animal but is not well suited for making comparisons between animals. The present studies, however, employed single- or few-fiber chemoreceptor preparations. Apart from considerations of species differences, it may be that chronic hypoxia from birth delays or reduces postnatal che-

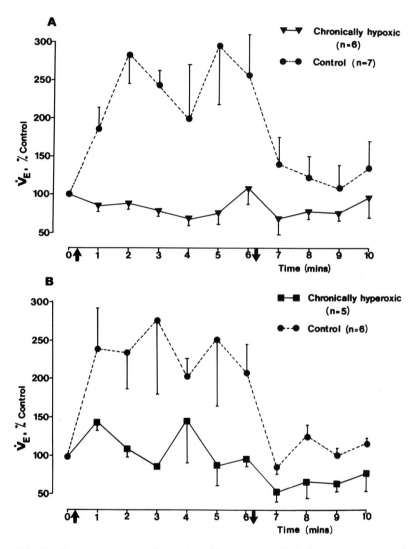

Fig. 12.2 Ventilatory responses of conscious kittens aged 12/13 days to acute hypoxia (F_IO_2 - 0.08) administered for the period between the arrows. The chronically hypoxic kittens breathed an F_IO_2 of 0.13–0.15, and the chronically hyperoxic kittens breathed an F_IO_2 of 0.30 from birth until the acute hypoxic trial. The normoxic control kittens in **A** breathed an F_IO_2 of 0.13–0.15 for 15 min before the acute hypoxic trial. The control kittens in **B** breathed an F_IO_2 of 0.30 for 15 min before the trial. The normoxic kittens showed a sustained $\dot{V}_E$ response to acute hypoxia; in contrast, the response of the hyperoxic kittens was variable and less prominent, and that of the hypoxic kittens was almost absent.

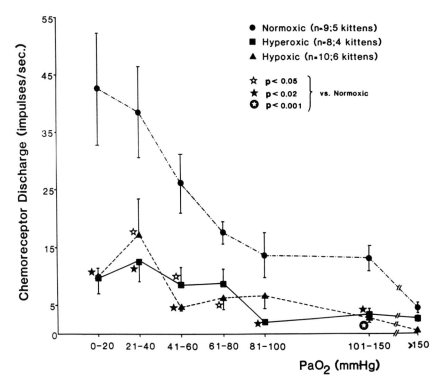

Fig. 12.3 Single- or few-fiber carotid chemoreceptor responses to isocapnic hypoxia for the three groups of kittens on postnatal days 12–23. (●) Normoxic ($P_a\text{CO}_2$ over the curve, 36.6 ± 1.4 mmHg, mean ± SE); (▲) chronically hypoxic ($P_a\text{CO}_2$, 40.2 ± 2.0 mmHg); (■) chronically hyperoxic ($P_a\text{CO}_2$, 36.9 ± 1.1 mmHg). For statistical comparison by unpaired t-test, the results have been grouped into $P_a\text{O}_2$ ranges. Over most ranges, the responses of the chemoreceptors from the chronically hypoxic and hyperoxic kittens were less than those from the normoxic kittens.

moreceptor resetting. It is interesting that this effect contrasts with that in the adult cat, in which Lahiri et al. (15) reported that chronic hypoxia produced an *increase* in the hypoxic sensitivity of the chemoreceptors recorded from the cut carotid sinus nerve. Further work is needed in this area.

Chronic hyperoxia from birth also appears to reduce drastically the sensitivity of the chemoreceptors to hypoxia. A similar observation has been made in the adult cat by Lahiri et al. (14), although in their study the animals were exposed to a higher $F_1\text{O}_2$ for a shorter period. At present, therefore, we do not know whether the effects we have seen are produced by oxygen toxicity or by some other means— for example, by changes in the carotid body vasculature.

ACKNOWLEDGMENTS

M.A.H. is a Wellcome Trust Senior Lecturer. We are grateful for the support of Servier Ltd., the Netherlands Organisation for the Advancement of Pure Research (ZWO), and Reading University Endowment Fund. We thank Pauline Carroll for technical assistance.

REFERENCES

1. Ahlfeld, F. von. Uber bisher noch nicht beschriebene intauterine Bewegungen des Kindes. In: *Verhandlungen der deutschen Gesellschaft der Gynakologie.* Leipzig: Breitkopf and Hartel, 1888, pp. 203–210.

2. Blanco, C. E., G. S. Dawes, M. A. Hanson, and H. B. McCooke. The response to hypoxia of arterial chemoreceptors in fetal sheep and newborn lambs. *J. Physiol (Lond.) 351:* 25–37, 1984.

3. Blanco, C. E., C. B. Martin, M. A. Hanson, and H. B. McCooke. Determinants of the onset of breathing at birth. *Pediatr. Res. 19:* 1343, 1985.

4. Boddy, K., G. S. Dawes, R. Fisher, S. Pinter, and J. S. Robinson. Foetal respiratory movements, electrocortical and cardiovascular responses to hypoxaemia in sheep. *J. Physiol. (Lond.) 243:* 599–618, 1974.

5. Brown, E. R., E. E. Lawson, A. Jansen, V. Chernick, and H. W. Taeusch. Regular fetal breathing induced by pilocarpine infusion in the near-term fetal lamb. *J. Appl. Physiol. 50:* 1348–1352, 1981.

6. Dawes, G. S. The central control of fetal breathing and skeletal muscle movements. *J. Physiol. (Lond.) 346:* 1–18, 1984.

7. Dawes, G. S., W. N. Gardner, B. M. Johnston, and D. W. Walker. Breathing in fetal lambs: the effects of brainstem section. *J. Physiol. (Lond.) 335:* 535–553, 1983.

8. Eden, G. J., and M. A. Hanson. Effect of hyperoxia from birth on the carotid chemoreceptor and ventilatory responses of rats to acute hypoxia. *J. Physiol. (Lond.) 374:* 24P, 1986.

9. Eden, G. J., and M. A. Hanson. Maturation of the respiratory response to acute hypoxia in the newborn rat. *J. Physiol (Lond.) 392:* 1–9, 1987.

10. Eden, G. J., and M. A. Hanson. Effects of chronic hypoxia from birth on the ventilatory response to acute hypoxia in the newborn rat. *J. Physiol. (Lond.), 392:* 11–19, 1987.

11. Gluckman, P. D., and B. M. Johnston. Lesions in the upper lateral pons abolish the hypoxic depression of breathing in unanaesthetized fetal lambs in utero. *J. Physiol. (Lond.), 382:* 373–383, 1987.

12. Hanson, M. A. Maturation of the peripheral chemoreceptor and central nervous components of respiratory control in perinatal life. In: *Neurobiology of the Control of Breathing,* ed. C. von Euler and H. Lagercrantz. New York: Raven Press, 1987, pp. 59–65.

13. Ioffe, S., A. H. Jansen, and V. Chernick. Effects of hypercapnia and hypoxemia on fetal breathing after decortication. *J. Appl. Physiol. 61:* 1071–1076, 1986.

14. Lahiri, S., E. Mulligan, A. Mokashi, S. Andronikou, and M. Shirahata. Altered function of cat carotid body chemoreceptors in prolonged hyperoxia. In: *Chemoreceptors in Respiratory Control,* ed. J. A. Ribeiro and D. J. Pallot. London: Croom Helm, 1987, pp. 50–58.

15. Lahiri, S., N. Smatresk, M. Pokorski, P. Barnard, and A. Mokashi. Efferent inhibition of carotid body chemoreception in chronically hypoxic cats. *Am. J. Physiol. 245:* R678–R683, 1983.

16. McCooke, H. B., and M. A. Hanson. Respiration of conscious kittens in acute hypoxia and effect of almitrine bismesylate. *J. Appl. Physiol. 59:* 18–23, 1985.

17. Tenney, S. M., and L. C. Ou. Ventilatory responses of decorticate and decerebrate cats to hypoxia and CO_2. *Respir. Physiol. 29:* 81–92, 1977.

18. Van Vliet, M.A.T., C. B. Martin, Jr., J. G. Nijhuis, and H.F.R. Prechtl. The relationship between fetal activity, behavioural states and fetal breathing movements in normal and growth-retarded fetuses. *Am. J. Obstet. Gynecol. 88:* 582–588, 1985.

19. Wilds, P. L. Observations of intrauterine fetal breathing movements—a review. *Am. J. Obstet. Gynecol. 131:* 315–338, 1978.

13

Possible Mechanisms of Oxygen Sensing in the Carotid Body

H. ACKER, M. A. DELPIANO, AND F. PIETRUSCHKA

Oxygen sensing in tissues defines a process by which cells are able to respond to Po_2 changes by altering metabolic activities or membrane properties in order to regulate their cell-specific functions. These cell-specific functions include (a) the secretion of hormones to excite nerve endings for controlling respiration and circulation, as occurs in the carotid body (7); (b) the production and secretion of erythropoietin, to increase the number of red cells under hypoxia (26); (c) the response to hypoxia by endothelial cells which regulate the microcirculation, as clearly demonstrated in the carotid body (43); and also (d) the proliferation of tumor cells (2).

In order to elucidate the molecular mechanism of the oxygen-sensing process, different possibilities must be considered. Because oxygen interacts directly with the respiratory chain, the regulation of ATP production by this process could be a signal for the cell to alter its activity. Since the critical mitochondrial Po_2 has been reported to be far below 1 torr (46), steep Po_2 gradients in the cytosol are required for the respiratory chain to work as a Po_2 sensor under normal oxygen supply conditions. However, the investigations of Wilson et al. (50) and Mills and Jöbsis (35) reveal that the critical Po_2 for the respiratory chain might correspond to higher cytosolic Po_2 values. Wilson et al. (50) showed that cytochrome c was reduced continuously, beginning with a Po_2 of 100 torr, by interaction with the ATP/ADP ratio. Mills and Jöbsis (35) concluded, from spectrophotometric studies on the carotid body, that a specialized cytochrome a/a_3 with a low O_2 affinity existed in the carotid body.

A second candidate for the oxygen sensor is lactate dehydrogenase (LDH). This enzyme exists as five different isoenzymes which are tetramers of two subunits, H and M. The synthesis of the different forms of the enzyme, from LDH_1 to LDH_5, can be influenced by changes in oxygen content. In lymphocytes and chicken embryos, hypoxia induces the formation of the M type of the isoenzymes which has a higher affinity for pyruvate (32). The V_{max} of other enzymes of the glycolytic chain such as pyruvate kinase can be increased by hypoxia (24), resulting in a higher glucose flux into the cells.

In the case of the carotid body, a third candidate indicated by the presence of a specialized O_2-binding protein has been discussed (33). It has been suggested that this protein has a hemoglobin-like structure and changes its allosteric conformation with variations in P_{O_2}. An O_2-binding protein could serve as a signal protein, reacting with oxygen at P_{O_2} levels far above the low critical mitochondrial P_{O_2}.

A fourth candidate would be oxidases and oxygenases with $K_{m O_2}$ between 30 and 300 torr; about 28 different types are known (28). Glutathione peroxidase might be of special interest: It reduces peroxides with concomitant oxidation of reduced glutathione (GSH) to form the corresponding thiol and glutathione disulfide (GSSG) (30). The transition in the thiol redox state has profound effects on active and passive cation permeability as well as on the chemical stimulation of excitable cells (44).

METHODS

As shown in Figs. 13.1 and 13.2, the experiments were carried out in the cat carotid body both in vivo and in vitro. These preparations have been described in detail by Acker and O'Regan (6) and by Delpiano and Acker (19), respectively. Special consideration should be given to the microelectrodes used in the experiments: Oxy-

Fig. 13.1 Dependence of oxygen consumption (●), tissue pH (▲), and ATP level of the cat carotid body on P_{O_2}. Oxygen consumption values are related to tissue P_{O_2} values of the cat carotid body in vivo. The relationship between tissue pH values in the cat carotid body in vitro and the P_{O_2} in the superfusion medium is shown for two experiments. The arrows indicate the arterial blood P_{O_2} at which the carotid body was excised from the animals.

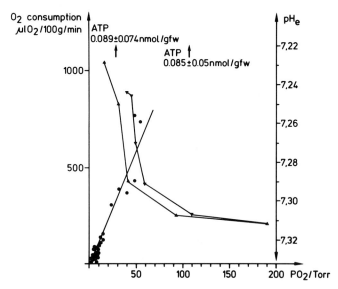

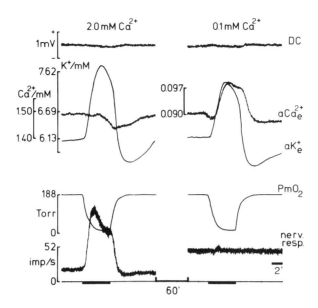

Fig. 13.2 Changes in extracellular potassium and calcium activity in the carotid body in vitro during hypoxia. From top to bottom, the traces represent the bioelectrical potential (DC), the extracellular calcium activity (aCa_e^{2+}), the extracellular potassium activity (aK_e^+), the oxygen pressure in the superfusion medium (P_mO_2), and chemoreceptor nervous activity (imp/s). The data in the left-hand column were obtained with 2.0 mM calcium in the medium; in the right-hand column, with 0.1 mM calcium in the superfusion medium.

gen tension within the carotid body was measured polarographically by use of microneedle electrodes (tip diameter, 2–5 μm) inserted into the organ through its ventromedial surface. When polarographic P_O_2 measurements are performed, oxygen molecules are reduced on a glass-isolated platinum wire surface which functions as a cathode. In the neutral and alkaline ranges, the chemical reaction is as follows:

$$O_2 + 2H_2O + 4e^- = 4OH^- \tag{13.1}$$

Electrochemical reduction generates the signal in the polarographic circuit. Because the cathode consumes oxygen continuously, a continuous flux of oxygen molecules develops toward the electrode. Under the assumption that at optimum polarization all the oxygen molecules are immediately reduced, the number of molecules on the cathode surface is zero. Under these boundary conditions, the P_O_2 in front of the electrode and the reduction current show a linear relationship. After the electrode is inserted into the carotid body, the position of the electrodes in vivo is tested by blowing oxygen over the surface of the carotid body. When the electrode is in a superficial position as opposed to a deep location, tissue P_O_2 increases during this test. In the in vitro preparation, the carotid body is supplied with oxygen by diffusion from the outside; thus the phenomenon of the "oxygen barrier" (5), as measured in vivo, is no longer measurable.

Measurements of different ion activities in the carotid body were performed with double- or triple-barreled ion-sensitive microelectrodes having a tip diameter between 1 and 3 μm (18,21). In principle, the ion activity measurement is a recording of an electrical potential that is generated in an ion-sensitive glass or in a liquid ion exchanger of a neutral ion carrier.

This process (22) can be described by the formula:

$$E = RT \ln \frac{a'_i + \Sigma k_{ij}a'_j}{a''_i + \Sigma k_{ij}a''_j} \qquad (13.2)$$

where

a',a'' = the activities of ions
k_{ij} = the selectivity constant for the jth ion with respect to the ith ion
i = the ion the electrode is expected to measure
j = the interfering ion
E = the electrical potential (V)
RT = the gas constant (8.3 joules/degree Kelvin/mol) $\times$ the absolute temperature.

The microelectrodes that were used for extracellular ion activity measurements in the carotid body are described below.

1. For extracellular pH measurements, a double-barreled pH microelectrode was used. One channel filled with 150 mM NaCl served as a DC electrode. A tip of pH-sensitive glass was introduced into the second channel toward the microelectrode tip, until a recess of about 30 μm long was formed. The pH glass was then fixed in the second channel by a high-atomic epoxy glue mixed with glass powder, giving an additional constant recess. The electrodes had a steepness of about 53 mV/pH unit at room temperature and a response time of about 20–30 s.

2. Triple-barreled ion-sensitive microelectrodes were prepared on the day of experimentation. We used simultaneously (a) channels containing the K^+ ion exchanger, valinomycin, to measure potassium activities; (b) the neutral ion Ca^{2+} carrier, D-nitro-phenyl-n-octyl ether, to measure calcium activities; and (c) 1 M magnesium acetate, to measure local DC potentials.

Signals recorded from the channel monitoring DC potentials were used to compensate the potentials recorded by the ion-sensitive microelectrodes so that these electrodes measured only ion activities. Slopes ($\pm$ SD) per decade change in ion concentrations were 55 mV and 27 mV for the K^+ and Ca^{2+} microelectrodes, respectively. A linear relationship existed between the logarithm of the ion activity and the potential recorded by the ion-sensitive microelectrodes. The mean response time (99%) for both microelectrodes was about 200 ms. Potentials from the ion-sensitive microelectrodes were differentially recorded by use of an amplifier (Burr Brown 3527 BM) with a high-input impedance. All microelectrodes were calibrated before and after insertion. If drifts of more than 4% per hour occurred between these calibrations, results obtained in the experiments were discarded.

In some experiments, we performed an analysis of the ATP content of the carotid bodies (in vivo). The tissue was frozen by liquid nitrogen. After homogenization of the frozen tissue in 0.1 N HClO$_4$, the probes were centrifuged for 10 min at 34,000 $\times$ g, and the supernatant was used for ATP determination. The bioluminescence method according to Strehler (47) was used for ATP determination. In brief, the method follows the scheme:

$$ATP + luciferin + O_2 \xrightarrow[\text{luciferase}]{\text{Mg}^{2+}} oxyluciferin + PP_i + AMP + CO_2 + light \quad (13.3)$$

The quantity of emitted light was measured with the bioluminescence analyzer SKAN XP 2000 (Skan AG, Basel). The quantity of emitted light is proportional to the amount of ATP present in the sample.

RESULTS AND DISCUSSION

The mechanism of the carotid body chemoreception transduction process from the sensing of the P_{O_2} level to the generation of the nerve impulse is still a matter of discussion. A generally accepted concept defines this process as a P_{O_2}-dependent release of transmitter from type I cells. This transmitter then is hypothesized to generate action potentials in the postsynaptic afferent nerve endings. It is known that in secretory cells (42), the level of cytosolic calcium activity determines the amount of transmitter that is released. This has been suggested also for the carotid body by Grönblad et al. (23). Using electron microscopy, these investigators demonstrated an increase in the exocytosis of transmitter-containing vesicles of type I cells after external application of ionophore A23187, which is known to increase cytosolic calcium activity. Bernon et al. (13) assigned cytosolic calcium a key role in the chemoreceptive process. These authors showed that an increase in chemoreceptive discharges was induced by calcium-containing lysosomes. These liposomes are capable of penetrating cell membranes and can thereby load the cytosol of type I and type II cells with calcium. To propose a working hypothesis for the chemoreceptor in the carotid body that would encompass these observations requires that one search for a link or interconnection between variations in oxygen pressure, and changes in cytosolic calcium activity that result in a transmitter-induced nervous excitation. This interconnection can be expressed by the following sequential steps:

$$P_{O_2} + S = \overline{P_{O_2} \cdot S} \quad (13.4)$$
$$\overline{P_{O_2} \cdot S} + E = P_{O_2} \cdot S \cdot E \quad (13.5)$$

where P_{O_2} = oxygen partial pressure in the tissue, S = sensor, and E = effector. Equations 13.4 and 13.5, deduced from schematic drawings of hormone–receptor interactions (29), indicate that oxygen is reacting with a sensor, forming a complex which then interacts with an effector, such as calcium, as described in detail below.

Tissue Oxygen Tension (P_{O_2})

The tissue oxygen tension in the carotid body, which is most likely the specific stimulus for chemoreception, has been measured with microelectrodes by two groups. The tissue P_{O_2} displayed in the form of a histogram by Acker et al. (5), for the cat carotid body, and Weigelt et al. (48), for the rabbit carotid body, was found to be in the range of 0–100 torr with a mean value of about 20 torr. In contrast, Whalen et al. (49) found mean P_{O_2} values of 40 and 50 torr and top values up to 100 torr at an arterial P_{O_2} of about 100 torr.

Degner and Acker (16) calculated the P_{O_2} histogram of the carotid body on the basis of a microscopical serial reconstruction, published physiological data, and a mathematical model. The calculation was made for glomoids as the subunit of the carotid body and the total organ by varying the following parameters: arterial P_{O_2}, oxygen consumption, hematocrit, diameter of vessels, perfusion pressure, and capillary length. The results explain the differences in the literature regarding the tissue P_{O_2} distribution in the cat carotid body. Changing the values for capillary length in the carotid bodies resulted in changes in the histograms similar to those seen in the literature (5, 50). Furthermore, local flow velocities in the carotid body were shown to be in the range of local flow velocities of other organs. Direct measurement in the carotid body by means of hydrogen clearances (25) showed local flow velocities to be in the range of 0.01–0.1 cm/s. With a total flow of the carotid body of about 2000 ml/100g/min, these local flow velocities signify local blood flow values of less than 10% of the total flow, which is in agreement with estimations of the local flow by Acker and O'Regan (6).

Sensor

In addition to flow and vascular arrangement of the tissue, oxygen consumption in the respiratory chain determines the P_{O_2} distribution in the carotid body. The respiratory chain of the carotid body mitochondria has often been considered to be the most probable candidate for a P_{O_2} sensor. Anichkov and Belenkii (12), as well as Joels and Neil (27), have hypothesized that chemosensory excitation, especially under hypoxia, is caused by a decrease in ATP levels in the carotid body tissue. Biscoe (14) proposed that energy depletion under hypoxia triggers the nerve discharge by producing membrane instability in the sensory nerve endings. Using several inhibitors and uncouplers of the respiratory chain, Mulligan et al. (37) gave further support to the idea that oxidative phosphorylation is involved in carotid body chemoreception. The mitochondria of the carotid body seem to be specialized, since the carotid body demonstrates P_{O_2}-dependent oxygen consumption (4, 31,41,49). Figure 13.1 shows the linear dependence of oxygen consumption on tissue P_{O_2} in the carotid body in vivo (4); thus high oxygen consumption values correspond to high oxygen pressure and vice versa. Normally, mitochondria show an oxygen consumption that is independent of P_{O_2} until a P_{O_2} of 0.1 torr is reached (46). Concomitant with decreasing oxygen consumption under hypoxia in the carotid body, acidification of the tissue can be measured (see Fig. 13.1) (19), which favors the participation of aerobic glycolysis in this organ. The question arises as to how the interconnection between the glycolytic pathway and the respiratory chain under different P_{O_2} conditions can be explained. The following three equations will help to clarify this question:

$$\text{Glucose} + 2\,\text{NAD}^+ + 2\,\text{ADP} + 2\,\text{Pi} \rightarrow 2\,\text{Pyruvate} \\ + 2\,\text{ATP} + 2\,\text{NADH, H}^+ + 2\,\text{H}_2\text{O} \quad (13.6)$$

$$\text{Pyruvate} + \text{NADH, H}^+ \rightarrow \text{Lactate} + \text{NAD}^+ \quad (13.7)$$

$$\text{Pyruvate} + 18\,\text{ADP} + 18\,\text{P}_i + 3\,\text{O}_2 \rightarrow 3\,\text{CO}_2 + 18\,\text{ATP} + 21\,\text{H}_2\text{O} \quad (13.8)$$

Equations 13.6 and 13.7 describe ATP generation and lactate formation in the glycolytic pathway, whereas Eq. 13.8 describes ATP production in the respiratory chain. Under the assumption that there is an excess of ADP, oxygen consumption remains independent of the P_{O_2} down to very low values while there is increased glycolytic ADP turnover and increased lactate formation. However, if the available ADP is in a critical range, oxygen consumption becomes linearly dependent on P_{O_2} since the glycolytic system competes with the respiratory chain for ADP. This simple consideration may provide the connecting link between oxygen consumption and tissue pH, as shown in Fig. 13.1. In attempting to explain the basic phenomenon, however, the question arises as to the nature of the "switch-on mechanism" for ADP turnover in the glycolytic pathway under sufficient oxygen supply. For this purpose, the carotid body needs an additional mechanism that would allow P_{O_2} changes under sufficient oxygen supply conditions to mediate changes in LDH activity. As demonstrated in Fig. 13.1, this is a surprisingly sensitive mechanism since it is initiated already at P_{O_2} values of 100 torr. Such sensitivity is in agreement with findings of Petrova (38), who showed that 20 min of hypoxia induced in the carotid body a distinct increase of an LDH isoenzyme mostly composed of M subunits; these M subunits have a higher affinity for pyruvate (32).

These results suggest that it is necessary to consider whether an O_2-binding protein is involved in this process as a mediator. Acker and Eyzaguirre (3) measured characteristic light absorbances at the wavelengths 540 and 580 nm in the mouse carotid body. The amount of absorbance at these wavelengths was very sensitive to P_{O_2} changes far above the critical mitochondrial P_{O_2}. Further experiments would have to verify whether these changes in light absorbance are associated with a specialized protein.

Effector

Having examined different possibilities for an O_2 sensor mechanism, it seems reasonable to assume that there is a specialized mechanism for the carotid body, whereby this organ is made so sensitive to P_{O_2} changes. Because mitochondria and cytosolic pH are involved in the regulation of cytosolic calcium levels (15,36), a decreasing oxygen consumption and an increasing acidification of the carotid body tissue associated with a decreasing P_{O_2} would provide an ideal mechanism to interconnect oxygen pressure variations and chemoreceptor nervous activity via calcium activity changes that could control transmitter release. This assumption is supported by our findings (1,18), showing that extracellular calcium activity decreases under hypoxia with a concomitant increase in extracellular potassium activity. We observed that calcium influx into carotid body cells is enhanced under hypoxia (18). Our finding was confirmed by Pietruschka and Acker (40), who measured a hypoxia-induced calcium influx into cultured type I cells. This hypoxia-induced calcium influx may activate potassium channels. Figure 13.2 describes this phenomenon more precisely. By using tribarreled ion-sensitive microelectrodes to measure the extracellular potassium and calcium activities in the in vitro superfused carotid body simultaneously with the bioelectrical potential of the tissue, it was possible to demonstrate the typical decrease in calcium along with the biphasic change in potassium under hypoxia. To analyze the relationship between the changes in calcium and potassium more intensively, the calcium content of the superfusion medium was lowered to 0.1 mM Ca^{2+} from the normal value of 2.0 mM Ca^{2+}. Under these conditions, hypoxia induced an extracellular calcium increase of about 0.007 mM combined with a smaller increase in potassium activity as compared to the control. In addition to the hypoxia-stimulated calcium influx, a hypoxia-related calcium efflux seemed to exist (17), as shown in Fig. 13.2 by the increase in extracellular Ca^{2+} activity under the 0.1 mM Ca^{2+} condition. In further experiments, addition of 1 mM $CoCl_2$ to the superfusion medium under low calcium conditions (0.1 mM Ca^{2+}) induced a total block of the hypoxia-induced calcium changes (18). These experiments suggest that a calcium ATPase is regulating the cytosolic calcium content in glomus cells under hypoxia. The cytosolic calcium content itself may regulate the degree of activation of potassium channels as well as the amount of transmitter released, as indicated by the unresponsiveness of chemoreceptor activity to hypoxia under a calcium concentration of 0.1 mM in the superfusion medium (Fig. 13.2).

The efferent sympathetic innervation of the carotid body is able to interact with ion exchanges across the cell membrane of the carotid body cells, since preganglionic sympathetic stimulation leads to a decrease in extracellular calcium simultaneously with an increase in extracellular potassium (8) and probably serves as an efferent controller of the effector.

To explain these different experimental findings, a simple model should depict the chemoreceptive process in the carotid body as an interaction between the different cellular elements in the carotid body. Figure 3.3 is a schematic drawing that attempts to integrate some of the experimental findings. The question mark (?) in Fig. 3.3 represents the Po_2 sensor, whose structure, at this time, is unknown. Future experiments should concentrate on the possible candidates that were mentioned in the introduction. This Po_2 sensor should be able to induce Po_2-dependent aerobic glycolysis in the carotid body, resulting in decreased oxygen consumption and a decreased intracellular pH; efferent nerve fibers of the carotid sinus nerve provide an additional control. Electrical stimulation of these different fibers leads to activation of the respiratory chain, which is measured as NADH oxidation (34). Acidification of the tissue during hypoxia could include two events: (a) an increase in cytosolic calcium due to liberation of calcium bound to protein, and (b) an impairment of the metabolic state of the respiratory chain by a reduction in the pH gradient across the inner mitochondrial membrane, according to Mitchell's chemiosmotic theory (36).

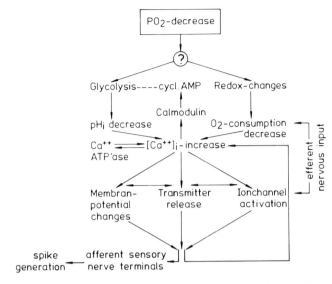

Fig. 13.3 Hypothetical pathway of chemoreception in the carotid body.

In the carotid body, total ATP content remains constant under hypoxia (10); this suggests that sufficient ATP production is maintained by glycolysis. The cyclic AMP content increases in the cat carotid body under hypoxia, and therefore might regulate the glycolytic pathway (20). An altered metabolic state would impair the calcium buffer capacity of the mitochondria, permitting a higher cytosolic calcium activity to be sustained. This higher cytosolic calcium level, which might be controlled by a specialized Ca^{2+}-ATPase as described by Starlinger (45), could induce a transmitter release with two consequences: first, the generation of nerve impulses in the afferent sensory nerve terminals, and second, further uptake of calcium leading to additional transmitter release. Thus Pietruschka (39) showed acetylcholine-induced calcium influx in cultured type I cells. The enhanced calcium uptake induced activation of potassium channels which resulted in membrane hyperpolarization, as measured in cultured type I cells (9). Thus calcium uptake might act as a set controller for transmitter release. The enhanced extracellular potassium level might contribute to the generation of nerve impulses in nerve terminals (11) or induce exocytosis in type I cells (23). The nervous efferent input enhanced under these circumstances might regulate oxygen consumption (34) or ion-channel activation (8). The role of the type II cells in this process could involve the clearance of the extracellular potassium that has been accumulated, since these cells possess glialike properties.

The scheme presented should be helpful in planning future experiments to clarify the mechanism of the Po_2 sensor, a mechanism that is certainly important for other organs as well. As research progresses, this scheme undoubtedly will have to be modified. However, as a working hypothesis, it can lead to better understanding of the processes involved.

REFERENCES

1. Acker, H. The meaning of tissue P_{O_2} and local blood flow for the chemoreceptive process of the carotid body. *Fed. Proc. 39:* 2641–2647, 1980.

2. Acker, H., J. Carlsson, R. Durand, and R. M. Sutherland, eds. Spheroids in cancer research. In: *Recent Results in Cancer Research,* Vol. 95. Berlin: Springer, 1984, pp. 1–179.

3. Acker, H., and C. Eyzaguirre. Light absorbance changes in the mouse carotid body during hypoxia and cyanide poisoning. *Brain Res., 409:* 380–385, 1987.

4. Acker, H., and D. W. Lübbers. The kinetics of local tissue P_{O_2} decrease after perfusion stop within the carotid body of the cat in vivo and in vitro. *Pflügers Arch. 369:* 135–140, 1977.

5. Acker, H., D. W. Lübbers and M. J. Purves. Local oxygen tension field in the glomus caroticum of the cat and its change at changing arterial P_{O_2}. *Pflügers Arch. 329:* 136–155, 1971.

6. Acker, H., and R. G. O'Regan. The effects of stimulation of autonomic nerves on carotid body blood flow in the cat. *J. Physiol. 315:* 99–110, 1981.

7. Acker, H., and R. G. O'Regan, eds. *Physiology of the Peripheral Arterial Chemoreceptors.* Amsterdam: Elsevier, 1983, pp. 1–491.

8. Acker, H., and R. G. O'Regan. Extracellular K^+ and Ca^{++} activities in the cat carotid body during chemoreceptor excitation and inhibition. *J. Physiol. (Lond.) 355:* 45, 1984.

9. Acker, H., and F. Pietruschka. Membrane potential of cultured carotid body glomus cells under normoxia and hypoxia. *Brain Res. 311:* 148–151, 1984.

10. Acker, H., and H. Starlinger. Adenosine triphosphate content in the cat carotid body under different arterial O_2 and CO_2 conditions. *Neurosci. Lett. 50:* 175–179, 1984.

11. Acker, H., H. Weigelt, D. W. Lübbers, D. Bingmann, and H. Caspers. Effect of changes in Ca^{++} and K^+ activity upon tissue P_{O_2} and chemoreceptor activity of the cat carotid body. In: *Morphology and Mechanism of Chemoreceptors,* ed. A. S. Paintal. New Delhi: Navchetan Press, 1976, pp. 103–112.

12. Anichkov, S. K., and M. L. Belenkii, eds. *Pharmacology of the Carotid Body Chemoreceptors.* Oxford: Pergamon Press, 1963.

13. Bernon, R., L. M. Leitner, M. Roumy, and A. Verna. Effects of ion-containing liposomes upon the chemoafferent activity of the rabbit carotid body superfused in vitro. *Neurosci. Lett. 35:* 289–295, 1983.

14. Biscoe, T. Carotid body: structure and function. *Physiol. Rev. 51:* 437–495, 1971.

15. Carafoli, E., and M. Crompton. The regulation of intracellular calcium. *Curr. Top. Membr. Transport 10:* 151–216, 1978.

16. Degner, F., and H. Acker. Mathematical analysis of tissue P_{O_2} distribution in the cat carotid body. *Pflügers Arch. 407:* 305–311, 1986.

17. Delpiano, M. A., and H. Acker. O_2 chemoreception of the cat carotid body in vitro. *Adv. Exp. Med. Biol. 169:* 705–717, 1984.

18. Delpiano, M. A., and H. Acker. The extracellular Ca^{++} and K^+ activities in the cat carotid body in vitro and their relationship to chemoreception. In: *The Peripheral Arterial Chemoreceptors,* ed. D. J. Pallot. London: Croom Helm, 1984, pp. 101–110.

19. Delpiano, M. A., and H. Acker. Extracellular pH changes in the superfused cat carotid body during hypoxia and hypercapnia. *Brain Res. 342:* 273–280, 1985.

20. Delpiano, M. A., H. Starlinger, and H. Acker. Changes in the cAMP content of the superfused cat carotid body produced by initial P_{O_2} decrease in the medium. *Pflügers Arch. 405:* R37, 1985.

21. Dufau, E., H. Acker, and D. Sylvester. Triple-barrelled ion sensitive microelectrode for simultaneous measurements of two extracellular ion activities. *Med. Proc. Technol. 9:* 33–38, 1982.

22. Durst, R. A. *Ion-Selective Electrodes.* Natl. Bur. Stand. Special Publicn. No. 314, 1969.

23. Grönblad, M., K. E. Akerman, and O. Eränko. Induction of exocytosis from glomus cells by incubation of the carotid body of the rat with calcium and ionophore A23187. *Anat. Res. 195:* 387–395, 1979.

24. Hance, A. J., E. D. Robin, L. M. Simon, S. Alexander, L. A. Herzenberg, and J. Theodore. Regulation of glycolytic enzyme activity during chronic hypoxia by changes in rate-limiting enzyme content. *J. Clin. Invest. 66:* 1258–1264, 1980.

25. Hilsmann, J., F. Degner, and H. Acker. Local flow velocities in the cat carotid body tissue. *Pflügers Arch. 410:* 204–211, 1987.

26. Jelkmann, W. Renal erythropoietin: properties and production. *Rev. Physiol. Biochem. Pharmacol. 104:* 140–215, 1986.

27. Joels, N., and E. Neil. The excitation mechanism of the carotid body. *Br. Med. Bull. 19:* 21–24, 1963.

28. Jones, D. P. Renal metabolism during normoxia, hypoxia, and ischemic injury. *Annu. Rev. Physiol. 48:* 33–50, 1986.

29. Kahn, C. R. Membrane receptors for hormones and neurotransmitters. *J. Cell Biol. 70:* 261–268, 1976.

30. Lash, H. L., D. P. Jones, and St. Orrenius. The renal thiol (glutathione) oxidase subcellular localization and properties. *Biochim. Biophys. Acta 779:* 191–200, 1984.

31. Leitner, L. M., and M. J. Liaubet. Carotid body oxygen consumption of the cat in vitro. *Pflügers Arch. 323:* 315–322, 1971.

32. Lindy, S., and M. Rajasalin. Lactate dehydrogenase isoenzymes of chicken embryo: response to variations of ambient oxygen tension. *Science 153:* 1401–1403, 1966.

33. Lloyd, B. B., D.J.C. Cunningham, and R. Goode. Depression of hypoxic hyperventilation in man by sudden inspiration of carbon monoxide. In: *Arterial Chemoreceptors,* ed. R. W. Torrance. Oxford: Blackwell, 1968, pp. 145–148.

34. Mills, E. Spectrophotometric and fluorometric studies on the mechanism of chemoreception in the carotid body. *Fed. Proc. 31:* 1394–1398, 1972.

35. Mills, E., and F. F. Jöbsis. Mitochondrial respiratory chain of carotid body and chemoreceptor response to changes in oxygen tension. *J. Neurophysiol. 35:* 405–428, 1972.

36. Mitchell, P., ed. *Chemiosmotic Coupling in Oxidative and Photosynthetic Phosphorylation.* Bodmin, UK: Glynn. Res., 1966.

37. Mulligan, E., S. Lahiri, and B. T. Storey. Carotid body O₂ chemoreception and mitochondrial oxidative phosphorylation. *J. Appl. Physiol. 51:* 438–446, 1981.

38. Petrova, N. V. Effect of hypoxia on the lactate dehydrogenase isoenzyme composition in the rat carotid body. *Bull. Exp. Biol. Med. 78:* 1005–1006, 1974.

39. Pietruschka, F. Calcium influx in cultured carotid body cells is stimulated by acetylcholine and hypoxia. *Brain Res. 347:* 140–143, 1985.

40. Pietruschka, F., and H. Acker. Membrane potential and Ca^{++} influx in hypoxic and normoxic carotid body type I cells. *Adv. Exp. Med. Biol. 191:* 727–735, 1985.

41. Purves, M. J. The effect of hypoxia, hypercapnia and hypotension upon carotid body blood flow and oxygen consumption in the cat. *J. Physiol. (Lond.) 209:* 395–416, 1970.

42. Schulz, J., and H. H. Stolze. The exocrine pancreas: the role of secretagogues, cyclic nucleotides and calcium in enzyme secretion. *Annu. Rev. Physiol. 42:* 127–156, 1980.

43. Seidl, E., H. Acker, and L. Teckhaus. Quantitative Erfassung des Gefäßvolumens des Glomus caroticum der Katze unter den Bedingungen der Normoxie, Hyperoxie und Hypercapnie. *Microsc. Acta 3:* 185–189, 1979.

44. Sies, H. Peroxisomal enzymes and oxygen metabolism in liver. In: *Tissue Hypoxia and Ischemia,* ed. M. Reivich, R. Coburn, S. Lahiri, and B. Chance. New York: Plenum, 1977, pp. 51–65.

45. Starlinger, H. ATPases of the cat carotid body and of the neighbouring ganglia. *Z. Naturforsch. 37C:* 532–539, 1982.

46. Starlinger, H., and D. W. Lübbers. Polarographic measurements of the oxygen pressure performed simultaneously with optical measurements of the redox state of the respiratory chain in suspension of mitochondria under steady state conditions at low oxygen tension. *Pflügers Arch. 341:* 15–22, 1973.

47. Strehler, P. L. Adenosin-5′-triphosphat und Creatin Phosphat-Bestimmung mit Luciferase. In: *Methoden der Enzymatischen Analyse,* Bd. II, ed. H. U. Bergmeyer. Weinheim: Verlag Chemie, 1974, pp. 2163–2177.

48. Weigelt, H., E. Seidl, H. Acker, and D. W. Lübbers. Distribution of oxygen partial pressure in the carotid body region and in the carotid body (rabbit). *Pflügers Arch. 388:* 137–142, 1980.

49. Whalen, W. J., P. Nair, T. Sidebotham, J. Spanda, and M. Lacerna. Cat carotid body. Oxygen consumption and other parameters. *J. Appl. Physiol. 50:* 129–133, 1981.

50. Wilson, D. F., C. S. Owen, and M. Erecinska. Quantitative dependence of mitochondrial oxidative phosphorylation on oxygen concentration: a mathematical model. *Arch. Biochem. 195:* 494–504, 1979.

14

Single-Channel Recordings from Isolated Carotid Body Cells

J.M.M. O'DONNELL, F. M. ASHCROFT, H. F. BROWN, AND P.C.G. NYE

Everyone accepts the concept that the carotid body (CB) "tastes" the blood. De Castro originally suggested that this is the case because one pole of each glomus cell is close to the blood whereas the other is in contact with an afferent nerve fiber. Heymans soon showed that it is hypoxia and hypercapnia to which the afferent responds. Thus it was assumed that the cell did the sensing and then fired the fiber.

Now, half a century later, we do know that the sensitivity of the nerve fiber depends upon its contact with a carotid glomus cell, but we do not yet know the cellular mechanisms underlying these responses. Are both the cell and the fiber phasically active in response to a stimulus, or does the cell act trophically on the nerve ending to make it able to respond without another cell first intervening as a transducer?

Recording the electrical activity of glomus cells should help to resolve this issue, but conventional microelectrodes have not yet revealed any consistent responses of glomus cells to their physiological stimuli. The resting membrane potentials recorded average only -20 mV, although occasionally a signal of -60 mV has been obtained (3,6). This is perhaps not surprising as the cells are very small (~ 10 μm in diameter), and the CB contains a large amount of connective tissue. Indeed, because conventional microelectrodes can reduce the resting membrane potential of cardiac myocytes (which are about 20 times the size of glomus cells) from -80 to -25 mV (8), we suspect that the resting potential of -20 mV and the mean input resistance of 40 megohm (MΩ) reported for glomus cells (2) may also be a consequence of microelectrode damage.

We have therefore applied the less traumatic patch-clamp method which enables more accurate measurement of input resistance and resting membrane potential. This approach allows us to explore more directly whether the type 1 cell is the site of chemotransduction and to elucidate the identity and role of intracellular second messengers. The patch-clamp method requires "clean" cell membranes; thus we developed a suitable method of isolating single CB cells and maintaining them in short-term culture. We report here preliminary cell-attached patch-clamp recordings from these isolated cells.

METHODS

Both carotid bodies were removed from six 7- to 10-day-old rats and placed in phosphate-buffered saline (PBS) + 0.5% glucose at 4°C. They were then cut into four pieces and gently teased apart in preincubated dissociation medium which consisted of 0.1% collagenase and 0.1% trypsin (5). Digestion, carried out at 37°C, was terminated after 50 min by addition of a few drops of fetal calf serum (FCS). Cells spun down were resuspended in 500 μl of culture medium, plated onto poly-lysine-coated glass cover-clips and maintained in short-term tissue culture for up to 5 days; however, most of the cells were used on days 2 and 3. The culture medium, which was renewed on day 3, was Ham's F-12 supplemented with 10% FCS, 80 U/l insulin, and 100 U/ml penicillin/streptomycin.

Our isolation method yielded two types of cells. The most numerous type had a diameter of approximately 10 μm and were phase bright. A smaller number of cells had diameters of 15–25 μm and extended processes within the first 2 days of culture. It is likely that the smaller 10-μm cells corresponded to the type 1 cells (5), and only these were used for the patch-clamp studies.

Standard patch-clamp methods (7) were used to record single-channel currents from cell-attached membrane patches. In this configuration, the potential across the patch membrane (V_m) is given by the difference between the resting potential of the cell (R_p) and any potential applied to the inside of the pipette (V_p):

$$V_m = R_p - V_p \qquad (14.1)$$

Currents were recorded by use of a List EPC5 patch-clamp amplifier and stored on FM tape (bandwidth 10 kHz at -3 dB) for later analysis with a PDP 11/73 micro-computer (1). All records are displayed using the normal sign conventions—that is, potentials relative to 0-mV external and inward currents across the membrane as downward deflections of the current trace. To record K-currents at the cell resting potential, the patch pipette contained a 140 mM K solution, which contained also 5 mM $CaCl_2$, 5 mM $MgCl_2$, and 5 mM NaHEPES (pH 7.4). The bath solution contained either this 140 mM K solution or a 5 mM K solution in which 135 mM Na replaced K^+. All experiments were carried out at room temperature in solutions equilibrated with air.

RESULTS

Single-channel currents recorded from a cell-attached patch on a CB cell immersed in 5 mM K solution and equilibrated with air are illustrated in Fig. 14.1A,C. As

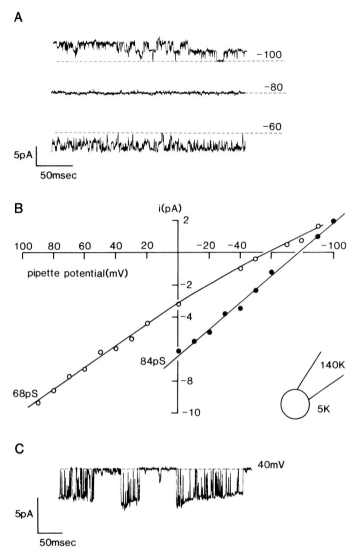

Fig. 14.1 (**A**) Single-channel currents recorded at different pipette potentials (indicated to the right of each trace) from a cell-attached patch on a cell in a 5 mM K solution. The closed state of the channel is indicated by the dotted line. Two channels were present in this patch. (**B**) Relationship between current amplitude (i; y axis) and pipette potential (V_p; x axis) for one of the channels shown in A (●) and for a channel from another patch (○). The line drawn through the filled circles is a linear regression (correlation coefficient, $r = .99$), with a conductance of 84 pS and a reversal potential of -78 mV. The line drawn through the lower nine open circles ($+100$ to 0 mV) is also a best-fit linear regression ($r = .99$) with a conductance of 65 pS and a reversal potential of -56 mV. Like K currents that we have observed in many carotid body cells, the I/V relation showed some inward rectification. (**C**) Single-channel currents showing relaxation in a cell that has a high input resistance.

135

shown in A, these currents are inward (i.e., into the cell) for pipette potentials positive to -60 mV; they reverse at a pipette potential of about -80 mV.

Current–voltage (I/V) relationships for 12 cells in the cell-attached configuration were recorded. Two representative examples of the relationship between the single-channel current amplitude and the pipette potential are given in Fig. 14.1B. The filled circles represent the channel currents illustrated in A, and the open circles are taken from another patch. The single-channel conductances were 84 and 65 picosiemens (pS), respectively, and the corresponding reversal potentials were -78 and -56 mV. In cell-attached recordings from cells immersed in 5 mM K solution all reversal potentials lay within this range. Because it is likely that under our recording conditions K^+ is the major charge carrier, this result is consistent with the resting potential of the CB cells lying within this range (cf. Eq. 14.1; we make the assumption that the K equilibrium potential (Ek) for the patch membrane lies close to 0 mV).

Figure 14.1C shows that the amplitude of single-channel currents recorded from cell-attached patches in 5 mM K^+ solution often showed a time-dependent decay. As discussed by Fenwick, Marty, and Neher (4), this relaxation is indicative of a high cell input resistance: Because the input resistance is high, current flowing through the open channel is sufficient to depolarize the cell, thereby bringing the patch membrane potential closer to E_K and reducing the single-channel current. A rough approximation to the cell input resistance can be obtained from the amplitude of the current decay (4) and yields values of around 15 gigohm (GΩ).

We found a range of single-channel conductances (35–140 pS; 12 patches) from cell-attached recordings on cells immersed in 5 mM K solution. It is possible that at least some of this variation results from the time-dependent current decay which precludes accurate measurement of current amplitude. This becomes a particular problem at positive pipette potentials where amplitudes are larger. Nevertheless, the results suggest the presence of more than one type of K-permeable channel.

In an attempt to overcome this problem, we also carried out experiments using bath solutions containing 140 mM K, a concentration that should substantially depolarize the cell. In high-K solution, single-channel current amplitudes showed no decay (Fig. 14.2A); this is as expected when the cell input resistance is decreased by K-depolarization. The I/V relation obtained for the records shown in Fig. 14.2A was linear, with a slope conductance of 140 pS (Fig. 14.2B) and a reversal potential of -12 mV (V_p). If we assume a resting potential of 0 mV in 140 mM K^+ solution, this corresponds to a membrane potential of $+12$ mV (Eq. 14.1) which is consistent with the channel's being permeable primarily to K^+ under our recording conditions. There are three possible explanations for the fact that the I/V relationship did not reverse at 0 mV: (a) The channel is not completely K-selective; (b) there is incomplete exchange of the bath solution; or (c) the intracellular K^+ concentration is greater than 140 mM.

We were unable to measure accurately the conductance of the channel illustrated in Fig. 14.2 when the cell was exposed to 5 mM K^+, because of the problem of current decay. It was clear, however, that in this solution the currents reversed at a pipette potential negative to -60 mV in this solution. There is therefore a shift in the reversal potential of more than 50 mV on changing from 5 mM K to 140 mM K, which suggests that the resting potential must be at least -50 mV for the CB cell in standard extracellular solution (5 mM K).

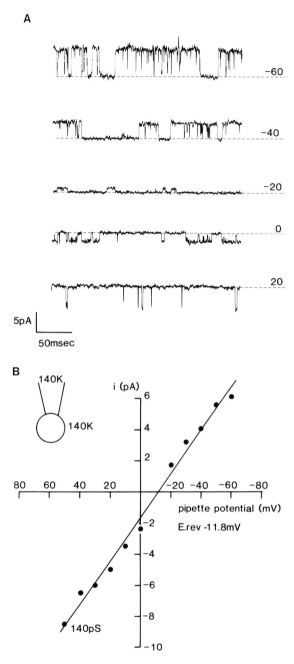

Fig. 14.2 (A) Single-channel currents recorded at the pipette potentials indicated from a cell-attached patch on a cell in 140 mM K solution. The closed state of the channel is indicated by the dotted line. (B) Corresponding current–voltage (I/V_p) relation for the channel shown in A. The line is a linear regression through the data points ($r = .99$) and has a slope of 145 and a reversal potential of -11.8 mV (V_p).

DISCUSSION AND CONCLUSIONS

These preliminary patch-clamp results demonstrate, for the first time, that it is possible to obtain single-channel current recordings from suitably prepared isolated carotid body cells. We feel that it is unlikely that the cells are damaged by the isolation method for three reasons: First, they survive in short-term culture. Second, they have a high-input resistance (>15 GΩ), as expected for a cell of 10-μm diameter. Finally, although we have not yet succeeded in obtaining good whole-cell recordings and thus a direct measurement of the resting potential, the difference in the reversal potentials of the single-channel currents in 5 mM K and 140 mM K solutions is consistent with resting potentials of at least -50 mV.

We believe that the application of patch-clamp methods to isolated carotid body cells will prove useful in investigating ionic mechanisms underlying the response of the carotid body to hypoxia and hypercapnia.

ACKNOWLEDGMENTS
    We thank the Wellcome Trust for their support, J.O'D. is a Wellcome Scholar, F.M.A. is a Royal Society Research Fellow, H.M.B. is supported by the British Heart Foundation and P.C.G.N. is a Wellcome Senior Lecturer. We also thank Bob Torrance for his helpful comments on the manuscript.

REFERENCES

1. Ashcroft, F. M., S.J.H. Ashcroft, and D. E. Harrison. Effects of 2-ketoisocaproate on insulin release and single potassium channel activity in dispersed rat pancreatic B-cells. *J. Physiol. (Lond.) 385:* 519–529, 1987.
2. Eyzaguirre, C., and S. Fidone. Transduction mechanisms in carotid body: glomus cells, putative transmitters, and nerve endings. *Am. J. Physiol. 239:* C135–C152, 1980.
3. Eyzaguirre, C., and P. Zapata. Perspectives in carotid body research. *J. Appl. Physiol. 57:* 931, 1984.
4. Fenwick, E. M., A. Marty, and E. Neher. A patch-clamp study of bovine chromaffin cells and of their sensitivity to acetylcholine. *J. Physiol. (Lond.) 331:* 577–597, 1982.
5. Fishman, M., and A. E. Schaffner. Carotid body cell culture and selective growth of glomus cells. *Am. J. Physiol. 246:* C106–118, 1984.
6. Goodman, N., and D. I. McCloskey. Intracellular potentials in the carotid body. *Brain Res. 39:* 501–504, 1972.
7. Hammill, O. P., A. Marty, E. Neher, B. Sackmann, and F. J. Sigworth. Improved patch-clamp techniques for high resolution current recording from cell and cell-free membrane patches. *Pflügers Arch. 391:* 85–100, 1981.
8. Pelzer, D., S. Trube, and H. M. Piper. Low resting potentials in single isolated heart cells due to membrane damage by the recording microelectrode. *Pflügers Arch. 400:* 197–199, 1984.

15

Effects of Substance P on the Carotid Chemoreceptor Responses to Natural Stimuli

M. SHIRAHATA

Substance P is present in the carotid body (3). Its amount has been reported to decrease in this organ as a result of hypoxic exposure (2). These observations led to the hypothesis that SP is a putative neurotransmitter for the hypoxic chemo-transduction. If this is the case, exogenous SP would elicit a prompt chemosensory excitation at any level of arterial oxygen tension (P_aO_2), and the effect would be independent of P_aO_2. Furthermore, a specific SP antagonist would block the hypoxic chemosensory response. The effect of SP on the chemoreceptor response to CO_2 would not necessarily be the same as its effect on the chemoreceptor response to O_2. To answer these questions, I examined the effects of exogenous SP on the chemosensory responses to natural stimuli, and of anti-SP infusion on the chemoreceptor responses to O_2 and CO_2. The responses to natural stimuli have been sufficiently characterized (1,4).

METHODS

Fifteen female cats, weighing 2.26–3.98 kg, were anesthetized with pentobarbital sodium (19–57 mg/kg, i.p.), and α-chloralose (total 20–120 mg, iv), paralyzed with gallamine triethiodide (3–4 mg/kg/h), and artificially ventilated. A fine catheter was inserted into the lingual artery or the thyroid artery for administering SP and pharmacological agents. Rectal temperature was controlled at about 38°C with a warm water blanket. For recording carotid chemoreceptor activity, a single or a few carotid chemoreceptor afferents were identified by their sporadic discharge pattern and by their responses to hypoxia or hypercapnia. The impulses of carotid chemoreceptor were displayed on an oscilloscope, selected by a window discriminator, and counted per second. Tracheal gas was sampled continuously, and tidal O_2 and CO_2 levels were monitored with a polarographic O_2 analyzer (Beckman, OM-11) and an infrared CO_2 analyzer (Beckman LB-2), respectively. Carotid chemoreceptor afferent activity, tracheal O_2 and CO_2 partial pressure, and arterial blood pressure were monitored and recorded continuously with an oscillographic recorder (Honeywell, Viscorder Model 1858). Arterial blood pH, P_aCO_2 and P_aO_2 were measured with a blood gas analyzer (Radiometer, BGA3 Blood Gas Analyzer).

Group A

Responses of carotid chemoreceptor activity to SP at several levels of P_aO_2 and P_aCO_2 were examined in six cats. End-tidal O_2 was changed in three steps at a constant level of end-tidal CO_2, and each level of end-tidal Po_2 was maintained for 30 min to test the carotid chemoreceptor response to substance P. End-tidal CO_2 was raised during hyperoxia, and maintained for 30 min. At each steady-state level of end-tidal Po_2 and Pco_2, arterial blood samples (0.5 ml) were taken. SP (10 μg) was given intraarterially, close to the carotid body, and the chemoreceptor response was observed for 20 min.

Group B

The effects of SP infusion on the carotid chemoreceptor responses to P_aO_2 and P_aCO_2 were examined in five cats. To obtain control responses, saline was infused at a rate of 0.5 ml/min with a pump through the thyroid artery. Five minutes after infusion was begun, end-tidal O_2 was changed in several steps at a constant level of end-tidal Pco_2, and each end-tidal Po_2 was maintained for 3–5 min for steady-state measurements. Then end-tidal CO_2 was raised and maintained for 3–5 min during hyperoxia. The carotid chemoreceptor activity was counted for 30 s during the steady-state period, and arterial blood samples (0.5 ml) were taken. Substance P was dissolved in saline and infused at the same rate as saline with the pump (10 μg/ml). Carotid chemoreceptor responses to P_aO_2 and P_aCO_2 were examined in the same manner as during the saline perfusion.

Group C

The effects of SP-antagonist infusion on the chemoreceptor responses to O_2 and CO_2 were examined in seven cats. As control, saline (0.5 ml/min) was infused through the thyroid artery, and steady-state chemoreceptor responses to O_2 and CO_2 were tested in the same manner as described for group B. Then, either [D-Pro^2, D-Phe^7, D-Trp^9]-SP or [D-Pro^2, D-Trp^{7,9}]-SP was infused (20 μg/min) and the chemoreceptor responses to O_2 and CO_2 were measured again.

Data are reported as mean ± SEM. To determine the significance of the differences among treatments, analysis of variance and Duncan's multiple arrangement test were used (11). A p value of $<.05$ was considered to be statistically significant.

RESULTS

Group A

Table 15.1 shows the changes in carotid chemoreceptor activity after substance P administration at different levels of P_aO_2 and P_aCO_2. During normoxia, SP produced a transient decrease and then a gradual and long-lasting but small increase in carotid chemoreceptor activity. The response varied from cat to cat, and maximum increases were observed between 1 and 4 min. The response to SP was significantly enhanced during hypoxia. During hyperoxia, SP still tended to increase chemoreceptor activity, although the change was not significant.

During hyperoxic hypercapnia, SP did not cause any significant change in chemoreceptor activity (Table 15.2).

Group B

As shown in Fig. 15.1, carotid chemoreceptor activity in response to O_2 and CO_2 showed characteristic increases during saline infusion. SP infusion increased the baseline activity of the carotid chemoreceptor and slightly enhanced the response to hypoxia but not to hypercapnia.

Group C

The SP antagonists, [D-Pro^2, D-Phe^7, D-Trp^9-SP] and [D-Pro^2, D-Trp^{7,9}]-SP, did not produce any consistent effects on the baseline chemoreceptor activity. These antagonists decreased the carotid chemoreceptor responses to SP, but did not fully abolish the response. The curves show that the chemoreceptor response to O_2 and CO_2 during the infusion of the SP antagonists did not differ significantly from the corresponding control curves.

DISCUSSION

As suggested in this study, SP did not produce a prompt chemoreceptor excitation. A small, variable, and prolonged effect of SP on the chemoreceptor activity is consistent with other reports. McQueen (5) showed a long-lasting chemoreceptor response to SP in vivo. Monti-Bloch and Eyzaguirre (6) observed variable effects of SP using an in vitro technique. The effect of SP is remarkably different from the hypoxic response of chemoreceptors, which is prompt and large. If SP is the immediate neurotransmitter for the hypoxic response, exogenous SP should mimic the hypoxic chemosensory response at any P_aO_2; possibly, during hypoxia it may cause less excitation, because of the occlusion principle which would predict partial occupation of the receptors by endogenous SP. However, this study showed that during mild hypoxia the SP effect was enhanced. It is unlikely but possible that the affinity of exogenous SP for the receptors was increased by hypoxia, thereby increasing the

Table 15.1 Changes in Carotid Chemoreceptor Activity (Δimp/s) After Substance P Administration at Three Levels of P_aO_2

P_aO_2 (torr)	P_aCO_2 (torr)	n	Control (imp/s)	Minutes after SP administration						
				0	0.5	1	2	3	4	5
59	31	5	10.29	−0.81	−0.27	*1.16	*†1.67	*†2.35	*†1.71	*†1.73
±1	±3		±1.89	±0.56	±0.53	±0.34	±0.41	±0.64	±0.43	±0.36
81	30	5	4.82	−0.21	0.10	*0.93	0.75	0.65	0.77	0.29
±1	±3		±1.04	±0.14	±0.49	±0.82	±0.35	±0.35	±0.36	±0.32
362	31	5	0.65	0.15	0.07	0.09	0.23	0.19	0.11	0.27
±22	±3		±0.21	±0.04	±0.08	±0.02	±0.07	±0.05	±0.05	±0.08

Note: The control chemoreceptor activity before each SP administration was counted for 30 s. Chemoreceptor activity after SP was sampled for 30 s at 0, 0.5, 1, 2, 3, 4, and 5 min from the beginning of SP administration. The differences in chemoreceptor activities after SP versus each control were calculated and are expressed as Δimp/s; data are reported as mean ± SEM.
*Significantly different from control; † significantly different from values during normoxia (P_aO_2 = 81).

Table 15.2 Changes in Carotid Chemoreceptor Activity Following Substance P Administration at Two Levels of P_aCO_2

P_aO_2 (torr)	P_aCO_2 (torr)	n	Control (imp/s)	Minutes after SP administration						
				0	0.5	1	2	3	4	5
346 ±31	31 ±3	5	0.79 ±0.17	0.17 ±0.04	0.15 ±0.10	0.13 ±0.04	0.19 ±0.08	0.19 ±0.05	0.10 ±0.05	0.23 ±0.10
333 ±26	52 ±2	5	4.06 ±0.79	−0.19 ±0.11	0.13 ±0.09	0.05 ±0.16	0.24 ±0.24	0.03 ±0.24	0.11 ±0.18	0.11 ±0.19

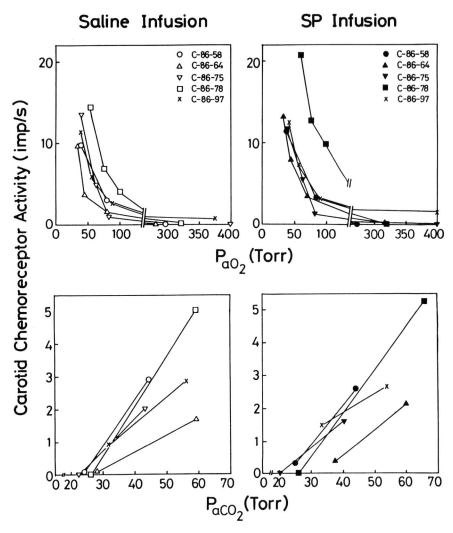

Fig. 15.1 Effect of SP infusion on steady-state responses of carotid chemoreceptor activity to P_aO_2 at constant P_aCO_2, and to P_aCO_2 during hyperoxia. Each symbol represents a different cat ($n = 5$).

response. A more likely explanation is that SP augmented the release of a putative excitatory neurotransmitter during hypoxia. For example, SP has been reported to release acetylcholine, prostaglandins, and histamine (9).

Prabhakar and colleagues reported that the administration of [D-Arg, D-Trp[7,9], Leu[1,2]]-SP (10 μg/kg) or [D-Pro[2], D-Phe[7], D-Trp[9]]-SP (10–15 μg/kg) blocked the hypoxic chemosensory excitation (7,8). In this study, I used proximal intraarterial infusion of two different types of SP antagonist—[D-Pro[2], D-Phe[7], D-Trp[9]]-SP and [D-Pro[2]-D-Trp[7,9]]-SP—which, however, did not affect chemoreceptor responses to hypoxia. Furthermore, the chemoreceptor response to SP was not completely blocked by these antagonists. One possible explanation is that the amount of SP antagonist employed was not sufficient for full antagonism of SP, although I used a far larger dose (i.e., 20 μg/min for more than 20 min) than Prabhakar et al. did (7,8). Another possibility is that these antagonists are not specific for the carotid body SP receptors, because SP analogues show different antagonistic effects for different tissues (10). The discrepancy between the results of the two studies is not due purely to technical differences either, and thus remains unexplained. It would have been ideal to be able to confirm the original observations of Prabhakar et al. (7,8; see also Prabhakar and Cherniack, Chap. 11, this volume) because SP could then be considered the neurotransmitter for the carotid chemosensory response to hypoxia.

All the observations made in this study strongly suggest that SP is unlikely to be the principal neurotransmitter for hypoxic stimulation of carotid body chemoreceptors. If SP plays a role in carotid chemotransduction, it may act as a neuromodulator for hypoxic excitation.

ACKNOWLEDGMENTS
I wish to thank Mr. A. Mokaski for his help. This study was supported in part by NIH Grant HL-19737-11.

REFERENCES

1. Fitzgerald, R. S., and D. C. Parks. Effect of hypoxia on carotid chemoreceptor response to carbon dioxide in cats. *Respir. Physiol. 12:* 218–229, 1971.

2. Hanson, G., L. Jones, and S. Fidone. Regulation of neuropeptide levels in sensory receptors and autonomic ganglia. In: Chemoreceptors in Respiratory Control, ed. J. A. Ribeiro and D. J. Pallot. London: Croom Helm, 1987, 169–177.

3. Jacobowitz, D. M., and C. J. Helke. Localization of substance P immunoreactive nerves in the carotid body. *Brain Res. Bull. 5:* 195–197, 1977.

4. Lahiri, S., and R. G. DeLaney. The nature of the response of single chemoreceptor fibers of carotid body to changes in arterial P_{O_2} and P_{CO_2}–H^+. In: *Morphology and Mechanisms of Chemoreceptors,* ed. A. S. Paintal. Delhi: Vallabhbhai Patel Chest Inst., 1976, pp. 18–24.

5. McQueen, D. S. Effects of substance P on carotid chemoreceptor activity in the cat. *J. Physiol. (Lond.) 302:* 31–47, 1980.

6. Monti-Bloch, L., and C. Eyzaguirre. Effects of methionine–enkephalin and substance P on the chemosensory discharge of the cat carotid body. *Brain Res. 338:* 297–307, 1985.

7. Prabhakar, N. R., J. Mitra, E. M. Adams, and N. S. Cherniack. Role of substance P in the hypercapnic excitation of carotid chemoreceptors [Abstract]. *Fed. Proc. 45:* 160, 1986.

8. Prabhakar, N. R., M. Runold, Y. Yamamoto, H. Langercrantz, and C. von Euler. Effect of substance P antagonist on the hypoxia-induced carotid chemoreceptor activity. *Acta Physiol. Scand. 121:* 301–303, 1984.

9. Regoli, D., P. D'Orleans-Juste, E. Escher, and J. Mizrahi. Receptors for substance P. I. The pharmacological preparations. *Eur. J. Pharmacol. 97:* 161–170, 1984.

10. Sandberg, B.E.B., and L. L. Iversen. Substance P. *J. Med. Chem. 25:* 1009–1015, 1982.

11. Steel, R.G.D., and J. H. Torrie. *Principles and Procedures of Statistics.* New York: McGraw-Hill, 1960, pp. 107–109.

Part III
OXYGEN-SENSING MECHANISMS

Introduction

B. B. LLOYD AND R. E. FORSTER

Physiologists still have much to learn about the mechanism by which reduced pressures of oxygen in different cells and tissues are sensed. In the first chapter in this section, Bauer elucidates the sequence of steps by which a fall in P_{O_2} in the kidney mesangial cells produces an increase in the synthesis of erythropoietin. The steps are a decrease in ATP, followed by an increase in arachidonic acid and a rise in prostaglandins. In the next three chapters, Tamura et al., Wilson et al., and Reynafarje are concerned largely with the changes in concentrations of cellular metabolites by which hypoxia might signal its presence without reference to a particular type of cell, tissue, or organ.

The chapter by Chance and colleagues provides some scintillating biochemical fireworks, utilizing as an end point phosphocreatine/phosphate (PCr/P_i) ratios determined by nuclear magnetic resonance. These investigators compare the relative reduction of cytochrome oxidase determined by near-infrared spectroscopy and blood oxyhemoglobin saturation determined by visible spectroscopy. As arterial P_{O_2} is reduced, PCr/P_i remains relatively constant until blood P_{O_2} reaches about 10 mmHg, when it suddenly falls; simultaneously, cytochrome oxidase becomes reduced.

The perenially favored candidate for the O_2-sensing molecule is cytochrome oxidase aa_3, located in mitochondria; however, it is difficult to explain how this enzyme, with a K_m of 1 μM (about 1 mmHg O_2 partial pressure) or less, can function in this capacity. Possible explanations for this contradiction have been proposed by Wilson and Reynafarje. Wilson et al. report a new, rapidly responding, and extremely sensitive instrument for measuring low $[O_2]$. Using this technique, these authors have determined that the reduction of mitochondrial cytochrome c begins at a P_{O_2} as high as 20–30 mmHg. Reynafarje reports that oxygen consumption of mitochondria varies considerably with P_{O_2} at this same level or higher.

In the final chapter of this section, Coburn discusses two ATP-linked mechanisms for transduction of the effect of a local decrease in P_{O_2}. The first involves an ATP-dependent potassium channel in cardiac myocytes; the channel opens when

ATP concentration falls, terminating the action potential. The second is a reduction in the activity of phosphoinositol phosphate (PIP) kinase in arterial smooth muscle, which results, through a cascade, in a lowering of calcium concentration and hence in relaxation. Coburn believes that the primary effect of a decreasing P_{O_2} is probably mediated through cytochrome oxidase.

16

Oxygen Sensing and Erythropoietin Formation in the Kidney: What Are the Prostaglandins Doing?

C. BAUER

Erythropoietin is a glycoprotein hormone with a molecular weight of 34,000. The carbohydrate part represents about 40% of the molecular mass (7), and it is this portion of the molecule that determines the biological fate of erythropoietin in the circulation. The terminal residues of the carbohydrate part are N-acetylneuraminic acid and the removal of even a small percentage of these residues reduces the biological half-life of erythropoietin from about 5–10 h to a few minutes (8,24).

The erythroid precursor cells in the bone marrow are the main target for erythropoietin (33). The hormone is thought to be a mitogen for specific pools of these erythroid precursor cells so that an increase in the concentration of erythropoietin leads to an enhanced formation of red blood cells. The normal concentration of erythropoietin in the serum of most mammals is about 20 mU/ml or about 10 pM under normal physiological conditions. Any decrease in the availability of oxygen leads to an increase in the concentration of erythropoietin by a factor of 2–300 (27). The main production site of erythropoietin is the kidney, as was first described by Jacobson and his colleagues (13,14). These workers surgically removed a number of organs including the spleen, a large part of the liver, the adrenals, and the thyroid and found that these interventions did not lessen the hypoxia-induced erythropoietin formation. Only removal of the kidneys, with ureter-ligated animals serving as controls, completely abolished the increase in erythropoietin production when the animals were exposed to hypoxia. Since then, these experiments have been confirmed and extended by a number of investigators (9,28,30). In all of the diverse experimental protocols, the kidneys were shown to be essential for hypoxia-induced erythropoietin formation.

For quite some time, the possibility was considered that the kidney did not generate erythropoietin directly but rather processed some kind of precursor molecule that was being produced at a different site within the body (cf. refs. 15,27 for a review of this topic). Recently, however, the gene for human erythropoetin has been isolated directly from a fetal liver cDNA library (12) and from a genomic DNA library (23). Furthermore, the monkey erythropoietin gene has been isolated from a kidney cDNA library (22) and the mouse erythropoietin gene from a mouse genomic library (25,32). It thus became possible to construct molecular probes that could be used to detect the existence of erythropoietin mRNA in different organs. With the help of these techniques it could be demonstrated that both bleeding and cobalt injection led to an accumulation of erythropoietin mRNA in the kidney but not in other organs, with the possible exception of the liver (4,5). These results prove, beyond any reasonable doubt, that the kidney produces authentic erythropoietin and furthermore show that the rate of production is probably transcriptionally regulated (4,5). Taken together, the results obtained with molecular probes have definitely settled the question regarding the organ in which erythropoietin is produced in response to hypoxia: The most important site is the kidney, with the liver being an auxiliary site. Furthermore, it has become clear that the erythropoietin mRNA is accumulated up to 200 times normal levels (5) in conditions of severe hypoxia—an increase similar to that observed for erythropoietin concentration (27).

WHY THE KIDNEY?

Anyone interested in the physiology of adaptation to hypoxia might wonder why the kidney should be the organ that elaborates erythropoietin as a function of oxygen availability. One reason is that the kidney appears to receive ample oxygen; this can be deduced from the fact that about one quarter of the cardiac output is being delivered to the kidney and that renal arteriovenous oxygen difference (AVD_{O_2}) is very low, amounting to only about 8% as compared to 20–25% for the body as a whole. On the other hand, it is known that erythropoietin formation is augmented by all forms of hypoxia, including hypobaric hypoxia, anemia, reduction of renal blood flow, carbon monoxide poisoning, as well as an increase of blood oxygen affinity (15,27). From these observations it clearly follows that the cell or cells within the kidney which "recognize" hypoxia should be situated in such a way that they are sensitive to a fall in both arterial P_{O_2} and venous P_{O_2}. Unfortunately, it is not known at present whether the same cell type within the kidney is engaged in both the "recognition" of hypoxia and the production of erythropoietin, or whether we are dealing with different cellular entities. Nevertheless, from physiological considerations it is possible to make some educated guesses on the cell type that functions as an oxygen sensor in the kidney.

The kidney is remarkable because it exhibits an unusually wide variation of P_{O_2} values despite the fact that oxygen flow is high in relation to oxygen consumption: First, even in the kidney cortex, there is a large variation in P_{O_2} values, ranging from the P_{O_2} in arterial blood to P_{O_2} values well below those found typically in venous blood (3,21). Second, there is a sharp fall in *average* P_{O_2} values as one passes the P_{O_2} electrode from the kidney cortex into the kidney medulla. The sharp corticomedullary gradient of oxygen is most easily explained by the vascular organization of the medulla. This arrangement allows countercurrent diffusion of oxygen between the arterial and venous branches of the hairpin loops of the vasa recta. This particular arrangement leads to Po_2 values in the medulla that are in the range of 10 torr (3,21). The steepest slope in the change of Po_2 occurs in the region of the juxtamedullary parts of the cortex and the outer stripe of the outer medulla. Would it not be logical to place the cellular structures involved in oxygen chemoreception in that region of the kidney where the largest drop of Po_2 occurs over a comparatively short distance? The tubular structures that appear to be most sensitive to hypoxia and that could therefore function as an oxygen chemoreceptor are the S3 segments of the straight part of the proximal tubules and the medullary thick ascending limb of Henle's loop (6,31,34). These cellular structures should, because of the arrangement of the vessels that supply them, be sensitive to a lowering of arterial as well as venous Po_2. Without having any further information at this point, it can be postulated that tubular structures at the corticomedullary boundary convey the chemosensitivity to the kidney.

WHAT KIND OF CHEMICAL SIGNALS MAY BE GENERATED IN RESPONSE TO RENAL HYPOXIA?

Any kind of renal hypoxia that eventually stimulates erythropoietin production is likely to act on the target cells by way of a specific chemical signal. I will consider here only those chemical signals that may be generated inside the kidney in response to renal hypoxia.

A wealth of biochemical reactions are dependent on the availability of oxygen (for review, see ref. 17). It seems useful in this context to distinguish between molecular oxygen sensors such as oxidases or oxygenases, and metabolic responses to hypoxia. A molecular oxygen sensor is an O_2-dependent enzyme (oxidase or oxygenase) and can be regarded as a primary sensor for physiological responses to hypoxia. A metabolic response defines the release of certain substances as result of hypoxia. Such substances may also be called *metabolic indicators* of hypoxia.

With regard to hypoxia-induced erythropoietin formation, the prostaglandins were shown to be such metabolic indicators. Certain criteria had to be met in order to substantiate that prostaglandins mediate the biological process within the kidney that leads to the production of erythropoietin. These criteria are as follows:

1. Perfusion of the isolated dog kidney with blood containing arachidonic acid, the rate-limiting substrate for prostaglandin synthesis, was found to enhance production of erythropoietin. This effect was blocked by indomethacin, a drug that interferes with prostaglandin formation (cf. ref. 10).
2. Hypobaric hypoxia led to an increased release of prostaglandin E_2 from the kidney (35).
3. Constriction of the renal artery as a means to induce kidney hypoxia led to the liberation of both prostaglandin E_2 and erythropoietin. Both of these effects could be suppressed by indomethacin (cf. ref. 10).

4. The rise in erythropoietin formation induced by hypobaric hypoxia, anemia, and exposure to carbon monoxide could be greatly lessened by indomethacin. However, when cobalt was used to induce erythropoietin formation, administration of indomethacin was without effect. This experiment was important because it clearly demonstrated that indomethacin itself does not interfere with erythropoietin production (16).

5. In cultures of mesangial cells taken from glomeruli of rat kidney, a hypoxia-induced formation of erythropoietin could be observed (18). This rise in erythropoietin could be completely abolished by indomethacin and restored by the addition of prostaglandin E_2, but not prostaglandin $F_{2\alpha}$. Such a specificity of prostaglandins with regard to erythropoietin formation was also observed in vivo (cf. ref. 10).

The entirety of these results justifies the conclusion that prostaglandins represent an important biochemical link in the mediation of hypoxia-induced erythropoietin formation. The possible pathway by which this relatively unspecific metabolic signal could eventually activate the gene that codes for erythropoietin has recently been delineated (2).

Although there is a substantial body of evidence on the relationship among hypoxia, prostaglandins, and erythropoietin formation, we have no information on the role of the prostaglandin system for the daily, normal regulation of erythropoietin formation. Apparently, anemia in humans occurs occasionally with prolonged use of indomethacin (cited after ref. 26) but this disorder is difficult to assess because no information is available on the erythropoietin concentration in the serum of such patients. In addition, local production of erythropoietin by macrophages in the bone marrow (29) may well be an important variable for the day-to-day control of erythropoiesis.

In the last part of this chapter, I briefly consider the possible mechanisms by which hypoxia may lead to an enhanced prostaglandin release in the kidney.

HYPOXIA AND PROSTAGLANDIN RELEASE: WHAT ARE THE CONNECTIONS?

The rate-limiting substrate for prostaglandin formation is arachidonic acid. The bulk of the arachidonate in mammalian cells is esterified in the fatty acyl chains of glycerophospholipids, almost exclusively in the 2-acyl position. The free fatty acid level in a tissue actually represents a balance between the liberation of arachidonate by hydrolysis and its reesterification into complex lipids by acyltransferases. Therefore, any increase in the availability of arachidonate can be brought about by activation of specific hydrolases such as phospholipases or by inhibition of reesterification.

We have conducted a set of experiments in order to discriminate between these two possibilities by using a permanent cell line from dog renal epithelial cells (high-resistance MDCK cells). These cells were shown to possess a furosemide- and ouabain-sensitive NaCl transport that could be stimulated by activation of adenylate cyclase (19,20). Activation of adenylate cyclase led to an immediate rise of both prostaglandin E_2 release and oxygen consumption. Both of these processes could be *reversibly* inhibited by furosemide. Furthermore, ouabain prevented the increase in prostaglandin E_2 formation and oxygen consumption. These data clearly point to a causal relationship among transport stimulation, prostaglandin release, and oxygen consumption because transport depends both upon a Na^+-K^+-$2Cl^-$ cotransport mechanism (which is inhibited by furosemide) and on the Na^+, K^+-ATPase (which is inhibited by ouabain).

We then searched for the possible mechanism by which stimulation of NaCl transport enhanced prostaglandin formation. The entirety of the results that were obtained led to the conclusion that (a) initiation of NaCl transport and increased oxygen consumption leads to (b) a local fall of the ATP concentration at or near the $(Na^+ + K^+)$-ATPase which, of course, is stimulated in this experimental condition. Such a local depletion of ATP results in (c) a stimulation of glycolysis, and most importantly (d) a decreased esterification of arachidonic acid into specific phospholipids, identified as diacylglycerol, phosphatidylinositol 4-monophosphate (PIP), and phosphatidylinositol 4.5-bisphosphate (PIP_2) (20).

The decreased reesterification of arachidonic acid finally results in enhanced availability of arachidonic acid and therefore enhanced formation of prostaglandin E_2. An increased rate of cleavage of arachidonate from phospholipids was not indicated in these experiments. The key element in this scheme is a local fall of ATP at the site where ATP is being consumed by the $(Na^+ + K^+)$-ATPase; this could inhibit arachidonoyl-CoA synthetase. A long-chain fatty acyl-CoA synthetase from rat liver microsomes has a K_m for ATP of 4.65 mM (1). Under the assumption that approximately the same K_m holds for arachidonoyl-CoA synthetase in MDCK cells, it follows that the enzyme is only half-maximally activated at normal intracellular concentrations of ATP. Once arachidonoyl-CoA is formed, it is transferred to the lysophosphoinositide by the appropriate acyltransferase. Until now, it has not been clearly established whether a separate acyltransferase for arachidonate actually exists (11). What seems to be true, however, is that the specificity of lysophosphoinositides for arachidonoyl-CoA is higher than for other phospholipids (11). This finding is in keeping with our observation that the rate at which arachidonate is incorporated into phosphoinositides is about 10 times higher than the rate of its incorporation into other phospholipids (20). The result is a high turnover rate of arachidonate with one specific pool of phospholipids, the phosphoinositides.

CONCLUSIONS

The oxygen-sensing mechanism in the kidney that was briefly described in the preceding section assumes a metabolic event involving prostaglandins as metabolic indicators. The initial step is a local fall in the concentration of ATP at a cellular site where the turnover rate of arachidonate is particularly high. This local fall of ATP concentration leads to decreased reesterification of arachidonic acid into phospholipids. Therefore, the availability of the rate-limiting substrate for prostaglandin formation increases, leading to enhanced prostaglandin formation. An increased cleavage of arachidonate from phospholipids by phospholipases cannot be excluded for the whole kidney. However, in our cellular model, we have not obtained evidence for enhanced hydrolysis of arachidonate under conditions of a mismatch between oxygen supply and oxygen consumption.

ACKNOWLEDGMENT
    I am grateful to Olga Stoupa for careful preparation of the manuscript. Supported in part by the Swiss National Science Foundation (grant 3.023-084).

REFERENCES

1. Bar-Tana, J., G. Rose, and B. Shapiro. Long chain fatty acyl-CoA synthetase from rat liver microsomes. In: *Methods in Enzymology,* ed. J. M. Lowenstein. New York: Academic Press, 1975, Vol. 35, pp. 117–122.
2. Bauer, C. Chemoreception of oxygen in the kidney and erythropoietin production. In: *Molecular and Cellular Aspects of Erythropoietin and Erythropoiesis,* ed. I. N. Rich. Berlin: New York: Springer Verlag, 1987, pp. 311–327.
3. Baumgaertl, H., H.-P. Leichtweiss, D. W. Luebbers, Ch. Weiss and H. Huland. The oxygen supply of the dog kidney: measurements of intrarenal Po_2. *Microvasc. Res. 4:* 247–257, 1972.
4. Beru, N., J. McDonald, C. Lacombe, and E. Goldwasser. Expression of the erythropoietin gene. *Mol. Cell. Biol. 6:* 2571–2575, 1986.
5. Bondurant, M. C., and M. J. Koury. Anemia induces accumulation of erythropoietin mRNA in the kidney and liver. *Mol. Cell. Biol. 7:* 2731–2733, 1986.
6. Brezis, M., S. Rosen, P. Silva, and F. H. Epstein. Renal ischemia: a new perspective. *Kidney Int. 26:* 375–383, 1984.
7. Dordal, M. S., F. F. Wang, and E. Goldwasser. The role of carbohydrate in erythropoietin action. *Endocrinology 116:* 2293–2299, 1985.
8. Emmanouel, D. S., E. Goldwasser, and A. I. Katz. Metabolism of pure human erythropoietin in the rat. *Am. J. Physiol. 247:* F168–F176, 1984.
9. Erslev, A. J. In vitro production of erythropoietin by kidneys perfused with a serum-free solution. *Blood 44:* 77–85, 1974.
10. Fisher, J. W. Prostaglandins and kidney erythropoietin production. *Nephron 25:* 53–56, 1980.
11. Irvine, R. F. How is the level of free arachidonic acid controlled in mammalian cells? *Biochem. J. 204:* 3–16, 1982.
12. Jacobs, K., C. Shoemaker, R. Rudersdorf, S. D. Neill, R. J. Kaufman, A. Mufson, J. Seehra, S. S. Jones, R. Hewick, E. F. Fritsch, M. Kawakita, T. Shimizu, and T. Miyake. Isolation and characterization of genomic and cDNA clones of human erythropoietin. *Nature 313:* 806–810, 1985.
13. Jacobson, L. O., E. Goldwasser, W. Fried, and L. Plzak. Role of the kidney in erythropoiesis. *Nature 179:* 633–634, 1957.
14. Jacobson, L. O., E. K. Marks, E. O. Gaston, and E. Goldwasser. Studies on erythropoiesis. XI. Reticulocyte response of transfusion-induced polycythemic mice to anemic plasma from nephrectomized mice and to plasma from nephrectomized rats exposed to low oxygen. *Proc. Soc. Exp. Biol. Med. 94:* 243–249, 1957.
15. Jelkmann, W. Renal erythropoietin: properties and production. *Rev. Physiol. Biochem. Pharmacol. 104:* 140–215, 1986.

16. Jelkmann, W., A. Kurtz, J. Seidl, and C. Bauer. Mechanisms of the renal glomerular erythropoietin production. In: *Atemgaswechsel und O₂-Versorgung der Organe,* ed. J. Grote and E. Witzleb. Mainz: Akademie der Wissenschaften und der Literatur, 1984, pp. 130–137.

17. Jones, D. P. Renal metabolism during normoxia, hypoxia, and ischemic injury. *Annu. Rev. Physiol. 48:* 33–50, 1986.

18. Kurtz, A., W. Jelkmann, J. Pfeilschifter, and C. Bauer. Role of prostaglandins in hypoxia-stimulated erythropoietin production. *Am. J. Physiol. 249:* C3–C8, 1985.

19. Kurtz, A., J. Pfeilschifter, C.D.A. Brown, and C. Bauer. NaCl transport stimulates prostaglandin release in cultured renal epithelial (MDCK) cells. *Am. J. Physiol. 250:* C676–C681, 1986.

20. Kurtz, A., J. Pfeilschifter, K. Malmstroem, R. D. Woodson, and C. Bauer. Mechanism of NaCl transport-stimulated prostaglandin formation in MDCK cells. *Am. J. Physiol., 252:* 6307–6314.

21. Leichtweiss, H.-P., D. W. Luebbers, Ch. Weiss, H. Baumgaertl, and W. Reschke. The oxygen supply of the rat kidney: measurements of intrarenal Po₂. *Pflügers Arch. 309:* 328–349, 1969.

22. Lin, F.-K., C.-H. Lin, P.-H. Lai, J. K. Browne, J. C. Egrie, R. Smalling, G. M. Fox, K. K. Chen, M. Castro, and S. Suggs. Monkey erythropoietin gene: cloning, expression and comparison with the human erythropoietin gene. *Gene 44:* 201–209, 1986.

23. Lin, F.-K., S. Suggs, C.-H. Lin, J. K. Browne, R. Smalling, J. C. Egrie, K. K. Chen, G. M. Fox, F. Martin, Z. Stabinsky, S. M. Badrawi, P.-H. Lai, and E. Goldwasser. Cloning and expression of the human erythropoietin gene. *Proc. Natl. Acad. Sci. U.S.A. 82:* 7580–7584, 1985.

24. Lukowsky, W. A., and R. H. Painter. Studies on the role of sialic acid in the physical and biological properties of erythropoietin. *Can. J. Biochem. 50:* 909–917, 1972.

25. McDonald, J., F.-K. Lin, and E. Goldwasser. Cloning, sequencing, and evolutionary analysis of the mouse erythropoietin gene. *Mol. Cell. Biol. 6:* 842–848, 1986.

26. Mujovic, V. M., and J. W. Fisher. The role of prostaglandins in the production of erythropoietin (ESF) by the kidney. II. Effects of indomethacin on erythropoietin production following hypoxia in dogs. *Life Sci. 16:* 463–473, 1975.

27. Powell, J. S., and J. W. Adamson. Hematopoiesis and the kidney. In: *The Kidney: Physiology and Pathophysiology,* ed. D. W. Seldin and G. Giebisch. New York: Raven Press, 1985, pp. 847–865.

28. Reissmann, K. R., T. Nomura, R. W. Gunn, and F. Brosius. Erythropoietic response to anemia or erythropoietin injection in uremic rats with or without functioning renal tissue. *Blood 16:* 1411–1423, 1960.

29. Rich, I. N., W. Heit, and B. Kubanek. Extrarenal erythropoietin production by macrophages. *Blood 60:* 1007–1018, 1983.

30. Schooley, J. C., and L. J. Mahlmann. Evidence for the de novo synthesis of erythropoietin in hypoxic rats. *Blood 40:* 662–670, 1972.

31. Schurek, H.-J., and W. Kriz. Morphologic and functional evidence for oxygen deficiency in the isolated perfused rat kidney. *Lab. Invest. 53:* 145–155, 1985.

32. Shoemaker, C. B., and L. D. Mitsock. Murine erythropoietin gene: cloning, expression, and human gene homology. *Mol. Cell. Biol. 6:* 809–818, 1986.

33. Till, J. E., and E. A. McCulloch. Hemopoietic stem cell differentiation. *Biochim. Biophys. Acta 605:* 431–459, 1980.

34. Venkatachalam, M. A., D. B. Bernard, J. F. Donohoe, and N. G. Levinsky. Ischemic damage and repair in the rat proximal tubule: differences among the S₁, S₂ and S₃ segments. *Kidney Int. 14:* 31–49, 1978.

35. Walker, B. J. Diuretic response to acute hypoxia in the conscious dog. *Am. J. Physiol.* *243:* F440–F446, 1982.

Recent experiments have revealed that the EPO-producing cells are located in the interstitial tissue of the kidney cortex and outer medulla (Lacombe, C. et al., *J. Clin. Invest.* 81:620-623, 1988; Koury et al., *Blood* 71:524-527, 1988) and that the renal oxygen sensor is associated with the proximal tubules of the kidney (Eckardt, K.-U. et. al., *Pflügers Arch. Eur. J. Physiol.* 411:R92, 1988).

17

Simultaneous Measurements of Tissue Oxygen Concentration and Energy State by Near-Infrared and Magnetic Resonance Spectroscopy

M. TAMURA, O. HAZEKI, S. NIOKA, B. CHANCE, AND D. S. SMITH

Tissue oxygen concentration is one of the critical determinants of the energy state of living tissue. The higher penetration of near-infrared light through bone into tissue can provide a method for measuring the oxygen concentration of the brain noninvasively, by determining the redox state of the oxygen acceptor, cytochrome aa_3 (1,4). However, considerable controversy exists concerning the hemoglobin admixture and contamination of the cytochrome aa_3 signal. In the present paper, we have attempted to differentiate the two signals (hemoglobin and cytochrome aa_3) by measuring the oxidation–reduction state of the copper ligand of cytochrome aa_3 (3) and to compare this to changes in the oxygen saturation of hemoglobin and in energy state as determined by ^{31}P magnetic resonance spectroscopy (MRS).

This approach to the measurement of cytochrome aa_3 differs from that of Jobsis (4), who chose isosbestic or equibestic wavelengths to allow cytochrome and hemoglobin to be differentiated. We chose instead a wavelength pair that optimally measures hemoglobin, with little interference from cytochrome, so that the hemoglobin contribution could be precisely determined and then subtracted from the combined cytochrome hemoglobin signal.

METHODS

Hemoglobin oxygenation and the redox state of cytochrome aa_3 were continuously monitored in brain by near-infrared spectrophotometry using a multichannel time-sharing spectrophotometer linked to the subject's skull by a 4-m flexible light guide (2). The hemoglobin absorbance was measured at the wavelength pair 700/730 nm, which has been found to be free from cytochrome aa₃ overlap, and the redox change of cytochrome aa₃ was measured at 780/830 nm (3). ³¹P MR spectra were obtained through a two-turn surface coil placed against the skull (after removal of skin and muscle) in a 25-cm, 2-Tesla, Oxford Magnet and a Phospho-energetics spectrometer. The surface coil and the end of the light guide were within 0.25 cm of each other so that they were measuring activity in similar regions of the brain.

Anesthetized, mechanically ventilated dogs and cats were used in this study. In some of the cats a fluorocarbon (20% Fluosol-DA, Green Cross) was used to partially replace hemoglobin as the oxygen carrier.

RESULTS

Figure 17.1, summarizes the data from the brain of one dog. The changes in the ratio of phosphocreatine to inorganic phosphate, PCr/P_i, and the absorbance at 780/830 nm are shown as a function of the degree of hemoglobin oxygenation. Despite a progressive fall in the fraction of O_2 in inspired air (F_iO_2) and a decreasing hemoglobin oxygenation, there was no change in PCr/P_i until hemoglobin oxygenation was reduced to 10%. At this point the PCr/P_i began to fall; below a hemoglobin oxygenation of 10%, this fall was rapid. The absorbance change at 780/830 nm was distinctly different. As hemoglobin oxygenation fell from 100% to 10% there

Fig. 17.1 The relationship among percent oxygenation of hemoglobin (700/730 nm), percent change of PCr/P_i (▲), and percent change of absorbance at 780/830 nm (○). The latter represents cytochrome oxidase and hemoglobin saturation in the dog brain. The dotted line corresponds to the maximal contribution of HbO_2 percent saturation in the absorbance change at 780/830 nm.

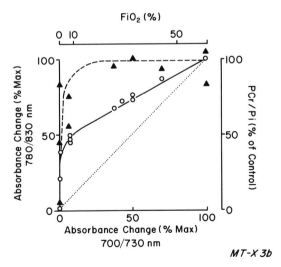

MT-X $3b$

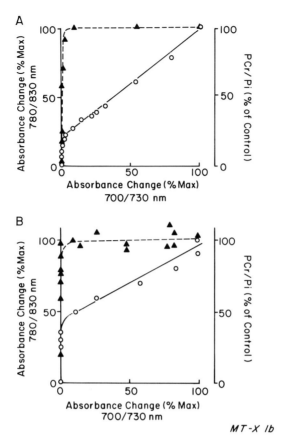

Fig. 17.2 The relationship among hemoglobin oxygenation, percent change of PCr/P$_i$, and percent change of absorbance at 780/830 nm in the normal cat brain **(A),** and after exchange transfusion with a fluorocarbon **(B).** See Fig. 17.1 for definition of symbols.

was a linear decrease in 780/830 nm absorbance, and as hemoglobin oxygenation reached 10% there was a marked increase in the rate of this fall. In fact, below this 10% breakpoint, the changes in PCr/P$_i$ and the 780/830 nm absorbance were very similar—a distinct contrast to their relationship when hemoglobin oxygenation was greater than 10%.

Figure 17.2A shows the relationship among hemoglobin oxygenation, 780/830 nm absorbance, and PCr/P$_i$ in the cat. The relationship among these three variables was similar to that found in the dog, except that the breakpoint was at a hemoglobin oxygenation of 8%. When the hemoglobin concentration was reduced by exchange transfusion with a fluorocarbon, the relationships between hemoglobin oxygenation and 780/830-nm absorbance changed (Fig. 17.2B). In this case, there was less of a fall in 780/830-nm absorbance above the breakpoint of 8% hemoglobin saturation. Below the breakpoint the decrease in 780/830-nm absorbance was similar to that seen in the cat with normal hemoglobin levels. Note that the reduction in hemoglobin and its replacement by a fluorocarbon did not affect the changes in PCr/P_i.

DISCUSSION

The rationale of this study was to observe the effects of hypoxia on brain hemoglobin oxygenation and cytochrome aa_3. Because hemoglobin can be measured without interference from cytochrome aa_3 at 700/730 nm, the absorbance changes in this wavelength pair can be used to determine the hemoglobin contribution to the absorbance changes at 780/830 nm, where the two signals are mixed. For example, if changes in hemoglobin oxygenation were the only contributor to the 780/830-nm signal, then a 45° line would be expected when this signal is plotted against the 700/730-nm signal (Fig. 17.1, dotted line). If, on the other hand, cytochrome aa_3 were the only contributor, then some other relationship would be expected unless cytochrome aa_3 affinity for oxygen exactly duplicated that for hemoglobin in that range of tissue oxygen tensions. If the affinity of cytochrome aa_3 in vivo is similar to that found in isolated mitochondria, then one would expect no change in cytochrome aa_3 absorbance at the higher tissue oxygen tensions, and a horizontal line would be expected when hemoglobin absorbance (700/730 nm) is plotted against the absorbance changes at 780/830 nm. The simultaneous measurement of absorbance and metabolic parameters via MRS allows critical metabolic states to be identified, in that the fall in PCr/P_i shows the point at which there is a fall in ATP production, pending energy failure.

In the present data (Figs. 17.1 and 17.2A), the fall in absorbance at 780/830 nm above the critical level of oxygen availability is slower than the changes in hemoglobin; after fluorocarbon exchange transfusion, which reduces hemoglobin concentration and thus decreases its contribution to the signal, it is slower still (Fig. 17.2b). This suggests that a major component of absorbance change above the breakpoint is related to hemoglobin change and that cytochrome aa_3 reduction is not detectable in this region. The rapid fall below the breakpoint, a fall that coincides with the fall in PCr/P_i, agrees with the changes as predicted from in vitro mitochondrial studies (5).

These data, though preliminary, provide confirmatory evidence for a new approach to the differentiation of hemoglobin and cytochrome signals in the brain. The approach uses hemoglobin absorbance at a "pure" hemoglobin wavelength pair to correct for changes at a mixed hemoglobin–cytochrome aa_3 band. In the present chapter, the correlation of optical change with metabolic parameters allows clearer delineation of the metabolic significance of these observations.

REFERENCES

1. Chance, B. A noninvasive biochemical assay and imaging of animal and human tissues by optical and nuclear magnetic resonance techniques. *Proc. Am. Philos. Soc. 127:* 1–25, 1983.

2. Chance, B., S. J. Legallais, and N. Graham. A versatile time-sharing multichannel spec-trophotometer, reflectometer, and fluorometer. *Anal. Biochem. 66:* 498–514, 1975.

3. Hazcki, O., and M. Tamura. Near-infrared spectroscopic monitoring of hemoglobin and cytochrome aa₃ in situ. *Adv. Exp. Med. Biol., 215:* 283–289, 1987.

4. Jobsis, F. F. Oxidative metabolic effects of cerebral hypoxia. *Adv. Neurol. 26:* 299–3182, 1979.

5. Oshino, N., T. Sugano, R. Oshino, and B. Chance. Mitochondrial function under hypoxic conditions. The steady state of cytochrome aa₃ and their relation to mitochondrial energy states. *Biochem. Biophys. Acta 368:* 298–330, 1974.

18

Intracellular Oxygen Concentration and Its Role in Energy Metabolism

D. F. WILSON, W. L. RUMSEY, T. J. GREEN, M. ROBIOLIO,
AND J. M. VANDERKOOI

In most tissues of higher animals, the primary source of metabolic energy for chemical and mechanical work is adenosine triphosphate (ATP). Most of this ATP is provided by mitochondrial oxidative phosphorylation which requires a continuous supply of oxygen. Delivery of oxygen to each region of the body at the necessary rate is accomplished primarily by alterations in vascular resistance, but the mechanisms by which vascular resistance is regulated remain obscure. The oxygen sensor(s) that are responsible for detecting tissue oxygen pressure and that provide the metabolic signal(s) for increasing and decreasing vascular resistance, although essential to the regulatory mechanism(s), remain incompletely identified. Mitochondrial oxidative phosphorylation, which uses more than 98% of the total oxygen consumed by the body, is the primary determinant of tissue oxygen needs. It is reasonable to suspect that mitocondrial oxidative phosphorylation is an important sensor of tissue oxygen pressure, but support for this hypothesis remains a matter of debate.

In the present work we have examined the effect of lowering oxygen pressure on mitochondrial oxidative phosphorylation using a new high-precision and rapid optical method for measuring oxygen. An instrument has been developed which allows these oxygen measurements to be made while monitoring the functional state of the mitochondrial respiratory chain via the reduction of cytochrome c. The results indicate that mitochondrial oxidative phosphorylation is sensitive to changes in oxygen pressure in the physiological range and can serve as an effective sensor of tissue oxygen pressure.

METHODS

Measurements of Oxygen Concentration and Cytochrome c Reduction

Oxygen concentration was measured using oxygen-dependent quenching of phosphorescence (see refs. 20,21 for details). Pd-coproporphyrin bound to bovine serum albumin was chosen as the phosphor because it is a water-soluble probe with a high quantum efficiency for phosphorescence and a relatively long phosphorescence lifetime in the absence of oxygen (0.4–1.2 ms). A flashlamp was used to generate the excited triplet state of the phosphor, and a red-sensitive photomultiplier was used to detect the light emitted from the sample. The photomultiplier output was digitized with a high-speed A/D board and the lifetime determined by fitting the decay of light emission to a single exponential (21). Cytochrome c reduction was measured with a dual-wavelength spectrophotometer which measured the difference in absorbance between 550 nm and 540 nm (A_{550} minus A_{540}). Time sharing permitted both measurements to be made in time intervals of 80–170 ms. The data processing operations required approximately 300 ms, allowing a set of measurements to be made approximately twice per second.

Calculation of the Oxygen Pressure

The oxygen pressure was calculated from the measured phosphorescence lifetime by use of the Stern–Volmer relationship:

$$T_0/T = 1 + k_q T_0 [O_2]$$

where T_0 and T are the lifetimes at oxygen concentrations of zero and any other oxygen concentration, respectively. The oxygen-dependent quenching constant (k_q) was 1×10^8 $M^{-1} \cdot s^{-1}$ for the selected probe and experimental conditions.

Miscellaneous

Mitochondria were prepared and assayed as previously described (26). The chemicals used were all reagent grade.

Data analysis was carried out with Asystant, a software program from Macmillan Software Co.

RESULTS

Measurements of the Oxygen Dependence of Mitochondrial Oxidative Phosphorylation in Suspensions of Isolated Rat Liver Mitochondria

Isolated rat liver mitochondria were suspended in a medium at pH 7.0, and succinate (8 mM) and glutamate (8 mM) were added to initiate respiration. A final concentration of 0.8 mM ATP was added to ensure that mitochondrial respiration occurred at a high phosphorylation-state ratio ([ATP]/[ADP][P_i]). Simultaneous measurements of oxygen pressure and reduction of cytochrome c were made as the oxygen in the medium was depleted. A representative set of experimental data is given in Fig. 18.1; approximately 450 points were taken in the 330 s shown in the figure. For convenience, reduction of cytochrome c is presented as a percentage of the total cytochrome c in the suspension. At high oxygen pressures, cytochrome c was approximately 16% reduced. Substantial additional reduction of cytochrome c occurred by the time the oxygen pressure had fallen to about 20 torr. In this experiment, after anaerobiosis an aliquot of hydrogen peroxide was added and, after its conversion to O_2 by catalytic activity in the preparation ($2\ H_2O_2 \rightarrow O_2 + H_2O$), measurements were made during a second cycle of oxygen depletion. The second cycle is included to indicate both the reversibility of the changes induced by lowering the oxygen pressure and the stability of the mitochondrial suspension. In other experiments, it was established that at any point in the experiment, raising the oxygen pressure caused cytochrome c to be reoxidized to its previous level of reduction at the higher oxygen pressure.

Fig. 18.1 The time dependence of oxygen pressure and cytochrome c reduction in suspensions of mitochondria at pH 7.0. Rat liver mitochondria were suspended at approximately 2 mg protein/ml in a mannitol (0.2 M), sucrose (0.07 M), ethyleneglycolbis(β-aminoethyl ether)-N,N,N',N'-tetraacetic acid, (EGTA, 0.4 mM) medium buffered with 15 mM morpholinopropane sulfonate adjusted to pH 7.0 with Trisma base. The medium contained 0.05% bovine serum albumin (Sigma type IV) and 0.5 μM Pd-coproporphyrin to permit oxygen measurement by phosphorescence lifetime. Succinate (8 mM) and glutamate (8 mM) were added as oxidizable substrates as well as ATP (0.8 mM) in order to ensure a high phosphorylation-state ratio during the experiment. Following anaerobiosis, a sufficient amount of H_2O_2, which was catalytically decomposed to O_2 and H_2O, was added to yield an oxygen pressure of approximately 60 torr. The difference in absorbance at 550 nm and 540 nm and the values for this absorbance at full oxidation and reduction were used to calculate the percentage of total cytochrome c reduced.

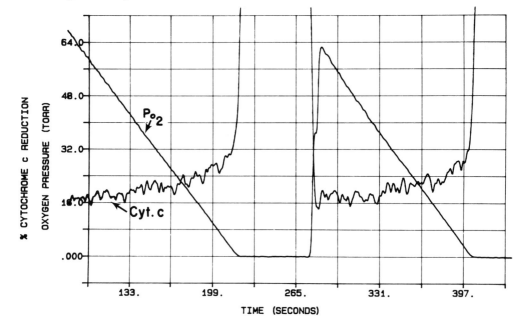

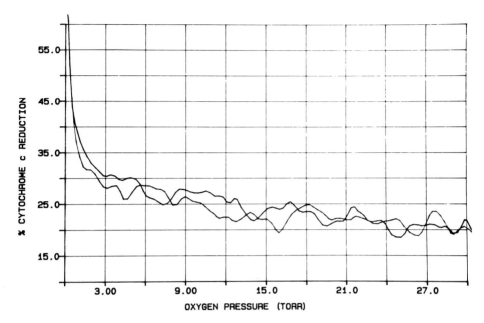

Fig. 18.2 Dependence of cytochrome c reduction on oxygen pressure. The data for Fig. 18.1 have been replotted as percent reduction of cytochrome c (ordinate) against oxygen pressure (abscissa).

In order to observe more clearly the dependence of reduction of cytochrome c on oxygen pressure, the data are presented in Fig. 18.2 as the percent reduction of cytochrome c plotted against oxygen pressure in the medium. Because the intracellular oxygen pressure in vivo is normally below 30 torr, only the data relevant to normal physiology are shown. Reduction of cytochrome c is biphasic. A moderate increase occurred as the oxygen pressure decreased to about 3 torr.

The Effect of pH on the Oxygen Dependence of Mitochondrial Oxidative Phosphorylation

It has been shown that oxidative phosphorylation is strongly pH dependent (e.g., see ref. 22). Comparison of Fig. 18.2 with Fig. 18.3 shows that cytochrome c was somewhat more reduced at high oxygen pressures when the pH was 7.8 (Fig. 18.3) than when it was 7.0 (Fig. 18.2). As the oxygen pressure was lowered, measurable reduction began at much higher oxygen pressures at pH 7.8 than was observed for pH 7.0.

The Apparent P_{50} for Oxygen as Measured from the Rate of Oxygen Consumption

The optical method for measuring oxygen pressure is sufficiently sensitive to measure the decrease in respiratory rate that accompanies the last phase of oxygen depletion (see Fig. 18.4). In well-coupled mitochondria respiring at a high [ATP]/

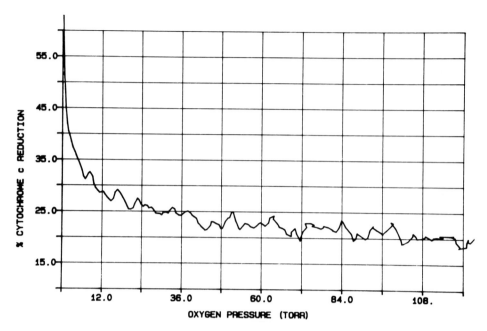

Fig. 18.3 The oxygen dependence of cytochrome c reduction in suspensions of mitochondria at pH 7.8. Mitochondria were suspended as described in the legend of Fig. 18.1 except that the pH was 7.8 and the substrate was ascorbate (8 mM) plus N,N,N',N'-tetramethyl-p-phenylenediamine (TMPD, 35 μM). This substrate donates reducing equivalents directly to cytochrome c.

[ADP][P_i], this value was 0.4–0.5 torr at pH 7.0. When the mitochondria were treated with uncoupler, the P_{50} value (the oxygen pressure required for 50% of maximal respiratory rate) decreased dramatically to values (less than 0.1 torr) that will require further development for accurate measurement. Moreover, when the mitochondria were uncoupled, the P_{O_2}-dependent reduction of cytochrome c did not become measurable until the oxygen pressure fell to less than 3% of the value for coupled mitochondria.

DISCUSSION

Oxygen enters tissue largely from the capillary bed, in which the oxygen pressure on the arterial side is greater than about 50 torr whereas on the venous side it is approximately 20 torr. Thus the oxygen pressure in the bloodstream ranges from 20 to over 50 torr, and oxygen transfer to the cell is in response to the oxygen gradient between the blood and the cell cytoplasm. It is, however, the *intracellular* oxygen pressure, not the oxygen pressure in the blood, that is important to tissue function. We must therefore have knowledge of both the dependence of cellular metabolism on the oxygen pressure in its immediate environment and the oxygen pressure in its environment under physiological conditions.

The only method that has yielded direct measurements of intracellular oxygen pressures in individual cells in tissue is that of Gayeski and Honig (7,8). These workers determined the oxygen saturation of myoglobin in individual cells of dog gracilis muscle. The muscles were rapidly frozen to trap myoglobin in its physiological state, and oxygenation was measured by cryospectrophotometric analysis of thin sections of the frozen tissue. The mean oxygen pressures inside myocytes of muscles working near maximal respiratory rate was calculated from the measured saturation of myoglobin and was reported to be in the range of 0.5 to 5 torr. Distribution of oxygen within individual cells showed relatively small oxygen gradients, usually less than 0.1 torr/μm. Furthermore, the oxygen pressure in small blood vessels also was estimated from the degree of oxygen saturation of the hemoglobin in red blood cells. From these data the authors concluded that the primary oxygen transfer barrier was from the red cell to the external surface of the capillary, but once inside the cell myoglobin facilitated diffusion resulted in relatively uniform oxygen pressure.

Other methods have been used to estimate the difference in oxygen pressure between the external medium and the cell cytoplasm in suspensions of isolated

Fig. 18.4 Fall in oxygen pressure with time (Δ), as calculated from phosphorescence lifetime measurements (O), a measure of O_2 consumption, in a mitochondrial suspension at low oxygen pressures. Mitochondria were suspended as described in the legend of Fig. 18.1, except that the mitochondrial protein content was decreased to 0.4 mg/ml. Each point is an independent measurement of phosphorescence lifetime, and thereby of the oxygen pressure, using the data averaged for 5 flashes (a period of 80 ms).

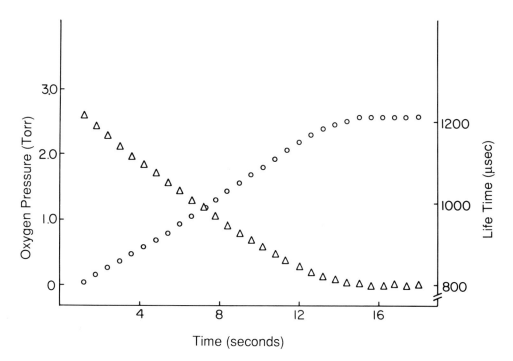

cells. Wittenberg and co-workers (5,27), for example, estimated the oxygen pressure at the outer mitochondrial membrane of isolated cardiac myocytes by the activity of monoamine oxidase. They varied the oxygen pressure in the suspending medium of isolated cardiac myocytes and provided evidence that the oxygen pressure difference between the extracellular medium and the mitochondria was small, not exceeding 2 torr. These results are in good agreement with those of Gayeski and Honig (7,8), and are also consistent with our observations indicating that both isolated mitochondria and mitochondria in cell suspensions have similar dependencies on oxygen pressure (refs. 22–24, and this chapter).

In the present experiments, it was observed that in suspensions of isolated mitochondria at pH 7.0 and high [ATP]/[ADP][P$_i$], the oxygen dependence of mitochondrial oxidative phosphorylation extends to at least 30 torr. This oxygen pressure range can be compared to the intracellular oxygen pressure of 0.5 to 5 torr measured in muscle working at near its maximal respiratory rate (8). At the range of oxygen pressures in the muscle cells, the oxygen dependence is large; that is, cytochrome c becomes reduced by more than two fold, as compared to the level of reduction at 30 torr. Such an increase in reduction of cytochrome c represents a substantial decrease in the phosphorylation state ratio that the mitochondria can maintain without changing their respiratory rate or reducing the intramitochondrial NAD pool (see refs. 2,23,25). Although mitochondria from rat liver were used in these studies, mitochondrial oxidative phosphorylation is similar for most tissues (see ref. 2). Differences in behavior arise from metabolic differences imposed by cellular metabolism. These metabolic differences account for the observation that different cell lines can have very different intramitochondrial NAD$^+$/NADH ratios and cytoplasmic [ATP]/[ADP][P$_i$] values. In general, the oxygen dependence increases with increasing [ATP]/[ADP][P$_i$] and increasing NAD$^+$/NADH (for further discussion, see ref. 25). Thus, the oxygen dependence of cells with high phosphorylation-state ratios (neurons, glia, muscle) is greater than for cells with low ratios (hepatocytes). In the present experiments with isolated mitochondria, the phosphorylation-state ratio was much higher than that of hepatocytes ($>5 \times 10^5$ M^{-1} compared to 3–6 $\times$ 10^3 M^{-1}), but the intramitochondrial NAD$^+$/NADH was substantially decreased relative to that of hepatocytes. As a result, the isolated mitochondria were as dependent on oxygen pressure as were mitochondria in intact hepatocytes (compare with ref. 4).

The kinetic pattern for the dependence of mitochondrial oxidative phosphorylation on oxygen pressure is markedly different from that predicted by simple Michaelis–Menten kinetics, the analytic method usually applied to such data (see refs. 1,17,18). The oxygen dependence of mitochondrial oxidative phosphorylation has a pronounced biphasic character, which can artificially be separated into (a) a higher oxygen region where cytochrome c is less than about 50% reduced, and (b) a low oxygen region where cytochrome c is greater than 50% reduced. Application of Michaelis–Menten analysis leads to serious errors if data from the low oxygen pressure region are extrapolated to the high oxygen pressure region because it incorrectly "cuts off" the high oxygen dependence. Computer modeling of possible mechanisms of oxygen reduction by cytochrome c oxidase has achieved good fit to the oxygen dependence observed in these experiments (e.g., see ref. 25).

Comparison of the Results in This Work with Those Obtained by Use of Other Methods

The data obtained at high oxygen concentrations are in good agreement with those obtained previously by this laboratory using oxygen electrodes to measure the oxygen concentration (22–24). Although the slow response times of the oxygen electrodes prevented accurate measurements from being made at low oxygen concentrations, the measurements above 3 torr are directly comparable. Thus the dependence of cytochrome c reduction on oxygen pressures above 3 torr are similar for the two methods. In addition, in each study the oxygen dependence increased markedly with increasing pH of the suspending medium. Equally importantly, the oxygen dependence decreased dramatically when the mitochondrial energy state was decreased, particularly when uncouplers were added.

Degn and Wohlrab (1) also measured the oxygen dependence of suspensions of isolated mitochondria, using a specially designed "respirograph." In these experiments, mitochondrial suspensions were made anaerobic and then the oxygen pressure was slowly raised by increasing the oxygen partial pressure of the gas phase above the stirred sample. As a result, the changes in the oxygen pressure in the suspending medium were slow enough that measurements could be made with an oxygen electrode. Both the oxygen pressure required for 50% oxidation of the cytochromes of the respiratory chain (P_{50}) and that for 50% of maximal rate of oxygen consumption were measured. Although only the low oxygen region of the mitochondrial responses (less than about 10 torr) was measured, in this region their data are in good agreement with ours. The P_{50} value for the respiration of well-coupled mitochondria was 0.6 μM (0.4 torr), and this value decreased to less than 0.05 μM (less than 0.03 torr) when uncoupled mitochondria were used. There was a similar decrease in P_{50} for cytochrome c oxidation. The absolute values for coupled mitochondria were equal within experimental error to those obtained in this laboratory, and the shift induced by addition of uncoupler was in the same direction (the direction of the uncoupler-induced change is particularly important, as will become apparent later in the discussion).

Chance and co-workers (17,18) made extensive measurements of the oxygen dependence of mitochondrial function, using the luminescence of a bacterium, *Photobacterium phosphoreum*, as a probe of oxygen pressure in the mitochondrial suspension. The method was similar to that of Degn and Wohlrab (1), except that a different oxygen indicator was used and stepwise changes were made in oxygen pressure in the gas phase instead of using a linear oxygen pressure gradient. The luminescence of *P. phosphoreum* is oxygen dependent below approximately 5 torr and is sensitive to oxygen pressure to less than 10^{-8} torr (17). The P_{50} for cytochrome c reduction in coupled mitochondria was reported by Chance and co-workers to be 0.04 μM (0.03 torr) (refs. 17,18) and 0.035–0.27 μM, depending on the substrate used. In addition, the P_{50} value increased with increasing rates of electron flow, and addition of uncoupler increased the P_{50} value for cytochrome c oxidation as compared to that for coupled mitochondria. It is difficult to reconcile the results of Chance and co-workers with those presented by ourselves and by Degn and Wohlrab. It is possible that the high chloride medium used to support the bacterial luminescence partially uncoupled the mitochondria. This would result in low P_{50} values for cytochrome c reduction, and this value may increase with increasing rates of electron transfer. Further experiments will be required to determine the reason for the differences and these are currently in progress.

Jones and co-workers (e.g., see refs. 9,10) have attempted to reconcile P_{50} values for mitochondrial respiration of 0.02–0.03 μM with experimental data for suspensions of isolated cells. This required them to postulate the existence of steep oxygen gradients within the cell, gradients requiring an oxygen diffusion constant of approximately 1.8×10^{-6} cm^2/s in the cell cytoplasm (9,10). The diffusion constant for oxygen in a 30% solution of hemoglobin, a reasonable approximation of the intracellular medium, is approximately 7.1×10^{-5} cm^2/s (6) whereas its effective diffusion constant in the plasma membrane of erythrocytes is approximately 3.2×10^{-5} cm^2/s (3). The latter value is 7.3×10^{-6} cm^2/s if a correction is made for an estimated partition coefficient of 4.4 for oxygen into the membrane. The higher concentration of oxygen in the membrane than in the surrounding aqueous medium contributes significantly to mass transfer through the membrane. These considerations indicate that the diffusion constants proposed by Jones and co-workers are likely to be underestimates. If the P_{50} value for mitochondrial respiration and cytochrome reduction measured by ourselves and by Degn and Wohlrab are used in the calculations, there is no need for the proposed steep oxygen gradients or low diffusion constants for oxygen.

It is more difficult to relate our work to that of Jobsis and co-workers (e.g., see refs. 11,19). These authors refer to measurements of cytochrome a, cytochrome a$_3$, and the copper atom measured by its absorption at 830 nm (low potential copper) as cytochrome a + a$_3$. Because the three components of cytochrome c oxidase have distinctly different functions and oxidation–reduction properties, lumping them together under one name leads to considerable confusion. Thus these authors consider that cytochrome a + a$_3$ is highly oxidized in isolated mitochondria under normoxic conditions, but this is true only for cytochrome a$_3$. For most metabolic conditions, cytochrome a and the 830-nm copper are near equilibrium with, and slightly more reduced than, cytochrome c. It appears that much of the data by these workers is consistent with the oxygen dependence of mitochondrial metabolism observed by ourselves. Interpretations of the data are different, however, and readers should compare the published papers for further information. It should be noted that we find no evidence for the presence of an additional cytochrome oxidase with a low affinity for oxygen in any cells or mitochondria examined to date. Such a low-affinity oxidase is not necessary to explain the oxygen dependence of cellular metabolism.

Are Mitochondria Important Tissue Oxygen Sensors?

The oxygen dependence of mitochondrial oxidative phosphorylation in the "high oxygen" region is of sufficient size to accurately measure the intracellular oxygen pressure and generate metabolic signals for tissue responses (such as vascular resistance) to changes in oxygen pressure. A detailed study has been made of the effect of modulators of mitochondrial oxidative phosphorylation on coronary flow in isolated perfused rat heart (14–16). These studies established that coronary resistance is dependent not on tissue oxygen pressure per se, but on the metabolic consequences of oxygen reduction by mitochondria. Thus inhibitors of the mitochondrial respiratory chain (14,16) and uncouplers of mitochondrial oxidative phosphorylation (15) both decrease coronary resistance, the decrease relating directly to their effect on the phosphorylation state ratio of the tissue.

In the cat carotid body, inhibitors of oxidative phosphorylation (i.e., inhibitors of the respiratory chain, ATP synthesis, and ATP and ADP translocation across the mitochondrial membrane) as well as uncouplers all mimic the effect of decreased oxygen pressure on electrical activity (12,13). That inhibitors and uncouplers have opposite effects on oxygen consumption implies that mitochondrial oxidative phosphorylation is important in sensing of oxygen pressure by the carotid body.

These observations, as well as many others in the literature, strongly support the view that mitochondrial oxidative phosphorylation is an important oxygen sensor for many of the physiological responses to changes in oxygen pressure. This appears to be true for regulation of local blood flow and of global responses such as respiratory activity.

ACKNOWLEDGMENTS
This work was supported by NIH grants GM-21524 and GM-36393.

REFERENCES

1. Degn, H., and H. Wohlrab. Measurement of steady-state values of respiration rate and oxidation levels of respiratory pigments at low oxygen tensions: a new technique. *Biochem. Biophys. Acta 245:* 347–355, 1971.
2. Erecinska, M., D. F. Wilson, and K. Nishiki. Homeostatic regulation of cellular energy metabolism: experimental characterization in vivo and fit to a model. *Am. J. Physiol. 234*(3): C82–C89, 1978.
3. Fischkoff, S., and J. M. Vanderkooi. Oxygen diffusion in biological and artificial membranes determined by the fluorochrome pyrene. *J. Gen. Physiol. 65:* 663–676, 1975.
4. Kashiwagura, T., D. F. Wilson, and M. Erecinska. Oxygen dependence of cellular metabolism: the effect of O_2 on gluconeogenesis and urea synthesis in isolated hepatocytes. *J. Cell. Physiol. 120:* 13–18, 1984.
5. Katz, I. R., J. B. Wittenberg, and B. A. Wittenberg. Monoamine oxidase, an intracellular probe of oxygen pressure in isolated cardiac myocytes. *J. Biol. Chem. 259:* 7504–7509, 1984.
6. Klug, A., F. Kreuzer, and J. W. Roughton. The diffusion of oxygen in concentrated hemoglobin solutions. *Helv. Physiol. Pharmacol. Acta 14:* 121, 1956.
7. Gayeski, T. E., and C. R. Honig. O_2 gradients from sarcolemma to cell interior in red muscle at maximal V_{O_2}. *Am. J. Physiol. 251:* H789–H799, 1986.
8. Gayeski, T.E.J., and C. R. Honig. Shallow intracellular O_2 gradients and the absence of perimitochondrial "wells" in heavily working red muscle. *Adv. Exp. Med. Biol. 200:* 487–494, 1986.
9. Jones, D. P. Intracellular diffusion gradients of O_2 and ATP. *Am. J. Physiol. 250:* C663–C675, 1986.

10. Jones, D. P., and F. G. Kennedy. Analysis of intracellular oxygenation of isolated adult cardiac myocytes. *Am. J. Physiol. 250:* C384–C390, 1986.

11. Mills, E., and F. F. Jobsis. Mitochondrial respiratory chain of the carotid body and chemoreceptor response to changes in oxygen tension. *J. Neurophysiol. 35:* 405–428, 1972.

12. Mulligan, E., and S. Lahiri. Dependence of carotid chemoreceptor stimulation by metabolic agents on P_aO_2 and P_aCO_2. *J. Appl. Physiol. 50*(4): 884–891, 1981.

13. Mulligan, E., S. Lahiri, and B. T. Story. Carotid body O_2 chemoreception and mitochondrial oxidative phosphorylation. *J. Appl. Physiol. 51*(2):438–446, 1981.

14. Nishiki, K., M. Erecinska, and D. F. Wilson. Energy relationships between cytosol metabolism and mitochondrial respiration in rat heart. *Am. J. Physiol. 234:* C73–C81, 1978.

15. Nuutinen, E. M., D. Nelson, D. F. Wilson, and M. Erecinska. Regulation of coronary blood flow: effects of 2,4-dinitrophenol and theophylline. *Am. J. Physiol. 244:* H396–H405, 1983.

16. Nuutinen, E. M., K. Nishiki, M. Erecinska, and D. F. Wilson. Role of mitochondrial oxidative phosphorylation in regulation of coronary blood flow. *Am. J. Physiol. 243:* H159–H169, 1982.

17. Oshino, R., N. Oshino, M. Tamura, L. Kobilinsky and B. Chance. A sensitive bacterial luminescence probe for O_2 in biochemical systems. *Biochim. Biophys. Acta 273:* 5–17, 1972.

18. Oshino, N., T. Sugano, R. Oshino, and B. Chance. Mitochondrial function under hypoxic conditions: the steady states of cytochrome a + a_3 and their relation to mitochondrial energy states. *Biochim. Biophys. Acta 368:* 298–310, 1974.

19. Sylvia, A. L., C. A. Piantadosi, and F. F. Jobsis-VanderVliet. Energy metabolism and in vivo cytochrome c oxidase redox relationships in hypoxic rat brain. *Neurochem. Res. 7:* 81–88, 1985.

20. Vanderkooi, J. M., G. Maniara, T. J. Green, and D. F. Wilson. An optical method for measurement of dioxygen concentration based upon quenching of phosphorescence. *J. Biol. Chem., 262:* 5476–5482, 1987.

21. Vanderkooi, J. M., and D. F. Wilson. A new method for measuring oxygen in biological systems. *Adv. Exp. Med. Biol. 200:* 189–193, 1986.

22. Wilson, D. F., and M. Erecinska. Effect of oxygen concentration on cellular metabolism. *Chest 88s:* 229s–232s, 1985.

23. Wilson, D. F., M. Erecinska, C. Drown, and I. A. Silver. The oxygen dependence of cellular energy metabolism. *Arch. Biochem. Biophys. 195:* 485–493, 1979.

24. Wilson, D. F., M. Erecinska, I. A. Silver, C. S. Drown, and K. Nishiki. Metabolic sensing of cellular oxygen tension. *Adv. Physiol. Sci. 10:* 391–398, 1981.

25. Wilson, D. F., C. S. Owen, and M. Erecinska. Quantitative dependence of mitochondrial oxidative phosphorylation on oxygen concentration: a mathematical model. *Arch. Biochem. Biophys. 195:* 494–504, 1979.

26. Wilson, D. F., C. S. Owen, and A. Holian. Control of mitochondrial respiration.: a quantitative evaluation of the roles of cytochrome c and oxygen. *Arch. Biochem. Biophys. 182:* 749–762, 1977.

27. Wittenberg, B. A., and J. B. Wittenberg. Oxygen pressure gradients in isolated cardiac myocytes. *J. Biol. Chem. 260:* 6548–6554, 1985.

19

Oxygen Modulation of Mitochondrial Energy Transduction

B. REYNAFARJE

The effect of O_2 concentration on the rates and extents of both O_2 uptake and energy-driven H^+ ejection by respiring mitochondria has been studied under well-defined metabolic states. Experimental evidence presented in this chapter shows the following novel aspects of mitochondrial energy transduction:

1. There is a lack of direct kinetic correlation between electron flow and H^+ ejection.
2. The H^+/O ratio is in fact variable and noninteger.
3. The rates of O_2 consumption measured at $t_{1/2}$ (the time required for one-half of the initial amount of O_2 to be consumed) decreases, rather than increases, when the initial concentration of O_2 greatly exceeds 5 μM.
4. The concentration of O_2 required for one-half the maximal rate of H^+ ejection (or ATP synthesis) in well-coupled mitochondria is in all probability higher than 20 μM O_2.

The word *respiration* has a broad meaning. It may express the visible physical process by which an organism takes air from its environment and conveys it to O_2-carrying systems, as well as the chemical process during which oxygen is finally reduced to water. The sole purpose of the respiratory process is, however, to supply the cells with the O_2 required for the generation of useful energy. Aerobic organisms, from bacterium to human, generate over 90% of this energy by reducing oxygen, with protons and electrons, to water. Some of the most relevant characteristics of this reaction are the following:

1. It is catalyzed by cytochrome c oxidase, an ubiquitous enzyme embedded in the ion-impermeable inner membrane of mitochondria.
2. Electrons and protons, two of the substrates of the reaction, are removed from respiratory substrates and transported by enzymes localized in the same membrane or in its immediate vicinity.

3. The free energy change (ΔG) of the downhill transport of electrons is trans-
formed into other forms of useful energy ($\Delta\mu_H^+$, ATP, etc.) by components
of the electron and H^+ transport system or by specific enzymes (ATPases)
all embedded in the same membrane.

Two fundamental questions regarding this reaction still remain unanswered up to
the present time, namely: (a) What is the nature of the initial form of useful energy
that is generated as the direct consequence of electron flow? That is, is it chemical,
conformational, electrochemical, or a combination thereof? And, (b) what is the
actual correlation in rates and extents between O_2 consumption and the generation
of useful energy? That is, what is the efficiency of energy transduction, classically
estimated by measuring the magnitude of the ATP/O or H^+/O stoichiometry?

The chemiosmotic hypothesis of Mitchell (6), the most commonly accepted at
the present time, postulates, first, that the initial event in the process of energy
conversion is the translocation of protons from the inner to the outer phase of the
mitochondrial membrane. It is assumed that the translocation of H^+ generates an
electrochemical gradient of H^+ ($\Delta\mu_H^+$) which actually constitutes the initial form
of energy used by the cell not only to synthesize ATP or transport ions and metabolites across membranes, but also to control the rates of electron flow and O_2 consumption. The electrochemical gradient of H^+ (or an equivalent form of chemical
energy such as the phosphorylation potential, ΔG_p) would control the rates of respiration by opposing the flow of electrons. The second postulate of Mitchell's
hypothesis is that exactly 2 H^+ are ejected per pair of electrons traversing each of
the three loops in which the components of the respiratory chain are arranged.
Cytochrome c oxidase was not considered part of these loops until recently (7). In
order to account for the increasing experimental evidence demonstrating that protons can also be ejected at the level of cytochrome c oxidase, Mitchell devised an
entire new loop at this level, postulating now that a maximum of 8 protons (not 6
as originally proposed) are ejected when a pair of electrons are transported from
NADH to O_2. The following results show novel aspects of mitochondrial energy
transduction.

RESULTS

The Kinetics of O_2 Consumption by Respiring Uncoupled Mitochondria

In order to allow the electrons to flow freely from the respiratory substrate to O_2 in
the absence of opposing forces ($\Delta\mu_H^+$ or ΔG_p), the mitochondrial membrane was
first disrupted by freezing and thawing. Under these conditions H^+ return to the
mitochondrial matrix immediately after they have been ejected, collapsing the electrochemical gradient of H^+ and releasing the free energy of electron transport as
heat. The effectiveness of the uncoupling procedure was tested by measuring the
extent of H^+ ejection in systems containing the disrupted mitochondria together
with charge-compensating cations—Ca^{2+} or K^+ plus valinomycin. Similar uncoupling effects were obtained using the unnatural protonophore FCCP*. Figure 19.1

---

*FCCP = carbonyl cyanide p-trifluoromethoxyphenylhydrazone

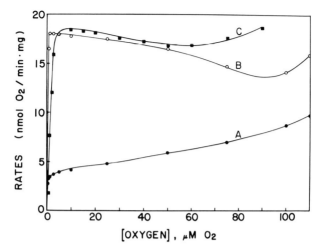

Fig. 19.1 Rates of O_2 consumption at different actual concentrations of O_2, as measured by the O_2 electrode. Respiration was initiated by adding uncoupled mitochondria to air-saturated medium at 25°C, containing glutamate + malate **(A)**, succinate **(B)**, or cytochrome c + ascorbate **(C)**.

shows the variations in the rates of O_2 consumption as the O_2 content (both measured with an O_2 electrode) of the supporting medium decrease from 100 μM O_2 to zero. Respiration was initiated by adding uncoupled mitochondria to a closed cell containing 240 μM O_2 and glutamate plus malate (A), succinate (B), or ascorbate plus cytochrome c (C), as respiratory substrates. Curve A shows that in the presence of glutamate plus malate, the rates of O_2 uptake declined continuously and gradually until the O_2 concentration of the medium fell below 1 μM O_2. At this point the rates declined, following an apparent first-order dependence on O_2 concentration. In the presence of either succinate or ascorbate plus cytochrome c (curves B and C), however, the rates of O_2 uptake neither remained constant nor decreased; rather, they increased as the O_2 content of the medium decreased down to 2 or 3 μM O_2, below which O_2 uptake decreased abruptly. To find out whether these unexpected changes in the rates of mitochondrial respiration were due only to experimental defects or indeed reflected the activity of the mitochondria, experiments were carried out in which the sensitivity of the equipment was increased 40–100 fold. Respiration was then initiated by adding small volumes of air-saturated medium to anaerobic suspension of uncoupled mitochondria supplemented with respiratory substrates in the presence and absence of inhibitors of electron flow. Figure 19.2A shows an experiment in which the reaction was initiated by adding 4.6 nmol O_2 to an anaerobic suspension of broken mitochondria in the presence of two potent inhibitors of mitochondrial electron flow: antimycin and myxothiazol (see ref. 14). Under these conditions, the O_2 added to the system was rapidly detected by the O_2 electrode and was recorded in full 200 ms after its addition. The O_2 added remained in the medium for an undetermined period of time without significant reduction in its concentration. The amount of O_2 physically bound to the mitochondria, however, was not detected because the process took place during the delay time of the recorder (= 200 ms). In Fig. 19.2B, the experimental condi-

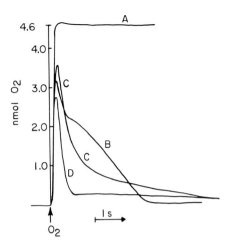

Fig. 19.2 Time course of O_2 consumption. Respiration was initiated by injecting pulses of O_2 into anaerobic suspensions of uncoupled mitochondria in the presence of antimycin + myxothiazol with succinate **(A)**, succinate **(B)**, glutamate + malate **(C)**, and cytochrome c + ascorbate **(D)** at 25°C.

tions were identical to those shown in A, except that the inhibitors were omittted and succinate was used as respiratory substrate. The time course of O_2 consumption in this experiment showed at least three phases of respiration. The initial phase took place at very fast rates, using over 25% of the O_2 added in less than 0.6 s. The first phase was followed, almost abruptly, by a second, much slower phase during which the rates of O_2 uptake gradually increased, rather than decreased, as the O_2 concentration of the medium decreased. Finally a third phase ensued, in which the rates of O_2 uptake decreased until the O_2 was totally exhausted. Curves C and D in Fig. 19.2 show the time course of O_2 consumption in experiments in which glutamate plus malate and ascorbate plus cytochrome c, respectively, were used as respiratory substrates instead of succinate. At the initial concentrations of O_2 used, more than 60% of the O_2 added was rapidly consumed during the first phase only. The second phase ensued at strikingly slow rates, particularly when ascorbate plus cytochrome c served as respiratory substrates.

The results of the experiments shown in Fig. 19.2B basically confirm those shown in Fig. 19.1B and C, indicating that the increased rates of respiration that occur as the O_2 concentration of the medium decreases may in fact be a functional characteristic of the mitochondria. These experiments, however, give no indication of the possible cause for this unusual and hitherto undescribed phenomenon. Table 19.1 collects the results of experiments in which the reactions were initiated by adding different amounts of O_2, ranging in concentration from 2.7 to 27 μM. The rates of respiration were then measured at different actual concentrations of O_2 along the course of the reaction from the beginning to the end of the second phase. It is evident that for the same concentration of O_2 in the system, the larger the amount of O_2 added to initiate the reaction, the slower the rate of respiration. At 1.5 μM O_2, for example, the rates of respiration decreased from 3.5 to 2.1 nmol O/ mg/min as the amount of O_2 initially added increased from 4 to 27 μM O_2.

Table 19.1 Rates of O_2 Consumption at Different Actual Concentrations of O_2

[O_2] added, μM	Actual [O_2], μM				
	0.5	1.0	1.5	2.5	5.0
2.7	4.3[a]	—	—	—	—
4.0	3.1	3.3	3.5	—	—
8.1	2.9	3.1	3.1	3.4	3.9
13.5	2.4	2.6	2.7	2.8	3.2
27.0	1.9	2.0	2.1	2.3	2.6

Note: The test system (1.65 ml; 25°C) contained 200 mM sucrose, 50 mM KCl, 3 mM Hepes (4-(2-hydroxyethyl)-1-piperazineethanesulfonic acid), frozen and thawed rat liver mitochrondria (3.0 mg protein) and 5 mM succinate as respiratory substrate. Rates are expressed in nmol O_2/min/mg mitochondrial protein. Reactions were initiated by adding different known amounts of O_2 (column 1) to anaerobic suspension of mitochondria respiring in the presence of succinate. Rates of respiration were measured during the course of each reaction at the actual five concentrations of O_2 remaining in the medium.

The Lack of Kinetic Correlation Between O_2 Consumption and H^+ Ejection in Coupled Mitochondria

The experimental results shown in Figs. 19.1 and 19.2 and in Table 19.1 were carried out in uncoupled mitochondria to study the uncontrolled rates of O_2 consumption. The function of mitochondria, however, is not to consume O_2 by reducing it with protons and electrons, but rather to generate useful energy, utilizing the free energy change of electron flow. It is therefore important to determine whether or not the polyphasic nature of O_2 uptake described for disrupted and uncoupled mitochondria also occurs in intact mitochondria where the energy of electron transport is used for the synthesis of ATP or the transport of ions and metabolites across the membrane. Figure 19.3 shows the time course of both O_2 consumption and H^+ extrusion in an experiment in which the energy of electron flow was coupled to the transport of Ca^{2+}. Three phases of O_2 consumption are also clear in this type of mitochondria, contrasting with the simple and monotonic time course of H^+ ejection. The difference is most clearly observed in the semilogarithmic plot shown in Fig. 19.3B. The computer-fitted regression lines were calculated assuming first-order kinetics (ln S = ln S_0 ± kt). In the presence of optimal concentrations of charge-compensating cations (Ca^{2+} or K^+ + valinomycin), the extrapolation of these lines to zero time should yield the H^+/O flow ratio at level flow, a condition where the maximal efficiency of energy transduction is most closely approached, that is, at the hypothetical instant at which the opposing force ($\Delta\mu_H^+$), which restricts and keeps under control the flow of electrons, is zero. Using this type of kinetic procedure, we have reported in the past (2,5,12) H^+/O stoichiometries near 8 and 4 for the oxidation of succinate and ferrocytochrome c, respectively. Other laboratories, however, have reported values that differed, in some instances, by more than 50%, particularly in regard to the oxidation of ferrocytochrome c (7,8,15). The discrepancies may be explained by considering that the translocation of H^+ may in fact be the *consequence,* rather than the *cause,* of an initial event in the process of energy transduction. The lack of strict correlation between O_2 consumption and H^+ ejection is illustrated in Table 19.2. The initial rates were cal-

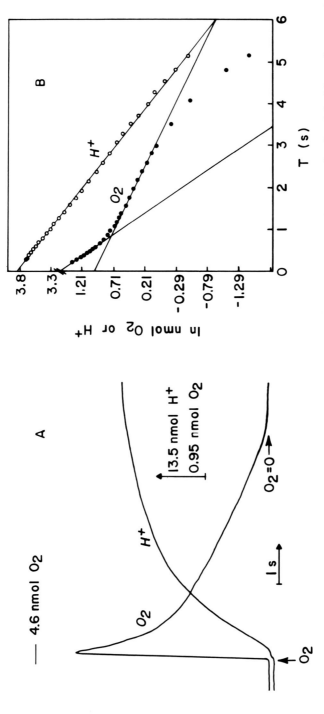

Fig. 19.3 (**A**) The simultaneous time course of O_2 uptake and H^+ ejection in coupled mitochondria. Conditions are as in Fig. 19.2 with succinate as substrate. (**B**) Semilogarithmic plot (see also text).

Table 19.2 Rates of O_2 Consumption and H^+ Ejection by Coupled Mitochondria Respiring at Different Initial Concentrations of O_2

Initial $[O_2]$, μM	O_2 consumption		H^+ ejection		H^+/O ratio		
	Rate in first phase	Rate at $t_{1/2}$	Initial rate	Extent (total)	In first phase	At $t_{1/2}$	Calc. from extent
0.28	52	—	56	5.4	1.1	—	5.8
0.42	61	—	77	6.1	1.3	—	4.3
0.56	74	—	121	8.6	1.6	—	4.6
0.70	100	—	138	12.8	1.4	—	5.5
0.84	126	—	174	14.2	1.4	—	5.1
1.13	143	—	225	17.2	1.6	—	4.6
1.41	163	135	291	24.8	1.8	2.1	5.3
2.11	175	122	377	34.6	2.2	3.1	4.9
2.82	183	92	532	43.9	2.9	5.8	4.7
4.23	200	78	521	57.6	2.4	6.7	4.1
5.63	236	56	667	66.5	2.8	11.9	3.6

Note: Experimental conditions as indicated in Table 19.1, except that intact, well-coupled rat liver mitochrondria were used. Rates are expressed in nmol H^+ or O (atoms)/min/protein.

culated by drawing lines along the apparent linear portions of H^+ ejection, and at $t_{1/2}$ of O_2 uptake. It is obvious that the H^+/O ratio varies greatly, depending on the method used for its evaluation. The dependence of the initial rates of H^+ ejection on O_2 concentration is, on the other hand, evident. The concentration of O_2 required for one-half the maximal rate of H^+ ejection is, in this experiment, 20 μM O_2 with a correlation of .989.

DISCUSSION

The results obtained compel us to wonder about the physiological significance of the different phases of O_2 uptake if they indeed happen to occur in vivo. Evidence has been obtained showing that the efficiency of energy transduction (H^+ ejection or Ca^{2+} uptake) depends directly on the first phase of respiration. It seems that the second phase represents a controlled state of the system, and the third phase is a transition between the controlled and the most active form of the respiratory enzyme(s).

The molecular mechanism of electron flow at the level of cytochrome c oxidase has been extensively studied (1,3,4,9–11,13) and recently described in an enlightening review by Naqui, Chance, and Cadenas (10). As a first approximation we can assume the following sequence of reactions:

$$E \underset{}{\overset{[e^-]}{\rightleftharpoons}} E' \cdot A \underset{}{\overset{[O_2]}{\rightleftharpoons}} E'' \cdot B \underset{}{\overset{[H^+]}{\rightleftharpoons}} E''' \cdot C \overset{H_2O}{\longrightarrow} E$$

where the entrance of the three substrates at specific points in the sequence results in the formation of enzyme–substrate complexes ($E' \cdot A$, $E'' \cdot B$, and $E''' \cdot C$) which, by undergoing redox and conformational changes in the protein, could affect the

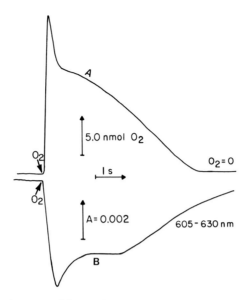

Fig. 19.4 Changes in the rates of O_2 uptake (**A**) and absorbance of cytochrome c oxidase (**B**) in parallel experiments. Conditions are as in Fig. 19.2, except that changes in absorbancy were measured at 10°C instead of 25°C (substrate, succinate).

net rates of electron flow, O_2 consumption, and energy transduction. From all these complexes the "oxy" and "peroxy" intermediates are, most likely, the determinants of the rates of O_2 consumption (9,10) at this level. Although all three substrates (e^-, O_2, and H^+) are essential for this control, it was shown here that the rates of O_2 consumption depend on O_2 in the entire range of concentrations between zero and 200 μM (16). Assuming unlimited availability of H^+ and electrons, it may be reasonably assumed that the rates of O_2 consumption depend on the following minimal number of factors:

$$-\frac{dO_2}{dt} = k_{E \cdot S} \times \frac{[CO_{red}]}{[CO_{ox}]} \times [O_2]$$

where $k_{E \cdot S}$ represents an undiscriminated aggregation of all the individual rate constants actually present in the sequence of respiratory reactions.

Figure 19.4 shows the time course of both O_2 consumption (A) and absorbancy changes in the redox state of cytochrome c oxidase (B), in two parallel experiments in which respiration was initiated by adding O_2 to anaerobic suspensions of uncoupled mitochondria in the presence of succinate. Under these conditions the oxidase is fully reduced, and the intial phase of O_2 consumption (Fig. 19.4A) coincides with the initial phase of net oxidation of the enzyme (Fig. 19.4B). If the "oxy" and "peroxy" forms of the oxidase are generated at rates that exceed their disappearance (e.g., when the availability of H^+ becomes limited and the concentration of O_2 is above 2 μM), the rates of O_2 consumption are greatly reduced (Fig. 19.4A) and the reduction of the oxidase exceeds its oxidation (Fig. 19.4B). Depending on the concentration of O_2, a true steady state in the redox state of the oxidase may ensue where the ratio of the reduced and oxidized forms of the oxidase is maintained constant, even when the net flow of electrons (and the rates of O_2 uptake) decreases. Below 2 μM O_2, respiration is limited solely by the availability of O_2, and the rates of O_2 uptake decrease despite the fact that the oxidase is mostly reduced (Fig. 19.4). The effect of the structural integrity of the membrane and its permeability to H^+ (the third substrate of the reaction) on the kinetics of O_2 consumption is currently under investigation.

REFERENCES

1. Antonini, E., M. Brunori, A. Colosimo, C. Greenwood, and H. Wilson. Kinetic behavior of an intermediate of cytochrome exodase. In: *Oxygen and Physiological Function,* ed. Frans F. Jobsis. Dallas: Professional Inf. Library, 1977, pp. 54–61.
2. Costa, L. E., B. Reynafarje, and A. L. Lehninger. Stoichiometry of mitochondrial H^+ translocation coupled to succinate at level flow. *J. Biol. Chem. 259:* 4802–4811, 1984.
3. Hill, B. C., and C. Greenwood. Kinetic evidence for the re-definition of electron transfer pathways from cytochrome c to O_2 within cytochrome oxidase. *FEBS Lett. 166:* 362–366, 1984.
4. Hill, B. C., and C. Greenwood. The reaction of fully reduced cytochrome c oxidase with oxygen studied by flow-flash spectrophotometry at room temperature. *Biochem. J. 218:* 913–921, 1984.
5. Lehninger, A. L., B. Reynafarje, R. W. Hendler, and R. I. Shrager. The H^+/O ratio of proton translocation linked to the oxidation of succinate by mitochrondria. *FEBS Lett. 192:* 173–178, 1985.
6. Mitchell, P. Translocations through natural membranes. In: *Adv. Enzymol.,* Vol. 29, ed. F. F. Nord. New York: Interscience, 1967, pp. 33–87.
7. Mitchell, P., R. Mitchell, A. J. Moody, I. C. West, H. Baum, and J. M. Wrigglesworth. Chemiosmotic coupling in cytochrome oxidase. *FEBS Lett. 188:* 1–7, 1985.
8. Mitchell, P., and J. Moyle. Respiration-driven proton translocation in rat liver mitochondria. *Biochem. J. 105:* 1147–1162, 1967.
9. Naqui, A., and B. Chance. Enhanced superoxide dismutase activity of pulsed cytochrome oxidase. *Biochem. Biophys. Res. Commun. 136:* 433–437, 1986.
10. Naqui, A., B. Chance, and E. Cadenas. Reactive oxygen intermediates in biochemistry. *Annu. Rev. Biochem. 55:* 137–166, 1986.
11. Naqui, A., C. Kumar, Y-C. Ching, L. Powers, and B. Chance. Structure and reactivity of multiple forms of cytochrome oxidase as evaluated by x-ray absorption spectroscopy and kinetics of cyanide. *Biochemistry 23:* 6222–6227, 1984.
12. Reynafarje, B., L. E., Costa, and A. L. Lehninger. Upper and lower limits of the proton stoichiometry of cytochrome c oxidation in rat liver mitoplasts. *J. Biol. Chem. 261:* 8254–8262, 1986.
13. Sone, N., A. Naqui, C. Kumar, and B. Chance. Pulsed cytochrome c oxidase from the thermophilic bacterium PS3. *Biochem. J. 223:* 809–813, 1984.
14. West, I. C., R. Mitchell, A. J. Moody, and P. Mitchell. Proton translocation by cytochrome oxidase in (antimycin $\pm$ myxothiazol)-treated rat liver mitochrondria using ferrocyanide or hexammineruthenium as electron donor. *Biochem. J. 236:* 15–21, 1986.
15. Wikstrom, M., and T. Penttila. Critical evaluation of the proton-translocation property of cytochrome oxidase in rat liver mitochondria. *FEBS Lett. 144:* 183–189, 1982.
16. Wilson, D. F., M. Erecinska, C. Drown, and I. A. Silver. The oxygen dependence of cellular energy metabolism. *Arch. Biochem. Biophys. 195:* 485–493, 1979.

20

ATP-Sensing Reactions and Oxygen Chemoreception

R. F. COBURN

It appears that oxygen chemoreception is one of the most poorly understood phenomena in biology. Questions regarding oxygen tension gradients in cells and in tissues, oxygen-dependent (O_2-sensing) reactions (8), and transduction and effector mechanisms in various oxygen chemoreception tissues and cells are still largely unanswered. This chapter reviews the status of some of these questions and explores possible mechanisms involved in O_2 chemoreception. I will use a broad definition of O_2 *chemoreception:* It is a mechanism by which changes in oxygen tension in cells result in an adaptive response. *Transduction* refers to the mechanism by which O_2-sensing reactions signal effector mechanisms. The term *effector mechanism* refers to the molecular mechanism directly involved in the physiological responses to altered cellular Po_2. How these terms are used will be clarified in the following examples.

Figure 20.1 shows two possible general mechanisms for O_2 chemoreception that we have discussed previously (8). The first schema (A) postulates an O_2 sensor that detects changes in Po_2 at some point in the cell or tissue. The O_2-sensing reaction in this schema is not cytochrome a_3. This reaction is linked to a transduction mechanism that generates signals which control effector mechanisms. In the second schema (B), the oxygen sensor is cytochrome a_3. This schema postulates that signals are transduced via a decrease in oxidative phosphorylation, which results in a decreased delivery of ATP or phosphorcreatine (PCr) to low-affinity, ATP-dependent reactions that control the effector mechanism and physiological response. These schemata are meant to indicate general pathways that may be involved in O_2 chemoreception. It may be that in some O_2 chemoreception cells there are cascades of transduction mechanisms leading to the physiological response to altered cellular Po_2. There may be multiple effector mechanisms determining physiological responses. And, as will be discussed later, the distinction between transduction and effector mechanisms may be blurred. However, the schemata shown in Fig. 20.1 give us a framework for discussing O_2 chemoreception mechanisms.

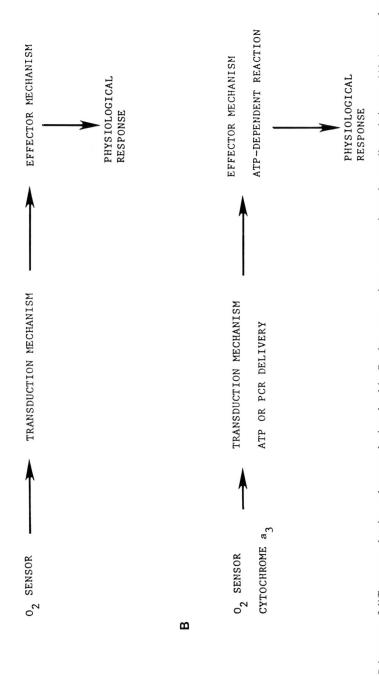

Fig. 20.1 Schemata of different mechanisms that may be involved in O₂ chemoreception responses in various cells and tissues. (**A**) A general mechanism; (**B**) a specific example with cytochrome a₃ as the sensor.

Evidence obtained in recent years is getting stronger for support of the second model, where the O_2 sensor is cytochrome oxidase, and at least part of the transduction mechanism involves decreased delivery of ATP or PCr (18,22,25,28,32 and unpublished data, S. Lahiri). There appear to be large differences in ATP affinities for various ATP-dependent reactions, and it is possible that ATP-dependent reactions involved in O_2 chemoreception have low ATP affinities—that is, they become limited with small decreases in [ATP]. Data suggest that ATP-dependent reactions essential to cell survival, or survival of the organism, have high ATP affinities (7,29,30,37) so that [ATP] at their location in the cell must decrease to very low levels before these reactions are inhibited.

It is possible that the transduction link between oxidative phosphorylation and the physiological response (metabolism–effector coupling) is produced by compounds, other than ATP or PCr, that operate by exerting allosteric control on components of the effector mechanism. Inorganic phosphate is a prime candidate for this role, and ADP and NADH/NAD also need to be considered. However, in this chapter my emphasis is on the possible ATP-dependent reactions and how they might be linked to effector mechanisms determining physiological responses.

It seems likely that effector mechanisms operating during O_2 chemoreception involve alteration of the time and frequency of ion channel opening, changes in cytosolic Ca concentration, or other second messengers. These, in turn, control such responses as secretion of neurotransmitters or mediators, contractility, or other processes. As indicated above, our definitions of transduction and effector may overlap. This can be illustrated by considering a hypothetical case where the physiological response to altered P_{O_2} involves a second messenger that activates a protein kinase, which results in phosphorylation of an ion channel, which in turn produces a change in the plasma membrane potential, the opening of voltage-gated Ca channels, an increase in cytosolic [Ca], and finally fusion of secretory granules and secretion. There is evidence for changes in the plasma membrane potential (15,17,31) during O_2 chemoreception responses in carotid body and vascular smooth muscle, and for the important of neurotransmitter or mediator secretion during the O_2 chemoreception response in carotid body (15).

The search for ATP-dependent reactions operative during O_2 chemoreception is complicated by ATP gradients, possible ATP compartmentation, PCr/free creatine shuttles, and other factors. In carotid body, there is little evidence for any of these. In vascular smooth muscle, there is evidence of ATP compartmentation where plasma membrane Na^+,K^+-ATPase preferentially utilize glycolytically produced ATP (21,24). In cells that contain the PCr/free creatine shuttle, it is still not proven whether energy can be supplied directly by phosphorylcreatine or whether ATP must be formed via the creatine kinase reaction (6).

The question of cellular ATP gradients has been approached in isolated rat hepatocytes by Awe and Jones (2). These investigators simultaneously studied, under conditions of altered energy metabolism, a cytosolic ATP-dependent reaction—sulfation of acetaminophen—which has an effective K_m for ATP of approximately 1 mM, and a plasma membrane ATP-dependent reaction—ouabain-inhibitable Rb^+ uptake. Cell ATP content was decreased in a graded manner by (a) an inhibition of ATP synthesis, (b) an increase in ATP utilization, or (c) a decrease in total phosphagen content. A decrease in cellular ATP content had a larger effect on Rb^+ uptake than on sulfation of acetaminophen. Complete inhibiton of ouabain-sensitive Rb^+ uptake occurred when estimated cytosolic [ATP] was decreased to about 1 mM, but acetaminophen sulfation still occurred at this ATP concentration. These data were interpreted in terms of ATP gradients between mitochondrial clusters (20) and plasma membrane Na^+,K^+-ATPase ATP binding sites. Calculations using previously determined ATP diffusion coefficients and an assumed geometry suggested that radial ATP gradients may occur during hypoxia so that ATP levels at the cytosolic face of the plasma membrane will reach nearly zero, a situation that could explain these investigators' experimental findings. However, during normoxia, ATP gradients are minimal. These data suggest a basis for considering that plasma membrane ATP-dependent reactions may be linked to O_2 chemoreception.

THE SEARCH FOR ATP-DEPENDENT REACTIONS LINKED TO OXYGEN CHEMORECEPTION

It seems most likely that control of effector mechanisms in O_2 chemoreception cells is located in the plasma membrane, because of data discussed above, and because the plasma membrane is a site of control of responses in many different cells. I have identified two plasma membrane ATP-dependent reactions that are candidates for ATP-sensors linked to O_2 chemoreception responses: (a) The ATP-dependent K channel, and (b) the phosphatidylinositol phosphate (PIP) kinase reaction, a component of the phosphoinositide transduction mechanism.

ATP-Dependent K Channel

The ATP-dependent K channel has been recently described in the myocardium (27). Figure 20.2 illustrates path-clamp data obtained with inside-out patches, which characterize this channel. A decrease in [ATP] on the cytosolic face of the patch resulted in increases in open times and in frequency of open times of this delayed rectifying channel. The effective K_m for ATP for this effect is about 0.2 mM. It is well known that the ventricular myocardial action potential shortens during "hypoxia," resulting in decreased force of ventricular contraction. It appears that a decrease in [ATP] results in an outward current which is responsible for shortening the action potential plateau. This appears to be an adaptation to hypoxia in that the decrease in force conserves ATP utilized by actomyosin ATPase, so that cytosolic [ATP] does not decrease to levels that would limit ATP-dependent reactions, such as the Ca^{2+}-ATPases, which are essential for cell survival. The attractiveness of the ATP-dependent K channel as a possible component of O_2 chemoreception responses is based on the high K_m for ATP and the central role of plasma membrane potential changes in controlling various cellular responses. The finding of ATP-controlled K channels allows us to speculate that there may be ATP control of other types of channels, as well.

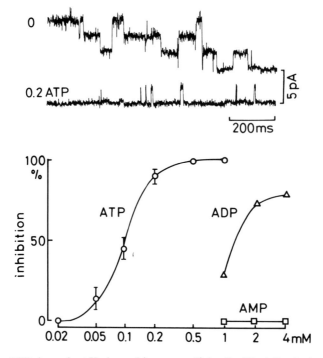

Fig. 20.2 The ATP-dependent K channel in myocardial cells. **(Top)** Patch-clamp data measuring K currents in inside-out patches at zero and 0.2 mM [ATP] at the cytoplasmic face of the plasma membrane. **(Bottom)** The relationship between [ATP] and open times of these K channels, expressed as percent inhibition. [Data are taken from Noma, 1983 (27).]

PIP Kinase

I was alerted to the possibility that PIP kinase could function as an ATP sensor under conditions of decreased ATP synthesis and delivery by the results of Lundberg et al. (23). These workers showed that phosphorylation of PIP to phosphatidylinositol bisphosphate (PIP$_2$) was inhibited in hepatocyte membrane preparations when [ATP] fell below 1 mM. The reaction by which PIP is phosphorylated to PIP$_2$ is part of a series of reactions that transduce and amplify signals generated by receptor binding to agonist, and provide the second messengers inositol trisphosphate (IP$_3$), inositol tetrakisphosphate (IP$_4$), and diacylglycerol (DAG) (5,19) (Fig. 20.3). Considerable evidence indicates that these second messengers are involved in the control of secretion, contractility, and other cellular processes (5). Thus, the appeal of the ideal that PIP kinase functions as an ATP sensor during O$_2$ chemoreception reactions is based on the high K_m for ATP, and the central role of the inositol phospholipid transduction system in control of secretion, contractility, and other cellular responses. The phosphoinositide transduction mechanism is expensive to the cell in that ATP is required for phosphorylation of phosphatidylinositol (PI), PIP, DAG, I(1,4,5)P$_3$, and phosphatidic acid. Further ATP is required for synthesis of cytidine triphosphate (CTP) utilized in PI resynthesis. The energy cost of this transduction mechanism has been estimated in canine trachealis muscle to be as great as 7% of the total increase in ATP flux (J_{ATP}) due to contraction (4).

Test of the Hypothesis that PIP Kinase Can Function as a ATP-Sensor During Oxygen Chemoreception

We chose to test this hypothesis using the isolated rabbit aorta. This tissue mounted in an organ bath and contracted by norepinephrine shows graded changes in mechanical tension with small changes in organ bath Po_2, which are maintained and completely reversible (10,11,14,17,26). The phenomenon studied in vitro in an organ bath may be a model for study of the mechanism of dilatation of peripheral vessels that occurs under conditions where there is a decreased O_2 content in arterial blood. We used the rabbit aorta model since data are available which partially define the state of energy synthesis and delivery during the O_2 chemoreception response. During hypoxia-induced relaxations, there is a large decrease in J_{ATP}, and a decrease in mean PCr/free creatine, without a change in mean ATP content (32–34).

Phosphorylation of PIP to PIP_2 was studied as follows (9): Resting aortic rings were incubated with [^{3}H]myoinositol, the precursor of PI, which labeled the intracellular free myoinositol pool without much label appearing in inositol phospholipids. We then contracted the tissue under two different conditions—during normoxia (organ bath Po_2 was approximately 250 mmHg), and during hypoxia (the organ bath fluid was bubbled with 95% N_2/5% CO_2, giving a Po_2 of approximately

Fig. 20.3 The phosphoinositide cycle. Note that the cycle includes degradation and resynthesis of the various inositol phospholipids and inositol phosphates. [Reproduced by permission from Berridge, 1986 (5).] The diagram does not show the recent finding that IP_3 is phosphorylated to IP_4, nor does it show other facets of degradation of inositol phosphates. It also fails to show the likely possibility that PI and PIP_2 may also be hydrolyzed to PI and to IP_2, respectively.

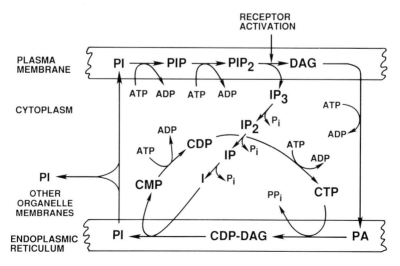

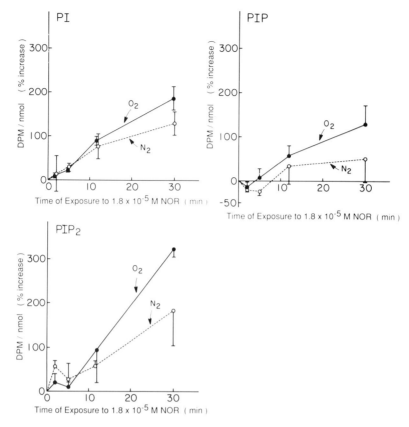

Fig. 20.4 Changes in specific radioactivity incorporated into phosphatidylinositol (PI), phosphatidylinositol phosphate (PIP), and phosphatidylinositol bisphosphate (PIP$_2$) in isolated rabbit aortic rings incubated with [$_3$H]myoinositol, during norepinephrine (NOR) activation under hypoxia and normoxia.

40 mmHg). Under both conditions, activation with norepinephrine resulted in myoinositol incorporation into inositol phospholipids and inositol phosphates. However, less myoinositol was incorporated when the tissue was activated during hypoxia. We computed flux rates from myoinositol incorporation rates under conditions of a 15- to 30-min exposure to norepinephrine. During hypoxia, flux rates were less than 50% of that observed during normoxia. Figure 20.4 illustrates this point by showing decreased rates of increase in specific activities of PI, PIP, and PIP$_2$. Total tissue pool size changes for PI, PIP$_2$, and phosphatidic acid during norepinephrine activation under hypoxia were similar to those seen during activation under normoxia. However, the increase in total tissue PIP pool size was much larger during activation under hypoxia than during activation under normoxia (Fig. 20.5). The same data, plotted as total pool PIP/total pool PIP$_2$, show a 300% increase when the tissue was activated during hypoxia as compared to normoxia. Inositol phosphate data were consistent with the above findings: The rates of incor-

poration of radioactivity into PI, PIP, and PIP$_2$ were significantly depressed at 2, 15, and 30 min after norepinephrine activation under hypoxia, as compared to normoxia.

These data support the hypothesis that PIP-kinase is limiting metabolic flux in the inositol phospholipid transduction system during hypoxia. Evidence includes the increase in PIP pool size and the decrease in the flux rate for inositol phospholipids when the tissue was activated by norepinephrine during hypoxia. The hypoxia-induced decreased metabolic flux in inositol phospholipids and the increase in the total PIP pool size occurred under conditions where total tissue PCr/ creatine was decreased but ATP content was unchanged from that determined during normoxic activation. This suggests that PCr/Cr is important in delivery of energy to PIP kinase. Glycolysis increases markedly under conditions of hypoxia in this tissue (33); thus it appears that ATP produced by glycolysis does not have access to PIP kinase, as occurs with Na$^+$,K$^+$-ATPase in vascular smooth muscle (24). Although the decrease in flux rate in the inositol phospholipids could be due to effects mediated at the receptor, or G proteins (5), the increase in PIP and PIP/ PIP$_2$ suggests that a rate-limiting step is the phosphorylation of PIP. Our data do not prove that the physiological response, relaxation during hypoxia, is due to a decrease in [IP$_3$] (resulting in a decreased release of Ca from the sarcoplasmic reticulum and reduced activation of myosin light chain kinase), since we measured flux rather than IP$_3$ pool sizes. Supporting this concept is considerable recent evidence suggesting that IP$_3$ exerts control over intracellular Ca in various tissues (5), including vascular smooth muscle (1,3,12,13,16,34–36). Hypoxia-induced relaxations could also result from decreased production of DAG or other second messengers generated by inositol phospholipid metabolism.

Fig. 20.5 Changes in total tissue pool size of phosphatidylinositol phosphate (PIP) resulting from activation of rabbit aortic muscle by norepinephrine (NOR) during hypoxia and normoxia.

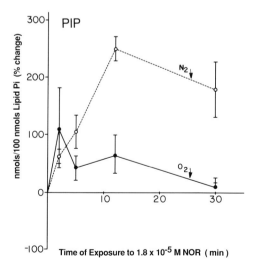

CONCLUSIONS

Evidence is now strong that cytochrome a_3 is an O_2 sensor involved in O_2 chemoreceptor in some mammalian cells. I have approached the topic of O_2 chemoreception by considering several ATP-sensors that could be involved in O_2 chemoreception responses.

ACKNOWLEDGMENTS
    The author acknowledges the assistance and advice of his collaborators and colleagues, Drs. C. Baron, S. Lahiri, and M. Papadopoulos.

REFERENCES

1. Alexander, R. W., T. A. Brock, M. A. Gimbrone, Jr., and S. Rittenhouse. Angiotensin increases inositol trisphosphate and calcium in vascular smooth muscle. *Hypertension* 7: 447–451, 1985.
2. Awe, T. Y., and D. P. Jones. ATP concentration gradients in cytosol of liver cells during hypoxia. *Am. J. Physiol. 249:* C385–C392, 1985.
3. Baron, C. B., M. Cunningham, J. F. Strauss, R. F. Coburn. Pharmacomechanical coupling in smooth muscle may involve phosphatidylinositol metabolism. *Proc. Natl. Acad. Sci. U.S.A. 81:* 6899–6903, 1984.
4. Baron, C. B., M. Pring, and R. F. Coburn. Synthesis and compartmentation of inositol phospholipids in unstimulated and carbamlylcholine-stimulated smooth muscle. (Submitted for publication)
5. Berridge, M. J. Agonist-dependent phosphoinostide metabolism: a bifurcating signal pathway. In: *New Insights into Cell and Membrane Transport Processes,* ed. G. Poste and S. T. Crooke. New York: Plenum, 1986, pp. 201–216.
6. Bessman, S. P., and P. J. Geiger. Transport of energy in muscle: the phosphorylcreatine shuttle. *Science 211:* 448–452, 1981.
7. Carafoli, E. Calmodulin-sensitive calcium-pumping ATPase in plasma membranes: isolation, reconstitution, and regulation. *Fed. Proc. 43:* 3005–3010, 1984.
8. Coburn, R. F. Oxygen tension sensors in vascular smooth muscle. In: *Tissue Hypoxia and Ischemia,* ed. M. Reivich. New York: Plenum, 1977, pp. 101–115.
9. Coburn, R. F., C. Baron, and M. T. Papadopoulos. Phosphoinositide metabolism in rabbit aorta is altered during hypoxia. (Submitted for publication)
10. Coburn, R. F., R. Eppinger, and D. P. Scott. Oxygen-dependent tension in vascular smooth muscle. Does the endothelium play a role? *Circ. Res. 58:* 341–347, 1986.
11. Coburn, R. F., B. Grubb, and R. D. Aronson. Effect of cyanide on oxygen tension-dependent mechanical tension in rabbit aorta. *Circ. Res. 44:* 368–378, 1979.
12. Cotecchia, S., L.M.F. Leeb-Lundberg, P. O. Hagen, R. J. Lefkowitz, and M. G. Caron. Phorbol ester effects on alpha$_1$-adrenoceptol binding and phosphatidylinositol metabolism in cultured vascular smooth muscle cells. *Life Sci. 37:* 2389–2398, 1985.
13. Danthuluri, N. R., and R. C. Deth. Phorbol ester-induced contraction of arterial smooth muscle and inhibition of alpha-adrenergic response. *Biochem. Biophys. Res. Commun. 125:* 1103–1109, 1984.
14. Detar, R., and D. F. Bohr. Oxygen and vascular smooth muscle contraction. *Am. J. Physiol. 214:* 241–244, 1968.

15. Eyzaguirre, C., R. S. Fitzgerald, S. Lahiri, and P. Zapata. Arterial chemoreceptors. In: *Handbook of Physiology, See. 2: The Cardiovascular System, Vol 3: Peripheral Circulation and Organ Blood Flow,* ed. J. T. Shepherd and F. M. Abboud. Bethesda: Am. Physiol. Soc., 1983, pp. 557–621.

16. Goldman, Y. E., G. P. Reid, A. P. Somlyo, A. V. Somlyo, D. R. Trentham, and J. W. Water. Activation of skinned vascular smooth muscle by photolysis of 'caged inositol trisphosphate' to inositol 1,4,5-trisphosphate. *J. Physiol. (Lond.) 377:* 100P, 1986.

17. Harder, D. R., J. Maddon, and C. Dawson. Hypoxia-induced activation in small isolated pulmonary arteries from the cat. *J. Appl. Physiol. 59:* 113–118, 1985.

18. Hellstrand, P., B. Johansson, and K. Norberg. Mechanical, electrical, and biochemical effects of hypoxia and substrate removal on spontaneously active vascular smooth muscle. *Acta Physiol. Scand. 100:* 69–83, 1977.

19. Hokin, L. E. Receptors and phosphoinositide-generated second messengers. *Annu. Rev. Biochem. 54:* 205–235, 1985.

20. Jones, D. P. Effect of mitochondrial clustering on O_2 supply in hepatocytes. *Am. J. Physiol. 247:* C83–C89, 1984.

21. Kutchai, H., and L. M. Geddis. Control of glycolytic rate in rat aorta. *Am. M. Physiol, 247:* C107–C114, 1984.

22. Lovgren, B., and B. Hellstrand. Graded effects of oxygen and respiratory inhibitors on cell metabolism and spontaneous contractions in smooth muscle of the rat portal vein. *Acta Physiol. Scand. 123:* 485–495 , 1985.

23. Lundberg, G. A., B. Jergil, R. Sundler, Subcellular localization and enzymatic properties of rat liver phosphatidylinositol-4-phosphate kinase. *Biochim. Biophys. Acta 846:* 379–387, 1985.

24. Lynch, R. M., and R. J. Paul. Compartmentation of glycolytic and glycogenolytic metabolism in vascular smooth muscle. *Science 222:* 1340–1344, 1983.

25. Mulligan, E., S. Lahiri, and B. Storey. Carotid body O_2 chemoreception and mitochondrial oxidative phosphorylation. *J. Appl. Physiol. 51:* 438–446, 1981.

26. Namm, D. H., and J. L. Zucker. Biochemical alterations caused by hypoxia in the isolated rabbit aorta. *Circ. Res. 32:* 464–472, 1972.

27. Noma, A. ATP-regulated K channels in cardiac muscle. *Nature 305:* 147–148, 1983.

28. Obeso, A., L. Almaraz, and C. Gonzalez. ATP content in the cat carotid body under different experimental conditions: support for the metabolic hypothesis. In: *Chemoreceptors in Respiratory Control,* ed. J. A. Ribeiro and D. J. Pallot. London: Croom Helur, 1987, 78–87.

29. Persechini, A., U. Mrwa, and D. J. Hartshorne. Effect of phosphorylation on the actin-activated ATPase activity of myosin. *Biochem. Biophys. Res. Commun. 98:* 800–805, 1981.

30. Philipson, K. D., and A. Y. Nishimoto. ATP-dependent Na transport in cardiac sarcolemmal vesicles. *Biochim. Biophys. Acta 733:* 133–141, 1983.

31. Roulet, M. J., and R. F. Coburn. Oxygen-induced contraction in the guinea pig neonatal ductus arteriosus. *Circ. Res. 49:* 997–1002, 1982.

32. Scott, M. P., and R. F. Coburn. Phosphagen levels in single rings of rabbit aorta during hypoxia-induced relaxations. *Fed. Proc. 44:* 458, 1985.

33. Scott, M. P., and R. F. Coburn. Effects of elevation of phosphorylcreatine on force and metabolism in rabbit aorta. *Am. J. Physiol. 253:* H461–H465, 1987.

34. Smith, J. B., L. S. Smith, E. R. Brown, D. Barnes, M. A. Sabir, J. S. Davis, and R. V. Farese. Angiotensin II rapidly increases phosphatidate–phosphoinositide synthesis and phosphoinositide hydrolysis and mobilizes intracellular calcium in cultured arterial muscle cells. *Proc. Natl. Acad. Sci. U.S.A. 81:* 7812–7816, 1984.

35. Somlyo, A. V., M. Bond, A. P. Somlyo, and A. Scarpa. Inositol trisphosphate-induced calcium release and contraction in vascular smooth muscle. *Proc. Natl. Acad. Sci. U.S.A. 82:* 5231–5235, 1985.

36. Suematsu, E., M. Hirata, T. Hasimoto, and H. Kuriyama. Inositol 1,4,5-trisphosphate releases Ca^{2+} from intracellular store sites in skinned single cells of porcine coronory artery. *Biochem. Biophys. Res. Commun. 120:* 481–485, 1984.

37. Walsh, M., R. Dabroska, S. Hindrens, and D. J. Hartshorne. Calcium ion-independent myosin light chain kinase of smooth muscle. *Biochemistry 21:* 1919–1925, 1982.

Part IV
PERIPHERAL CHEMORECEPTORS: ADAPTATION

Introduction

N. H. EDELMAN

Adaptation is a common, perhaps universal, characteristic of sensory receptor mechanisms. In respiratory physiology, adaptation ordinarily takes the form of attenuation; that is, receptor output declines with a constant stimulus. The three chapters in this section highlight the relatively recent discovery of what appears to be an unusual form of sensory adaptation shown by the carotid body: an increase of output with a constant hypoxic stimulus. The time course of this phenomenon is not fully worked out, but it appears to be such that it may play an important role in the ventilatory acclimatization to high altitude.

Each chapter provides important information on this characteristic of the carotid body. Weil and Vizek show that the phenomenon persisted after efferent denervation of the carotid body, thereby dissociating it from a more generalized autonomic nervous system effect. Bisgard and colleagues, using an elegant preparation of an isolated perfused carotid body in a behaving animal, report that the phenomenon was apparent after as little as 2 h of hypoxia and that it was not elicited by comparable stimulation with hypercapnia. Lahiri and associates show that it is part of a more generalized phenomenon which is represented over the broad spectrum of oxygen tensions; that is, prolonged hypoxia increases and prolonged hyperoxia attenuates carotid body responsiveness to acute hypoxia.

Thus the pursuit of the elusive factor or factors responsible for the ventilatory acclimatization to high altitude has taken a new turn. After a generation of essentially confining our explorations to the acid–base status and neurochemistry of the central nervous system, we now have good reason to return to the carotid bodies themselves. However, it is important to stipulate that an increasing sensitivity of the carotid bodies is unlikely to be fully responsible for ventilatory acclimatization to prolonged hypoxia. There is significant evidence from previous work, including that from the laboratories represented in this section, that the accompanying hypocapnia plays a role as well. Progress has been made, but the problem has not been simplified.

Another contribution of this work may be improved understanding of hypoxia-induced chemoreception itself. The discovery of this phenomenon certainly underscores the fact that the carotid chemoreceptors are likely to be more susceptible to modulation and therefore more complex than "simple" sensory organs such as mechanoreceptors or olfactory chemoreceptors.

21

Ventilatory Response to Hypoxia in High-Altitude Acclimatization

J. V. WEIL AND M. VIZEK

Fascination with the phenomenon of adaptation to high altitude has been an historically important stimulus to research concerned with the control of ventilation in general and with the hypoxic ventilatory response in particular (12). It seems clear that the increase in ventilation in response to the hypoxia of high altitude is important in the preservation of arterial oxygenation in the face of an altitude-induced fall in ambient oxygen tension (10). This chapter reviews evidence that optimal function at high altitude is vitally related to the extent of increase in ventilation, and that ventilation in turn reflects, at least in part, the interaction of the presumed stimulus—the hypoxia of high altitude—with the sensitivity to that stimulus—the hypoxic ventilatory response. Under circumstances where the hypoxic stimulus is relatively constant, as at a fixed altitude, variations in ventilatory sensitivity to hypoxia may be important determinants of both ventilation and performance. In this chapter, we review evidence suggesting that baseline or preascent hypoxic ventilatory response may be important in adjustment to high altitude but that, in addition, following ascent, during the period of acclimatization, there are further increases in the ventilatory response to hypoxia—increases that perhaps are attributable to changes within the carotid body—which may contribute to the progressive rise in ventilation that follows altitude ascent.

Several lines of evidence suggest that human performance at high altitude is in some way positively related to the ventilatory sensitivity to hypoxia measured at low altitude. First, in individuals selected for an ability to complete very high-altitude climbs, hypoxic ventilatory responses are found to be high relative to control subjects lacking such ability (14,18,19). This stands in stark contrast to the low hypoxic ventilatory responsiveness found in individuals possessed of another kind of physical prowess—long-distance running (3,19). The basis for an association between a relatively high hypoxic ventilatory response and the ability to climb (exercise) at high altitude may be in part attributable to the finding that high hypoxic ventilatory responsiveness is not surprisingly associated with a high level of ventilation and better preservation of arterial oxygenation during exercise at altitude (18). It also appears that high hypoxic ventilatory responsiveness may protect against altitude maladaptation. Symptoms of acute mountain sickness have been observed to be infrequent in individuals with a high hypoxic ventilatory responsiveness, and roughly four times more frequent in individuals with a low hypoxic ventilatory response (9).

Thus the hypoxic ventilatory response as measured at low altitude may be a predictor and perhaps a determinant of oxygenation at high altitude. As a result, a vigorous hypoxic ventilatory response may optimize the ability to exercise and minimize the occurrence of symptoms of maladaptation. However, it also seems clear that within the first few hours and days following altitude ascent, the ventilatory response to hypoxia is only partially expressed. It appears that there is a ventilatory dilemma of altitude ascent wherein the rise in ventilation stimulated by hypoxia may, improve oxygenation on the one hand, but also lead to development of inhibitory influences exemplified by, but not limited to, hypocapnic alkalosis, which act to limit the extent of the rise in ventilation produced by hypoxia. This is illustrated by findings illustrated in Fig. 21.1 which demonstrates the changing relationship between ventilation and its presumed stimulus (arterial oxygenation) over successive days in human subjects following ascent to the summit of Pikes Peak. The altitude data are shown in relation to the stimulus–response relationship generated prior to ascent during acute exposure to progressive isocapnic hypoxia (11). It is evident that on the first days following ascent the ventilatory response to the hypoxemia of high altitude fell well below that predicted from the acute isocapnic response. Acute measurements at low altitude suggested that this inhibition could be reproduced by the combined effects of the development of hypocapnia and sustained hypoxic exposure (11). Whatever its cause, this shortfall in ventilation seems to undergo progressive resolution with the passage of time at altitude such that after several days, ventilation at high altitude closely approximates values predicted from the acute isocapnic hypoxic response.

This resolution of the apparently inhibitory aspects of early altitude exposure on ventilatory responsiveness to hypoxia likely reflects the operation of the well-described but poorly understood phenomenon of ventilatory acclimatization to high altitude. Although its mechanism is uncertain, there is a consensus regarding its characteristics (5,20). Typically acclimatization is described as an increase in ventilation beginning within minutes to hours following ascent to high altitude, progressing over several days and perhaps persisting for many years. It is commonly measured as increased ventilation or decreased P_aCO_2 and is associated with a decline in bicarbonate concentration in blood and cerebrospinal fluid (CSF). There are also characteristic changes in the hypercapnic ventilatory response curve, which is both steepened and shifted to the left. There is also residual hyperventilation wherein acclimatization-associated increases in ventilation persist despite relief of hypoxemia by oxygen administration. Several theories have been proposed to explain acclimatization; these include (a) progressive resolution of alkalosis in blood, CSF, or brain interstitium; (b) progressive rise in ventilatory responsiveness, especially the hypercapnic response; (c) a general sensitization of the central nervous system to a variety of ventilatory stimuli; and (d) a progressive improvement

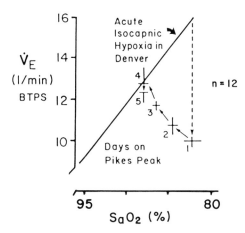

Fig. 21.1 Ventilation ($\dot{V}_E$) versus arterial oxygen saturation (S_aO_2) on 5 successive days following ascent to high altitude (Pikes Peak, 4300 m). The data are shown in relation to the ventilatory response to acute isocapnic hypoxia measured in these subjects prior to ascent (solid line). On the first few days following ascent, ventilation is considerably below values predicted from the acute hypoxic response, but increases progressively. At the end of the exposure period, ventilation closely approximates values measured during acute hypoxia. [Reproduced by permission from Huang, 1984 (11).]

in lung mechanics which would act to enhance the ventilatory expression of the drive to breathe. Although an extensive discussion of each of these theories is beyond the scope of this chapter, it is probably fair to say that although there is some evidence in support of each of these theories, none can be considered established by direct testing as a proven mechanism of ventilatory acclimatization to hypoxia.

It is possible that a progressive rise in ventilatory responsiveness to its stimulus—the hypoxia of high altitude—could contribute to increased ventilation during acclimatization. On the face of it, such an increase in the hypoxic ventilatory response seems probable during acclimatization. This is evidenced in the data displayed in Fig. 21.1, wherein the response, ventilation, increases over time at high altitude despite a progressive decrease in its presumed stimulus (hypoxemia) (11). Indeed if theoretical hypoxic ventilatory responses are constructed by relating stimulus–response points for ventilation and arterial oxygenation for each day at high altitude to the baseline low-altitude point, a fan of lines of increasing slope is generated (Fig. 21.2), which suggests a progressive steepening of the ventilatory response to hypoxia. Recent measurements in human subjects following ascent to the summit of Pikes Peak tend to confirm this prediction; a progressive steepening of the ventilatory response to isocapnic hypoxia over the 7 days following ascent is demonstrated (see Fig. 21.3) (22). This is all the more remarkable because it occurs in the face of hypocapnia, which in acute laboratory studies is a potent depressant of the ventilatory response to hypoxia (21). These findings add to an established controversy regarding the question of changes in the hypoxic ventilatory response during high-altitude acclimatization. Two studies have reported an

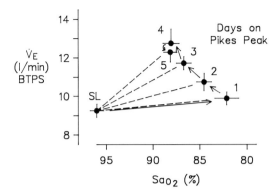

Fig. 21.2 Theoretical ventilatory responses to hypoxia on successive days at high altitude. Response lines were generated from the data shown in Fig. 21.1 by connecting each high-altitude point to the baseline, sea-level (SL) reference values. The increasing ventilatory response to decreasing hypoxemia suggests that the ventilatory response to hypoxia increases during altitude acclimatization.

increased hypoxic response during acclimatization (4,7), whereas four studies found no change (1,13,15,16). Reasons for the discrepant results are unclear, but substantial differences in study design and in techniques for measuring hypoxic ventilatory response probably contributed. However, even the finding of an unchanged hypoxic ventilatory response during altitude acclimatization suggests potentiation because, as mentioned previously, concomitant hypocapnia would have been expected to depress the hypoxic response.

In an attempt to clarify further the question of alterations in the hypoxic ven-

Fig. 21.3 Ventilatory responses to acute isocapnic hypoxia following ascent to the summit of Pikes Peak (4300 m). $\dot{V}_E$ BTPS: ventilation–body temperature and pressure, saturated. These measurements, in a group of 7 human subjects, show a progressive increase in the hypoxic ventilatory response despite the development of increasing hypocapnia. [Data taken from White, 1987 (22).]

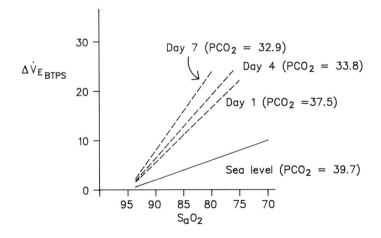

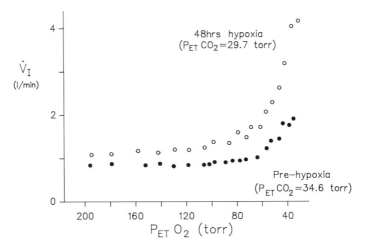

Fig. 21.4 Increased ventilatory response to acute isocapnic progressive hypoxia before and after exposure to hypobaric hypoxia in a single cat. This animal was illustrative of the entire group, showing an increase in the hypoxic ventilatory response following exposure to simulated altitude despite the development of hypocapnia.

tilatory response during acclimatization, we undertook a series of studies in cats exposed to simulated altitude in a hypobaric chamber with the goal of assessing changes in the hypoxic ventilatory response and to explore potential mechanisms of any changes that might be found. Cats were intubated under α-chloralose–urethan anesthesia with measurement of the isocapnic ventilatory response to progressive hypoxia with P_{CO_2} maintained at resting, baseline values. Anesthesia was carefully maintained to abolish pain stimulus-withdrawal but to preserve the corneal reflex and produce minimal ventilatory depression (i.e., P_{CO_2} below 38 torr or within ± 2 torr of unanesthtized baseline values). These initial screening measurements were used to assign animals to two groups comprised of seven animals each, one serving as a control and the other undergoing subsequent altitude exposure. Baseline measurements were then made in animals of both groups during anesthesia. Animals in the experimental group were then exposed to simulated altitude in a hypobaric chamber maintained at a barometric pressure of 440 torr, roughly equivalent to an altitude of 15,000 feet, for 48 h. Animals in the control group were maintained at ambient altitude. Immediately after the exposure, anesthesia was induced and preexposure measurements were repeated. In altitude-exposed animals, hypoxia was maintained with a low-oxygen inspiratory gas mixture, from the termination of hypobaric exposure to the time of measurement of the ventilatory responses. We found that hypocapnia developed in animals exposed to simulated altitude, evidenced by a fall in P_{CO_2} from 34.5 ± 0.9 to 28.9 ± 1.2 torr ($p < .05$), whereas no change was observed in the pre- and postexposure periods for the control group (34.8 ± 0.7 vs. 34.5 ± 0.7 torr). The decrement in P_{CO_2} that followed altitude acclimatization persisted during acute normoxia. Ventilatory responses to hypoxia were measured during progressive isocapnic hypoxia with P_{CO_2} maintained within 2 torr of baseline values. The ventilatory response to hypoxia was increased after simulated altitude exposure (see Fig. 21.4). When expressed as the shape parameter A, the hypoxic ventilatory response increased from 24.9 ± 2.6 to 35.2 ± 5.6 ($p < .05$), whereas no change was observed in the control group (25.7 ± 3.2 vs. 23.1 ± 2.7, $p = $ NS). Thus despite the development of hypocapnia, which, as mentioned above, acutely depresses the ventilatory response to hypoxia, we observed an increase in the ventilatory response to hypoxia in cats after 48 h of exposure to simulated altitude.

These observations raised the question of whether increases in the ventilatory response to hypoxia might be related to increased sensitivity of the carotid body to hypoxia. Several lines of evidence suggest that the carotid body may play a critical role in acclimatization. Most, although not all, studies suggest that peripheral chemoreceptor denervation blocks acclimatization (20). Further, in addition to the data already reviewed concerning the possibility of increased ventilatory responsiveness to hypoxia during acclimatization to altitude, acclimatization seems also to be associated with increased sensitivity to several other stimuli thought to be relatively selective for the peripheral chemoreceptors, including brief CO_2 exposure (17) and the administration of doxapram and cyanide (8). In addition, recent studies reviewed by Bisgard and colleagues (2; see also Chap. 22, this volume) suggest that hypoxia limited to the carotid body by isolated perfusion techniques produces a slow, progressive rise in ventilation which closely resembles acclimatization.

In order to determine whether development of acclimatization was associated with enhancement of the hypoxic sensitivity of the carotid body, we undertook measurements of the neural output of the carotid body in the control and altitude-exposed groups outlined above. These measurements could be made only once on each animal and were done for both groups at the time of the postexposure ventilatory measurements. The carotid sinus nerve was exposed just above the carotid body and stripped of surrounding tissue; we eliminated baroreceptor discharge by stripping the adventitia over the surface of the carotid sinus. Carotid body neural output was recorded from the uncut, whole desheathed nerve with platinum bipolar electrodes. Nerve signals were processed with a technique based on the principle that the number of active fibers and the activity of individual fibers are determinants of interspike amplitude summation (6). As a result, an increase in the number of active fibers or in the activity of individual fibers increases the variability or range of signal amplitude, which can be measured as amplitude variance of the whole-nerve signal. Because absolute values are confounded by differences in nerve geometry and electrode–nerve contact, the results are expressed as the ratio of observed to baseline variances in quantitations of responses to hypoxia. Carotid sinus nerve activity measured in this fashion is tightly correlated with oxygen tension, and the response has a configuration and magnitude comparable to that seen with ventilation (Fig. 21.5). Because the response could be measured on only one occasion, comparisons were made between control and altitude-exposed groups. Overall, carotid body responses to hypoxia were substantially greater in the altitude-exposed than in the control group: The sinus nerve response to hypoxia, measured as the shape parameter A, averaged 44.5 ± 8.2 after altitude exposure compared with a value of 24.2 ± 4.7 in the control group ($p < .05$). To eliminate the potential effects of afferent activity flowing from the central nervous system to the carotid body in the carotid sinus nerve, we repeated the hypoxic response measurement after sectioning the nerve and recording from the distal (carotid body)

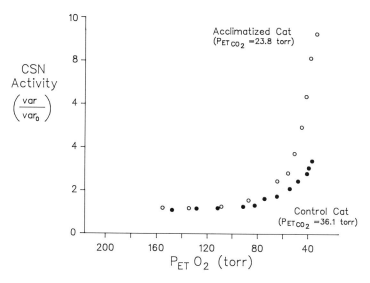

Fig. 21.5 The response of carotid sinus nerve (CSN) activity to progressive isocapnic hypoxia in a representative control cat, compared with the response in a cat after a 48-h exposure to hypobaric hypoxia. Peripheral chemoreceptor responses to hypoxia were increased in the acclimatized group in comparison with values measured in controls.

segment. This had a slight, nonsignificant attenuating effect on the shape parameter A in acclimatized animals, but the difference between control and acclimatized groups persisted, suggesting that descending sinus nerve activity did not account for the increased carotid sinus nerve response to hypoxia which was seen following acclimatization.

Because the ventilatory and carotid sinus nerve responses to hypoxia were measured simultaneously, it was possible to estimate the relationship between the hypoxia-induced increase in carotid sinus nerve input to the central nervous system and the resulting ventilatory output. Cross-plots of ventilation against carotid sinus nerve activity are linear, reflecting the similarity of shape of ventilatory and carotid sinus nerve responses to hypoxia; furthermore, the slope of this relationship may provide useful information concerning the characteristics of central translation of peripheral chemoreceptor into ventilatory activity. Plots of carotid sinus nerve activity versus ventilation produced lines of comparable slope for control and acclimatized groups (Fig. 21.6). This finding suggests that acclimatization did not enhance central translation of peripheral chemoreceptor activity into ventilation.

Thus, although the mechanism of ventilatory acclimatization to altitude remains to be elucidated, it is apparent that the phenomenon is characterized by a progressive increase in ventilation despite a decrease in the hypoxic stimulus to ventilation. This suggests that there may be a heightened ventilatory sensitivity to hypoxia, which is borne out by recent studies in humans, goats, and cats. The increased ventilatory sensitivity to hypoxia is paralleled by, and possibly attribut-

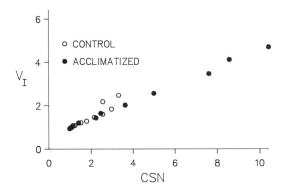

Fig. 21.6 A cross-plot of inspiratory ventilation (V_I) in relation to carotid sinus nerve (CSN) activity. This plot illustrates the characteristics of central nervous system (CNS) translation of input to the CNS via the carotid sinus nerve in relation to ventilatory output during progressive isocapnic hypoxia. Results shown here, for a single control and a single acclimatized cat, suggest that hypoxic exposure had no effect on the characteristics of central translation of chemoreceptor activity into ventilation.

able to, increased carotid body responsiveness to hypoxia. Thus the increasing ventilation during acclimatization may in part reflect a direct or indirect action of hypoxia on the carotid body which acts to heighten the sensitivity of the peripheral chemoreceptor to the hypoxic stimulus (see also Bisgard et al.; Lahiri et al., Chaps. 22 and 23, respectively). However, it must be kept in mind that the perpetuation of increased ventilation of acclimatization following restoration of normoxia by oxygen administration or following section of the carotid sinus nerves indicates that other factors must be invoked to explain the perpetuation, if not the genesis of, ventilatory acclimatization to high altitude.

ACKNOWLEDGMENT
    This work was supported by Program Project Grant HL-14985 from the National Heart, Lung, and Blood Institute.

REFERENCES

1. Astrand, P. The respiratory activity in man exposed to prolonged hypoxia. *Acta Physiol. Scand. 30:* 342–368, 1953.
2. Busch, M. A., G. E. Bisgard, and H. V. Forster. Ventilatory acclimatization to hypoxia is not dependent on arterial hypoxemia. *J. Appl. Physiol. 58:* 1874–1880, 1985.
3. Byrne-Quinn, E., J. V. Weil, I. E. Sodal, G. F. Filley, and R. F. Grover. Ventilatory control in the athlete. *J. Appl. Physiol. 30:* 91–98, 1971.
4. Cruz, J. C., J. T. Reeves, R. F. Grover, J. T. Maher, R. E. McCullough, A. Cymerman, and J. C. Denniston. Ventilatory acclimatization to high altitude is prevented by CO_2 breathing. *Respiration 39:* 121–123, 1980.
5. Dempsey, J. A., and H. V. Forster. Mediation of ventilatory adaptations. *Physiol. Rev. 62:* 262–346, 1982.

6. Dick, D. E., J. R. Meyer, and J. V. Weil. A new approach to quantitation of whole nerve bundle activity. *J. Appl. Physiol. 36*(3): 393–397, 1974.

7. Forster, H. V., J. A. Dempsey, M. L. Birnbaum, W. G. Reddan, J. Thoden, R. F. Grover, and J. Rankin. Effect of chronic exposure to hypoxia on ventilatory response to CO_2 and hypoxia. *J. Appl. Physiol. 31:* 586–592, 1971.

8. Forster, H. V., J. A. Dempsey, E. Vidruk, and G. DoPico. Evidence of altered regulation of ventilation during exposure to hypoxia. *Respir. Physiol. 20:* 379–392, 1974.

9. Hackett, P. H., J. T. Reeves, R. F. Grover, and J. V. Weil. Ventilation in human populations native to high altitude. In: *High Altitude and Man,* ed. J. West and S. Lahiri. Bethesda: Am. Physiol. Soc., pp. 179–191.

10. Houston, C. S., and R. L. Riley. Respiratory and circulatory changes during acclimatization to high altitude. *Am. J. Physiol. 149:* 565–588, 1974.

11. Huang, S. Y., J. K. Alexander, R. F. Grover, J. Mahler, R. E. McCullough, R. G. McCullough, L. G. Moore, J. B. Sampson, J. V. Weil, and J. T. Reeves. Hypercapnia and sustained hypoxia blunt ventilation on arrival at high altitude. *J. Appl. Physiol. 56:* 602–606, 1984.

12. Kellogg, R. Altitude acclimatization, a historical introduction emphasizing the regulation of breathing. *Physiologist 11:* 37–57, 1968.

13. Lahiri, S. Dynamic aspects of regulation of ventilation in man during acclimatization to high altitude. *Respir. Physiol. 16:* 245–285, 1972.

14. Masuyama, S., H. Kimura, T. Sugita, T. Kuriyama, K. Tatsumi, F. Kunitomo, S. Okita, H. Tojima, Y. Yuguchi, S. Watanabe, and Y. Honda. Control of ventilation in extreme-altitude climbers. *J. Appl. Physiol. 61*(2): 500–506, 1986.

15. Michel, C. C., and J. S. Milledge. Respiratory regulation in man during acclimatization to high altitude. *J. Physiol. (Lond.) 168:* 631–643, 1963.

16. Milledge, J. S., and S. Lahiri. Respiratory control in lowlanders and Sherpa Highlanders at altitude. *Respir. Physiol. 2:* 310–322, 1967.

17. Pande, J. N., S. P. Gupia, and J. S. Guleria. Ventilatory response to inhaled CO_2 at high altitude. *Respiration 31:* 473–483, 1974.

18. Schoene, R. B., and S. Lahiri, P. H. Hackett, R. M. Peters, Jr., J. S. Milledge, C. J. Maret, and J. B. West. Relationship of hypoxic ventilatory response to exercise performance on Mount Everest. *J. Appl. Physiol. 57:* 1478–1483, 1984.

19. Schoene, R. B., and R. Saxon. Control of ventilation in climbers to extreme altitude. *J. Appl. Physiol. 53:* 886–890, 1982.

20. Weil, J. V. Ventilatory control at high altitude. In: *Handbook of Physiology,* Sec. 3: *The Respiratory System,* Vol. 2: *Control of Breathing,* ed. N. S. Cherniack and J. G. Widdicombe. Bethesda: Am. Physiol. Soc., 1986, pp. 703–727.

21. Weil, J. V., E. Byrne-Quinn, I. E. Sodal, W. D. Friesen, B. Underhill, G. F. Filley, and R. F. Grover. Hypoxic ventilatory drive in normal man. *J. Clin. Invest. 49:* 1061–1072, 1970.

22. White, D. P., K. Gleeson, C. K. Pickett, A. M. Rannels, A. Cymerman, and J. V. Weil. Altitude acclimatization: influence on periodic breathing and chemoresponsiveness during sleep. *J. Appl. Physiol., 63:* 401–412, 1987.

22

Mechanisms of Ventilatory Acclimatization to Hypoxia in Goats

G. E. BISGARD, A. NIELSEN, E. VIDRUK, L. DARISTOTLE, M. ENGWALL, AND H. V. FORSTER

Previous studies have indicated the importance of the presence of the carotid chemoreceptors in the time-dependent hyperventilation on exposure to hypoxia, a phenomenon termed *ventilatory acclimatization* (VAH) (10,20). The role of the peripheral chemoreceptors has usually been considered to be necessary to initiate hyperventilation upon hypoxic exposure, but other mechanisms were thought to cause VAH. Some of these proposed mechanisms have included acidification of cerebral interstitial fluid in the environment of the central chemoreceptors (7), change in brain monoamine metabolism (16), and suprapontine facilitation of respiratory activity (18). All of these mechanisms, associated with the presence of cerebral hypoxia, may play some role in modulating the ventilatory response to sustained hypoxia. However, on the basis of studies we have carried out in the past few years, we believe that the carotid chemoreceptors play a major role in the mechanism of VAH.

We used a method to isolate and perfuse the carotid bodies of awake goats with hypoxic blood ($P_aO_2 = 39$ torr) in order to determine if brain hypoxia was a necessary component in the mechanism of VAH (3,5). We found that the early phase (the first 4–6 h) of VAH could proceed in the absence of brain hypoxia (Fig. 22.1). These results did not reveal the site of the increasing ventilatory drive; therefore, we decided to attempt to use another mode of carotid body stimulation in the awake goat perfusion model, namely hypercapnia. We reasoned that if CNS mechanisms were responsible for VAH, then the stimulus mode at the carotid body should not matter. The assumption in this case was that steady-state hypoxic or hypercapnic stimulation would cause a steady-state response from the carotid body and, further, that the CNS structures receiving afferent input from the carotid chemoreceptors could not distinguish between modes of stimuli at the carotid body. Unlike the response to hypoxia, we found that there was no time-dependent change

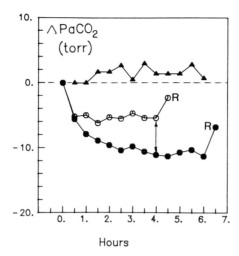

Fig. 22.1 Hyperventilation expressed as mean change in arterial P_{CO_2} during perfusion of the carotid body in awake goats: (▲) control normoxic–normocapnic perfusion ($n = 3$); (●) isocapnic–hypoxic perfusion ($P_{cb}O_2 = 40$ torr, $P_{cb}CO_2 = 39$ torr; $n = 6$); (O) hypercapnic–normoxic perfusion ($P_aCO_2 = 78$ torr, $P_{cb}O_2 = 100$ torr; $n = 6$). With hypoxic perfusion of the carotid body there was a time-dependent hyperventilation (acclimatization), whereas with hypercapnic perfusion no acclimatization occurred. R indicates a return to control conditions. [Adapted by permission from Bisgard et al. (2), 1986.]

in the ventilatory response to carotid body hypercapnia, that is, no acclimatization (Fig. 22.1) (2). These results suggested the possibility that the carotid body itself was increasing its activity in a time-dependent manner with hypoxic stimulation, but not with hypercapnic stimulation.

In order to explore further the responses of the carotid chemoreceptors to sustained hypoxic and hypercapnic stimuli, we have carried out the following studies in which chemoreceptor activity was recorded from single afferent fibers in anesthetized goats.

METHODS

Adult goats of several breeds were utilized. In each study the animal was anesthetized initially with intravenous thiamylal sodium (15 mg/kg) followed by continuous intravenous α-chloralose (5–15 mg/kg/h). Immediately after induction of anesthesia, femoral arterial and venous catheters were inserted to allow monitoring of arterial blood pressure, measurement of acid–base and blood gases, and administration of fluids. It was considered essential to maintain normal arterial blood homeostasis throughout the long period of dissection prior to neural recording. Thus, frequent blood sampling was carried out, and supplemental O_2 was administered and/or artificial ventilation was instituted as needed. End-tidal CO_2 was monitored continuously.

The carotid sinus nerve was dissected free and severed at its junction with the glossopharyngeal nerve. It was placed on a stainless-steel dissection platform, and the nerve sheath was removed. The nerve was split into small fibers by trial and error until a single chemoreceptor unit was isolated for study using unipolar recording methods. During neural dissection and recording, the animal was paralyzed with intravenous gallamine hydrochloride (1.5 mg/kg initially, followed by 0.75 mg/kg every 30 min) and artificially ventilated. Single units were identified by their typical brisk response to intravenous NaCN (50 μg/kg) and increasing activity with acute hypoxia.

Single-unit frequency was recorded for each steady-state measurement for 3 min, bracketing an arterial blood sample. The mean frequency was expressed as impulses per second (imp/s).

RESULTS

Hypoxia Data

Throughout the period of surgical preparation and control recording of single-unit activity, arterial acid–base and blood gases were controlled near levels in normoxic awake goats (pH = 7.39 $\pm$ 0.01, P_aO_2 = 96 $\pm$ 3 torr, P_aCO_2 = 39 $\pm$ 1 torr [mean $\pm$ SE]). During hypoxia, arterial blood gases were maintained at levels we had previously used in carotid body perfusion studies in awake goats (pH = 7.38 $\pm$ 0.01, P_aO_2 = 39 $\pm$ 1 torr, P_aCO_2 = 38 $\pm$ 1 torr).

Our goal was to record single-unit activity for 4 h in a given single chemoreceptor fiber. We obtained data from 7 fibers for at least 3.5 h, and in 3 other fibers for a minimum of 2 h. It required about 20 min to reach steady-state hypoxia in these studies. In the first 60 min of recording, it was apparent that there was a constant firing frequency. However, beyond the end of the first hour, the mean firing rate increased at the rate of 1.7 imp/s/h ($p < .01$, $r = .87$). Only one of 10 fibers failed to increase its firing frequency (Fig. 22.2). In two animals, blood gases were maintained in the normoxic control range during prolonged recording. There was no systematic change in their firing frequency (Fig. 22.2).

Hypercapnia Data

Control arterial blood gases and acid–base variables were similar to those achieved for the hypoxia studies (pH = 7.40 $\pm$ 0.01, P_aO_2 = 102 $\pm$ 2, P_aCO_2 = 40 $\pm$ 1). During steady-state hypercapnia, mean values were as follows: pH, 7.09 $\pm$ 0.02; P_aO_2, 105 $\pm$ 4; and P_aCO_2, 91 $\pm$ 3.

We recorded steady-state chemoreceptor frequency for more than 3.5 h of hypercapnia in 4 animals and for at least 2.3 h in 2 other animals. The response of single-unit chemoreceptor afferents to acute hypercapnia was brisk and was characterized by an overshoot relative to the steady-state response that followed. Throughout the sustained hypercapnia, mean chemoreceptor frequency remained elevated 3.5 fold above the normocapnic level; however, there was a moderate time-dependent reduction in chemoreceptor firing frequency (mean = 21.5%) in 3

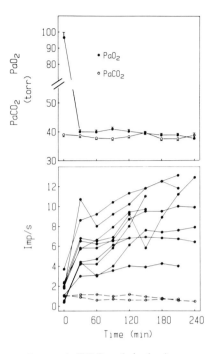

Fig. 22.2 Arterial blood gases (mean ± SEM) and single chemoreceptor unit frequency during a period (up to 4 h) of steady-state isocapnic hypoxia. Dashed lines in the lower panel indicate control studies in which normoxic–normocapnic conditions were maintained.

of the 4 fibers in which chemoreceptor activity was measured for more than 3.5 h. In the remaining fiber, frequency increased by 25% over the period (Fig. 22.3).

DISCUSSION

The data obtained indicate a clear difference between carotid chemoreceptor responses to sustained hypoxia and hypercapnia in the anesthetized goat. These results provide further evidence that the transduction processes within the carotid body for hypoxia and hypercapnia are different. Other investigators have described differing physiological and metabolic responses between these two stimuli (8,9,15). The chemoreceptor responses to hypoxia were compatible with the time course of ventilatory responses obtained in awake goats subjected to hypoxic perfusion of the carotid body (3,5) and ventilatory increase in goats subjected to hypobaric hypoxia (10,20). The response to sustained hypercapnia was also similar to the ventilatory response of the awake goat to hypercapnic carotid body perfusion (2), although results of the present studies suggest that some adaptation of afferent chemoreceptor activity may occur with sustained hypercapnia. The results of the present studies strongly support time-dependent increasing activity of the carotid chemoreceptors as contributing significantly to the early phase of VAH in goats.

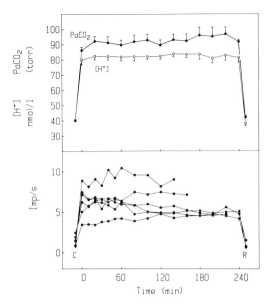

Fig. 22.3 Arterial blood gases (mean ± SEM) and single chemoreceptor unit frequency during a period (up to 4 h) of steady-state hypercapnic normoxia.

We are aware of only one other report of afferent carotid chemoreceptor activity recorded for a period of 4 or more hours of isocapnic hypoxia. In that study, no time-dependent change in afferent chemoreceptor activity was found in anesthetized cats (1). This may reflect a species difference in the time course of acclimatization which varies widely among species (6). The time course of VAH in cats during the first hours of hypoxia is not well described. After 3 or more weeks of hypoxia in cats, an increased carotid chemoreceptor firing rate has been found (14). In these studies the increased firing frequency in response to hypoxia occurred only after the whole carotid sinus nerve was severed, suggesting that efferent innervation of the carotid chemoreceptor modulated the increased activity (see also Lahiri et al., Chap. 23, this volume).

The possibility that hypoxic ventilatory chemosensitivity increases in human subjects during or after ventilatory acclimatization to hypoxia was examined previously (reviewed by Weil, ref. 21). There was no agreement as to the results of these studies. Some reported increased responses to acute hypoxia (11) whereas others found no change (13). Forster et al. found an increase not only in the ventilatory response to acute hypoxia (11), but also in the response to intravenous doxapram infusion, which suggested an effect mediated via the peripheral chemoreceptors (12). More recently, two reports indicate an augmented ventilatory response to acute hypoxia during altitude sojourn, providing new evidence to support that viewpoint (19,22). These studies did not reveal whether the increase was due to greater peripheral chemoreceptor responsivity or to an augmented CNS response to the input from the peripheral arterial chemoreceptors. Our data are compatible with an increase in ventilatory response to hypoxia and suggest that increased peripheral chemoreceptor afferent output contributes to this response.

What mechanisms could be responsible for time-dependent increases in carotid body activity during hypoxia? The mechanism remains unknown at the present time. The following possibilities may be considered: (a) time-dependent changes in efferent neural influences on the carotid body, which could include either diminished inhibitory activity of the carotid sinus efferent pathway or facilitation via sympathetic efferents (17); (b) facilitation via circulating agents such as catecholamines; or (c) intrinsic mechanisms within the carotid body itself, such as increased metabolism and activity of neurochemical facilitatory processes or diminished inhibitory mechanisms—for example, depletion of an inhibitory neurotransmitter.

Because the carotid sinus nerve was cut in the present studies, any possible inhibitory efferents via that pathway were eliminated; however, in the awake goat carotid body perfusion studies, all innervation of the carotid body was intact (2,3,5). These findings, taken together with our present neural recording data, would suggest that the presence of intact efferent pathways does not eliminate the time-dependent response of the carotid body to prolonged hypoxia.

We previously proposed that depletion of the putative inhibitory carotid body neurotransmitter, dopamine, could be responsible for the increasing activity associated with hypoxia (2). We tested this hypothesis by administering a peripheral dopamine antagonist, domperidone, to awake goats before and during hypoxic exposure (4). The data obtained indicated some increase in the acute response to hypoxia and a modified rate of acclimatization after drug treatment. However, the results were not clear enough to firmly support or refute the hypothesis. These findings encourage use of another approach to more adequately examine the potential role of carotid body dopaminergic mechanisms.

ACKNOWLEDGMENTS
We wish to express our thanks to Margaret Zuba, Gordon Johnson, and Kathleen Gilmore for their assistance. This study was supported by NIH Grant HL-15473.

REFERENCES

1. Andronikou, S., and S. Lahiri. Prolongation of isocapnic hypoxia did not alter carotid chemosensory response. *Fed. Proc. 45:* 160, 1986.
2. Bisgard, G. E., M. A. Busch, L. Daristotle, A. D. Berssenbrugge, and H. V. Forster. Carotid body hypercapnia does not elicit ventilatory acclimatization in goats. *Respir. Physiol. 65:* 113–125, 1986.
3. Bisgard, G. E., M. A. Busch, and H. V. Forster. Ventilatory acclimatization to hypoxia is not dependent upon cerebral hypocapnic alkalosis. *J. Appl. Physiol. 60:* 1011–1015, 1986.
4. Bisgard, G. E., N. A. Kressin, A. M. Nielsen, L. Daristotle, C. A. Smith, and H. V. Forster. The effects of carotid body dopamine receptor blockade on ventilatory acclimatization to hypoxia. *Fed. Proc. 44:* 1001, 1985.
5. Busch, M. A., G. E. Bisgard, and H. V. Forster. Ventilatory acclimatization to hypoxia is not dependent on arterial hypoxemia. *J. Appl. Physiol. 58:* 1874–1880, 1985.
6. Dempsey, J. A., and H. V. Forster. Mediation of ventilatory adaptations. *Physiol. Rev. 62:* 262–346, 1982.

7. Fencl, V., R. A. Gabel, and D. Wolfe. Composition of cerebral fluids in goats adapted to high altitude. *J. Appl. Physiol. 47:* 508–513, 1979.

8. Fitzgerald, R. S., and G. A. Dehghani. Neural responses of the cat carotid and aortic bodies to hypercapnia and hypoxia. *J. Appl. Physiol. 52:* 596–601, 1982.

9. Fitzgerald, R. S., P. Garger, M. C. Hauer, H. Raff, and L. Fechter. Effect of hypoxia and hypercapnia on catecholamine content of the cat carotid body. *J. Appl. Physiol. 54:* 1408–1413, 1983.

10. Forster, H. V., G. E. Bisgard, and J. P. Klein. Effect of peripheral chemoreceptor denervation on acclimatization of goats during hypoxia. *J. Appl. Physiol. 50:* 392–398, 1981.

11. Forster, H. V., J. A. Dempsey, M. L. Birnbaum, W. G. Reddan, J. S. Thoden, R. F. Grover, and J. Rankin. Comparison of ventilatory responses to hypoxic and hypercapnic stimuli in altitude-sojourning lowlanders, lowlanders residing at altitude, and native altitude residents. *Fed. Proc. 28:* 1274–1279, 1969.

12. Forster, H. V., J. A. Dempsey, E. Vidruk, and G. DoPico. Evidence of altered regulation of ventilation during exposure to hypoxia. *Respir. Physiol. 20:* 379–392, 1974.

13. Gabel, R. A., and R. B. Weikopf. Ventilatory interaction between hypoxia and [H$^+$] at chemoreceptors of man. *J. Appl. Physiol. 39:* 292–296, 1975.

14. Lahiri, S., N. Smatresk, M. Pokorski, P. Barnard, and A. Mokashi. Efferent inhibition of carotid body chemoreception in chronically hypoxic cats. *Am. J. Physiol. 245:* R678–R673, 1983.

15. Mulligan, E., and S. Lahiri. Separation of carotid body chemoreceptor responses to O$_2$ and CO$_2$ by oligomycin and antimycin A. *Am. J. Physiol. 242:* C200–C206, 1982.

16. Olson, E. B., Jr., E. H. Vidruk, D. R. McCrimmon, and J. A. Dempsey. Monoamine neurotransmitter metabolism during acclimatization to hypoxia in rats. *Respir. Physiol. 54:* 79–96, 1983.

17. O'Regan, R. G., and S. Majcherczyk. Control of peripheral chemoreceptors by efferent nerves. In: *Physiology of the Peripheral Arterial Chemoreceptors,* ed. H. Acker and R. G. O'Regan. Amsterdam: Elsevier, 1983, pp. 257–298.

18. Ou, L. C., W. M. St. John, and S. M. Tenney. The contribution of central mechanisms rostral to the pons in ventilatory acclimatization. *Respir. Physiol. 54:* 343–351, 1983.

19. Roach, R. C., R. B. Schoene, P. H. Hackett, H. Donner, and C. Woodland. Operation Everest II: Peripheral and central ventilatory chemosensitivity increases with exposure to hypobaric hypoxia. *Fed. Proc. 45:* 883, 1986.

20. Smith, C. A., G. E. Bisgard, A. M. Nielsen, L. Daristotle, N. A. Kressin, H. V. Forster, and J. A. Dempsey. Carotid bodies are required for ventilatory acclimatization to moderate and severe chronic hypoxemia. *J. Appl. Physiol. 60:* 1003–1010, 1986.

21. Weil, J. V. Ventilatory control at high altitude. In: *Handbook of Physiology,* Sec. 3: *The Respiratory System,* Vol. 2: *Control of Breathing,* ed. N. S. Cherniack and J. G. Widdicombe. Bethesda: Am. Physiol. Soc., 1986, pp. 703–727.

22. White, D. P., K. Gleeson, and J. V. Weil. The influence of altitude acclimatization on awake respiratory chemosensitivity and ventilation during sleep. *Fed. Proc. 45:* 1031, 1986.

23

Mechanisms of Carotid Body Responses to Chronic Low and High Oxygen Pressures

S. LAHIRI, E. MULLIGAN, N. J. SMATRESK, P. BARNARD,
A. MOKASHI, D. TORBATI, M. POKORSKI, R. ZHANG,
P. G. DATA, AND K. ALBERTINE

The carotid and aortic bodies (the peripheral chemoreceptors) monitor arterial blood gases and generate electrical activity in the chemoreceptor afferents (4–6). This activity is also influenced by arterial blood temperature, by arterial osmolarity, and by humoral substances (3–5). Part of the activity is dependent on local blood flow, which is also regulated by arterial blood gases (3–5). Thus, a dual chemosensing system determines carotid chemoreceptor activity.

Because the arterial blood gases oscillate with rhythmic respiration, the chemosensory discharges also oscillate, in turn influencing breath-by-breath respiration. Accordingly, these chemoreceptors came to be closely identified with the control of respiration. A less known integrative function of these chemoreceptors is their input into the control of autonomic nervous system and hence their indirect control of several other systems, particularly the cardiovascular system.

The peripheral chemoreceptor cells respond to arterial blood oxygen *tension* rather than *content*. The source of oxygen is the ambient air, and the atmospheric oxygen pressure is a determinant of arterial oxygen pressure. The other natural stimulus, CO_2, does not derive from the external environment. It is generated from within the internal environment, from oxidative metabolism. One may therefore advance the viewpoint that the peripheral chemoreceptors were originally designed to monitor arterial oxygen. Accordingly, the peripheral chemoreceptors might be expected to undergo cellular changes in conditions of chronic low and high arterial oxygen pressure, and the specific cellular expressions could possibly be used as a guide to investigate the oxygen-sensitive mechanisms. The hypothesis to be investigated here is that a lack of stimulus due to high chronic oxygen pressure and an increased stimulus to the chemoreceptors due to low oxygen pressure would cause changes in the structure and function of the oxygen-sensitive chemoreceptor cells.

In this study, we investigated the effects of chronic exposure of animals to low and high oxygen pressures on carotid body (a) chemosensory responses to natural arterial blood gas stimuli; (b) putative neurotransmitter metabolism; and (c) cellular ultrastructure.

METHODS

Cats and rats were used as experimental animals. For chronic hypoxia or hyperoxia, the animals were exposed to appropriate low (10%) or high (50% and 100%) concentrations of inspired oxygen at sea level. Each group of experimental animals was matched by appropriate controls.

Carotid body chemosensory responses were measured in anesthetized cats as described previously (9). Biogenic amines were measured by high-performance liquid chromatography or by mass fragmentography in rat and cat carotid bodies. For structural studies, carotid bodies were fixed in situ with buffered glutaraldehyde. Thin sections of the carotid body were made, and morphometry (13) was performed on electron micrographs for these sections.

RESULTS

Effects of Prolonged and Chronic Hypoxia

Carotid Chemosensory Responses

Cats were exposed to 10% inspired O_2 for 21–49 days. Carotid body chemoreceptor afferents were prepared without injuring the bulk of the nerve, and the chemoreceptor responses to hypoxia were measured at a constant level of P_aCO_2. These responses were compared with those in appropriate control cats which were maintained at sea level, breathing room air.

The results from these experiments are described under three categories: (a) activity of chemoreceptor afferents from an otherwise intact carotid sinus nerve (CSN); (b) efferent inhibition of the chemosensory discharge; and (c) mechanism of efferent inhibition.

The effects of chronic hypoxia of 28 days' duration on carotid body chemosensory responses to hypoxia are shown in Fig. 23.1. The mean of 16 afferents each from the chronically hypoxic and normoxic groups are compared. Arterial pH values were similar, although the P_aCO_2 levels in the chronically hypoxic cats were lower. Both of the responses were hyperbolic, but those of the chronically hypoxic group were significantly greater, despite a lower P_aCO_2 (2).

We also observed that with sectioning of the main trunk of the CSN, the hypoxic responses in the chronically hypoxic group were further augmented relative to the control (2, for review, see 6). These observations demonstrated that the chemosensory responses to hypoxia were partially suppressed by the carotid chemoreceptor efferent activity in chronic hypoxia. Dopamine receptor blockade by haloperidol (primarily a D_2 receptor blocker) augmented the chemosensory respon-

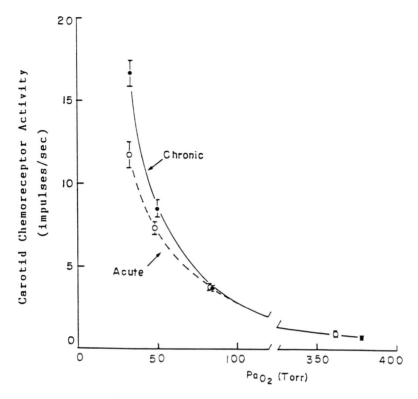

Fig. 23.1 Effects of chronic hypoxia (inspired P_{O_2} = 70 torr for 28 days) on carotid chemo-sensory responses (●————●) are compared with those of control cats (O---O). The discharge rates of single chemoreceptor afferents (n = 16) are given as means $\pm$ SEM. The arterial pH values were 7.373 $\pm$ 0.01 and 7.364 $\pm$ 0.03, and the P_aCO_2 values were 31.8 $\pm$ 1.0 and 23.3 $\pm$ 0.7 torr in control and chronically hypoxic cats, respectively.

ses to hypoxia in both control and chronically hypoxic groups. This augmentation was significantly greater in the latter group. Dopamine receptor blockade also eliminated the effect of sectioning the CSN on the chemosensory responses to hypoxia. These results strongly suggested that the augmented efferent inhibition during chronic hypoxia was dopaminergic (for review, see 6,11).

In summary, hypoxic sensitivity of carotid chemoreceptors increased after exposure to chronic hypoxia of several weeks' duration. Simultaneously, the efferent inhibition of the response also increased. Without this inhibition, the effect of chronic hypoxia on the chemosensory response would be even greater. The efferent inhibition was dopaminergic. The effect of chronic hypoxia on the cat carotid body required more than several hours to develop, which may be coincident with the synthesis and greater turnover rate of neurotransmitters and with cellular growth (see later).

An implication of the enhanced chemosensory response to chronic hypoxia is that it may be responsible for the ventilatory acclimatization to chronic hypoxia (see Weil and Visek; Bisgard et al., Chaps. 21 and 22, this volume). However, an increase in ventilation at a given inspired P_{O_2} also raises arterial P_{O_2} and lowers P_{CO_2} and [H^+]. Consequently, the chemosensory activity gained by the sensitivity increase may be substantially lost as a result of a concomitant increase in arterial P_{O_2} and a decrease in arterial P_{CO_2}. Without the increased sensitivity of the chemoreceptors to hypoxia, the contribution of the carotid body to ventilatory acclimatization would be diminished.

Neuromodulators

Chronic hypoxia led to striking increases in the levels of carotid body dopamine and norepinephrine in the rat (4–6). Acute hypoxia is known to release carotid body dopamine (5). If the release is dependent on the carotid body dopamine level, the total amount of dopamine release would increase in chronic hypoxia, and hence its effect on the chemosensory discharge would also increase. It is known that exogenous dopamine suppresses chemosensory responses to moderate hypoxia in the cat (4,6). Thus, the augmented efferent inhibition, which is dopaminergic, may be related to the enhanced dopamine release in chronic hypoxia.

The carotid body also contains neuropeptides (4). If these putative neurotransmitters are in the same vesicles as the dopamine, as occurs in the vesicles in the adrenal medullary cells, they may be released during hypoxia by the same processes as dopamine. Indeed, it has been reported that the neuropeptide substance P, is released from the carotid body during hypoxia (see Fidone et al., Chap. 10, this volume). It is not known, however, whether the turnover rate and content of the neuropeptides are increased during chronic hypoxia (4).

Acetylcholine, another putative neurotransmitter, is also released from the carotid body during acute hypoxia (4). However, the effect of chronic hypoxia on acetycholine metabolism in the carotid body is not known.

In summary, acute hypoxia may generally augment the release of all the putative neurotransmitters in the peripheral chemoreceptors, and chronic hypoxia may cause a general effect on neurotransmitter metabolism. Accordingly, all of these neurochemicals may be considered cotransmitters for the hypoxic chemosensory response.

Carotid Body Structure

It is abundantly clear that the carotid body is enlarged during chronic hypoxia in many species (4,5,13). This enlargement consists of carotid body parenchyma and small blood vessels. Rats exposed to an inspired P_{O_2} of 70 torr for 3 weeks or longer show glomus cells that are enlarged four fold. The mechanism of this growth is not known. However, we have observed that chronic exposure to carbon monoxide (700 ppm in air) for 4 weeks, a condition that stimulates erythropoiesis (hematocrit, about 75%) to the same extent as does chronic hypoxia (inspired P_{O_2} = 70 torr for 4 weeks), does not appear to promote carotid body growth (S. Lahiri, D. Penney, and K. Albertine, unpublished observations). These results suggest that carotid body growth during chronic hypoxia is due to a local P_{O_2}-sensitive mechanism. This growth mechanism may be linked to an augmented neurotransmitter metabolism and the chemosensory excitation. It is known that inhalation of 0.05% carbon monoxide in air, which results in 40% carboxyhemoglobinemia at an arterial P_{O_2} of 80–90 torr in the cat, does not increase chemosensory discharge (4,6). The lack of stimulation correlates with the lack of carotid body growth due to carboxyhemoglobinemia. This means that the carotid body tissue P_{O_2} during carboxyhemoglobinemia was not low enough to stimulate the oxygen-sensitive mechanism, and hence a growth response of the carotid body was not elicited. The erythropoietic response to chronic CO inhalation, on the other hand, must mean that the carboxyhemoglobinemia diminished the erythropoietic tissue P_{O_2} to stimulate erythropoietin output. One may infer that the local tissue P_{O_2} is critical for the growth response of the carotid body tissue. The fact that a substantial carboxyhemoglobinemia does not augment the respiratory chemoreflex was demonstrated early by Comroe and Schmidt (see ref. 3). Carboxyhemoglobinemia decreases arterial blood O_2 content and increases O_2–hemoglobin affinity. This combination of effects is expected to reduce strikingly the venous P_{O_2} of an organ with normal oxygen consumption and blood flow, as well as to reduce tissue P_{O_2}. Obviously the carotid body is an exception, probably because of the very high blood flow to the carotid body (see McDonald; O'Regan et al.; Mulligan et al.; Chaps. 1–3, this volume). Because of this high flow, the tissue P_{O_2} was not sufficiently decreased by the carboxyhemoglobinemia at a normal level of arterial P_{O_2}.

The foregoing evidence indicates that chronic tissue hypoxia elaborates a local factor or factors that stimulate carotid body cells to grow. This factor seems to be specific for the carotid body since similar growth is not obvious in the adrenal gland which also contains similar cells with similar neurochemicals. Presumably, the stimulus for growth is linked with the carotid body neurotransmitters and their receptors.

The hypoxia-induced growth raises several interesting questions (8). First, the hypoxia-induced growth did not lead to mitotic division of glomus cells. However, the number of cytoplasmic organelles increased with the increase in cell volume. Thus, the factor that initiated the growth clearly includes synthetic activity. Whether this is a direct effect of hypoxia or is due to a trophic interaction between the neural activity and the glomus cell is not known. This interaction could be tested by examining the effects of chronic hypoxia on the carotid body with and without intact innervation.

Another interesting structural effect of chronic hypoxia concerns the synaptic contact between the glomus cells and the nerve endings. Figure 23.2 compares these synaptic contact zones in the carotid bodies in the chronically hypoxic and control cats. The nerve ending in the chronically hypoxic cat contained more numerous clear-core vesicles, and the vesicles seemed to be participating in an activity at the contact zone. A quantitative study of these features may substantiate the idea that the incidence of active zone (8) is increased during chronic hypoxia and that these structures are the basis of the augmented chemosensory response to hypoxia.

Effects of Prolonged Normobaric Hyperoxia

Carotid Chemosensory Responses

Cats were exposed to normobaric hyperoxia ($F_IO_2 = 1$) for 60–70 h, and carotid chemoreceptor responses to hypoxia and hypercapnia and to intravenous administration of cyanide (20–50 μg), nicotine (25–50 μg), and dopamine (20–50 μg) were measured. The responses to hypoxia and hypercapnia of the carotid chemorecep-

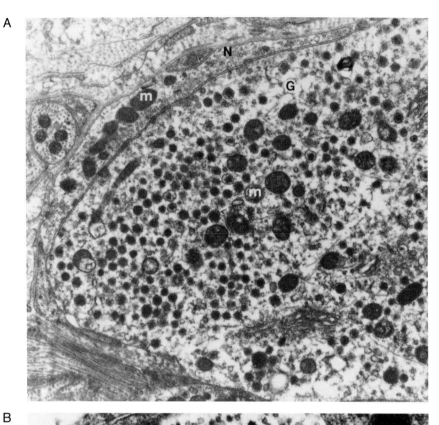

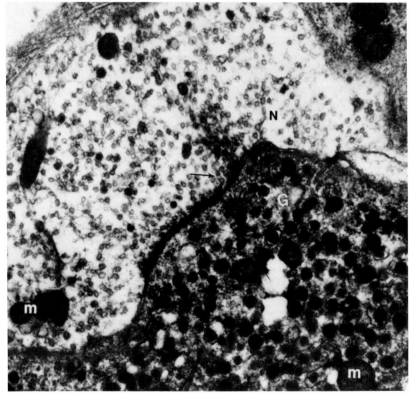

tors in the cats that were exposed to normobaric hyperoxia are shown in Fig. 23.3. Lowering the end-tidal P_{O_2} from 116 torr to 70 torr did not stimulate the discharge rate (panel A), whereas changes in the end-tidal P_{CO_2} changed the chemoreceptor activity (panel B). The initial depression in end-tidal P_{CO_2} (in B) resulted in a decreased chemoreceptor activity (compare the activity in first part of panel B with that in panel A). A rise in end-tidal P_{CO_2} was followed by a prompt rise in the dynamic and steady-state chemoreceptor activity (panel B). The steady-state carotid chemoreceptor responses to hypoxia in control and chronically hyperoxic cats are compared in Fig. 23.4. Normobaric hyperoxia severely attenuated the hypoxic responses. This diminished hypoxic response is consistent with a blunted response to cyanide. However, the responses to nicotine and dopamine were intact (10).

These results show that the chemoreceptor responses to hypoxia and hypercapnia are separable, and that their mechanisms of responses are not the same. Also, the intact responses to nicotine and dopamine indicated that the nicotine and dopamine receptors were fully functional. That is, the neural responses to these putative neurotransmitters were intact, suggesting that perhaps the release of putative neurotransmitters was blocked by exposure to chronic hyperoxia, or that the putative neurotransmitters due to hypoxia were depleted.

Putative Neurotransmitters

After exposure to normobaric hyperoxia, the contents of dopamine and norepinephrine were not depleted; in fact, both increased significantly. It is possible that the release of these neurotransmitters during acute hypoxia was blocked after chronic hyperoxic exposure.

Ultrastructure

We also examined the effects of prolonged hyperoxia on the ultrastructure of the carotid body, in collaboration with Donald McDonald. The most visible effect was on the mitochondria of the glomus cells. The space between the mitochondrial cristae increased and the cristae appeared thicker than normal. The dense-core granules were at least as abundant as in the control, and some of them appeared fused together. The structural change noted suggests that the mitochondria of the glomus cells may be a possible site of the hyperoxic effects. Consequently, oxidative metabolism and phosphate potential—and hence, neurotransmitter release and chemosensory excitation—were presumably no longer affected by hypoxia.

Effects of Hyperbaric Oxygen

The effects of normobaric hyperoxia could have been due to oxygen radicals. Because the formation and concentration of oxygen radicals in tissues are expected to be greater in hyperbaric oxygenation, we also tested carotid chemoreceptor

←_____

Fig. 23.2 Ultrastructure of carotid bodies showing "synaptic" contact between nerve ending and glomus cells in **(A)** normal ($\times 20,000$) and **(B)** chronically hypoxic ($\times 25,000$) cats. N = nerve ending; G = glomus cells; m = mitochondrion. The nerve ending (N) in the hypoxic carotid body shows a large number of clear vesicles converging at the "active zone."

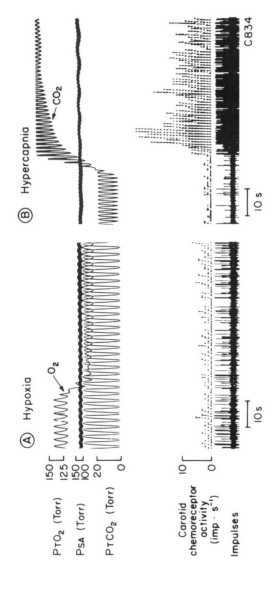

Fig. 23.3 Effects of acute hypoxia (**A**) and hypercapnia (**B**) on the same carotid chemoreceptor afferents in a cat that was exposed to chronic hyperoxia. The cat was anesthetized, paralyzed, and ventilated artificially. Note that the cat was initially hyperventilated to reduce end-tidal P_{CO_2} in B relative to that in A. The low P_{CO_2} reduced the chemoreceptor discharge rate. Induction of hypercapnia was accompanied by vigorous responses with an initial overshoot.

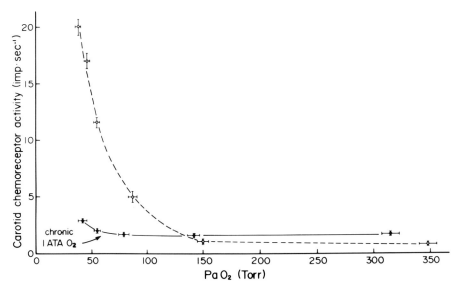

Fig. 23.4 Steady-state activity of carotid chemoreceptors (means $\pm$ SEM; $n = 9$) at several levels of arterial P_{O_2} in control and chronically hyperoxic cats at constant levels of pH (7.380 $\pm$ 0.03 and 7.362 $\pm$ 0.01, respectively) and P_{CO_2} (28.6 $\pm$ 0.03 and 26.6 $\pm$ 1.3 torr, respectively). Control cats (O) showed the usual hyperbolic response to hypoxia, whereas chronically hyperoxic cats (●) showed a severely attenuated response.

responses to hypoxia and hypercapnia before and after exposure of anesthetized cats to 100% O_2 at 5 atm for 90–135 min. The hyperbaric oxygenation attenuated the chemoreceptor responses to hypoxia, but the effect was not nearly as striking as in chronic normobaric hyperoxia. The results suggested that oxygen radicals could have initiated the process attenuating the oxygen-sensitive mechanism, but it did not proceed far enough within the exposure period.

Effects of Prolonged Exposure to an Inspired P_{O_2} of 350 Torr

Cats were exposed to an F_IO_2 of 0.5 at sea level for 14 days. These cats were then anesthetized, and the responses of single carotid chemoreceptor afferents to hypoxia were measured as in the control cats. The chemoreceptor activity at high P_aO_2 was significantly greater in these chronically hyperoxic cats than in the control cats, but the hypoxic response curve was shifted to the left of the control. A one-way analysis of variance showed that there was a significant diminution of the hypoxic response of the carotid chemoreceptors in the chronically hyperoxic group.

DISCUSSION

The chemosensory response to hypoxia was used as an expression of oxygen chemoreception in the carotid body. If the normalized hypoxic responses between the

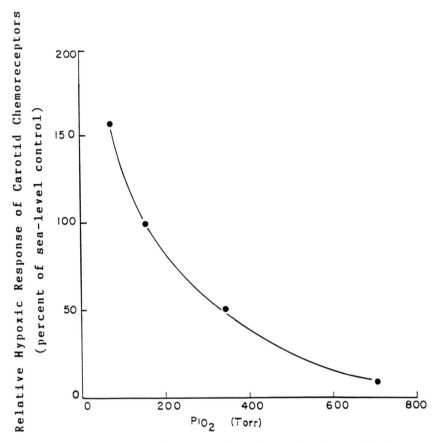

Fig. 23.5 Effects of chronic hypoxia and normobaric hyperoxia on the carotid chemoreceptor responses to hypoxia relative to cats breathing room air at sea level. Four levels of chronic inspiratory Po_2 were used: 70, 150, 350 and 700 torr. The responses to acute hypoxia in each group of cats were calculated by taking the ratio of the chemoreceptor activities at P_aO_2 of 40 and 300 torr. The ratios were expressed relative to an assigned value of 100 to the sea-level cats. These values are plotted as a function of the chronic inspired Po_2.

groups of cats—chronically hypoxic, normoxic, and hyperoxic—are compared, it becomes clear that chronic hypoxia increased and chronic hyperoxia diminished the responsiveness in a nonlinear, dose-dependent fashion (see Fig. 23.5). These effects seem to represent a continuum.

The continuum of the chronic oxygen effect may indicate that the basic mechanisms for the effects of different levels of O_2 are the same, or closely related. A clue to the mechanisms derives from the similarities between the effects of chronic hyperoxia and those of inhibitors of oxidative phosphorylation. We have shown previously (14) and confirmed recently (15) that oligomycin in appropriate doses blocks the chemosensory response to hypoxia but not to hypercapnia, dopamine, and nicotine. This similarity suggests that chronic hyperoxia may have caused specific damage to the sites of mitochondrial oxidative metabolism which may mediate oxygen sensing. Whether it is the cellular phosphate potential or other indicator of energy metabolism is not yet known (see Acker et al.; Tamura et al.; Wilson et al.; Reynafarje; Coburn, Chaps. 13,17–20, this volume). The possibility that some mechanisms (12) other than oxidative phosphorylation are involved in attenuating the chemosensory response to hypoxia has not been ruled out.

Chemosensory discharge in the normal carotid body increases when arterial P_{O_2} decreases from 200 torr to 100 torr which may or may not influence O_2 metabolism. This is a crucial issue, and a section of this volume is devoted to it (see Tamura et al.; Wilson et al.; Reynafarje; Coburn, Chaps. 17–20, this volume).

Another issue with regard to metabolic O_2-sensing is that of the ATP concentration gradient between the mitochondrion, the site of ATP production, and the site of ATP utilization such as the plasma membrane or vesicle membranes. Because of this gradient (1), a small change in ATP concentration at the source may assume critical importance at the active site.

Hyperoxia generates highly reactive oxygen radicals (7) which could act at any specific stage of this proposed pathway between energy metabolism and the site of the neurotransmitter action. Dopamine and nicotine receptors were not damaged nor were the biogenic amines depleted after exposure to chronic hyperoxia. It is suggestive that release of the putative neurotransmitters was blocked after chronic hyperoxia. We also found that a brief exposure to hyperbaric oxygenation did not block the oxygen chemoreception. These results suggest that the attenuating effect of hyperoxia on oxygen chemosensitivity is time dependent. Time may be required for a gradual transformation of the mitochondrial function after the initial effect of the oxygen radicals.

The same metabolic hypothesis does not readily apply to the augmented hypoxic chemosensory response after chronic hypoxia. It is possible, however, that the same strength of hypoxic stimulus causes release of the neurotransmitters in larger quantum because of their greater amounts in the carotid body as a result of chronic hypoxia.

Ultrastructural studies did not show changes in the glomus cell mitochondria in chronically hypoxic animals. However, the contrast in comparison with controls shows that the observed change in the mitochondria of the glomus cells after exposure to chronic hyperoxia was probably not an artifact.

A trophic interaction between the chemoreceptor neural activity and glomus cell structure and function is an important consideration in the context of these results. The growth of the carotid body during chronic hypoxia and a possible decrease in the carotid body size during chronic hyperoxia clearly indicate that oxygen chemosensing may be related to carotid body growth. Whether this change occurs without intact chemosensory fibers has not been tested. Intact glomus cells are present in the carotid body even after chronic denervation of the carotid body (4). Also, after denervation the carotid sinus nerve grows back into the carotid body at a rate faster than reinnervation by another nerve (4). It is quite possible that oxygen has an effect on the carotid body even without intact carotid chemosensory nerves. However, a normal feedback relationship between the cells and the nerves may assume critical importance under chronic conditions of low and high chemosensory activity.

In summary, chronic states of low and high oxygen environment exert profound effects on the structure, chemistry, and function of the carotid body. These cellular responses provide us with an opportunity to sort out the relationship between the oxygen-sensitive cellular components and functions of the carotid body. These results also show that the peripheral chemoreceptor function and chemoreflexes can change strikingly in health and disease.

ACKNOWLEDGMENTS
    This work was supported in part by NIH grants R01 NS 21068-03, HL-08899-15, HL-19737-11, and 5-T32-HL-070270. We thank Ms. Gail K. Stevens for her secretarial assistance.

REFERENCES

1. Awe, T. Y., and D. P. Jones. ATP concentration gradients in cytosol of liver cells during hypoxia. *Am. J. Physiol.* 249: C385–C392, 1985.
2. Barnard, P., S. Andronikou, M. Pokorski, N. Smatresk, A. Mokashi, and S. Lahiri. Time-dependent effect of hypoxia on carotid body chemosensory function. *J. Appl. Physiol.* 63: 685–691, 1987.
3. Comroe, J. H. The peripheral chemoreceptors. In: *Handbook of Physiology, Sec. 3: The Respiratory System,* Vol. 1: *Circulation and Nonrespiratory Functions,* ed. A. P. Fishman and A. B. Fisher. Washington, DC: Am. Physiol. Soc., 1964, pp. 557–583.
4. Eyzaguirre, C., R. S. Fitzgerald, S. Lahiri, and P. Zapata. Arterial chemoreceptors. In: *Handbook of Physiology, Sec. 2: The Cardiovascular System,* Vol. 3: *Peripheral Circulation and Organ Blood Flow,* ed. J. T. Shepherd and F. M. Abboud. Bethesda: Am. Physiol. Soc., 1983, pp. 557–621.
5. Fidone, S. J., and C. Gonzalez. Initiation and control of chemoreceptor activity in the carotid body. In: *Handbook of Physiology, Sec. 3: The Respiratory System,* Vol. 2: *Control of Breathing,* ed. N. S. Cherniack and J. G. Widdicombe. Bethesda: Am. Physiol. Soc., 1986, pp. 247–312.
6. Fitzgerald, R. S., and S. Lahiri. Reflex responses to chemoreceptor stimulation. In: *Handbook of Physiology, Sec. 3: The Respiratory System,* Vol. 2: *Control of Breathing,* ed. N. S. Cherniak and J. G. Widdicombe. Bethesda: Am. Physiol. Soc., 1986, pp. 313–362.
7. Fridovitch, I. Superoxide radical: an endogenous toxicant. *Annu. Rev. Pharmacol. Toxicol.* 23: 239–257, 1983.
8. Goss, R. J. *The Physiology of Growth.* New York: Academic Press, 1978.
9. Lahiri, S., and R. G. DeLaney. Stimulus interaction in the responses of carotid body chemoreceptor single afferent fibers. *Respir. Physiol.* 24: 349–366, 1975.
10. Lahiri, S., E. Mulligan, S. Andronikou, M. Shirahata, and A. Mokashi. Carotid body chemosensory function in prolonged normobaric hyperoxia in the cat. *J. Appl. Physiol.* 62: 1924–1931, 1987.
11. Lahiri, S., N. J. Smatresk, and E. Mulligan. Responses of peripheral chemoreceptors to natural stimuli. In: *Physiology of the Peripheral Arterial Chemoreceptors,* ed. H. Acker and R. G. O'Regan. Amsterdam: Elsevier, 1983, pp. 221–256.
12. Lundberg, G. A., B. Jergil, and R. Sundler. Subcellular localization and enzymatic properties of rat liver phosphatidylinositol-4-phosphate kinase. *Biochim. Biophys. Acta* 846: 379–387, 1985.
13. McGregor, K. H., J. Gil, and S. Lahiri. A morphometric study of the carotid body in chronically hypoxic rats. *J. Appl. Physiol.* 57: 1430–1438, 1984.

14. Mulligan, E., and S. Lahiri. Separation of carotid body chemoreceptor responses to O_2 and CO_2 by oligomycin and by antimycin A. *Am. J. Physiol. 242 (Cell Physiol. 11):* C200–C206, 1982.
15. Shirahata, M., S. Andronikou, and S. Lahiri. Differential effects of oligomycin on carotid chemoreceptor responses to O_2 and CO_2 in the cat. *J. Appl. Physiol. 63:* 2084–2092, 1987.

Part V
CENTRAL EFFECTS OF HYPOXIA

Introduction

F. L. ELDRIDGE

It is well known that hypoxia leads to depression of neuronal function in the central nervous system. It has also become clear that respiratory neurons are similarly depressed by severe enough hypoxia, the phenomenon becoming readily apparent in the absence of facilitatory input from the peripheral chemoreceptors. The purpose of this section is to examine the thus elusive mechanism that leads to the depression of breathing with hypoxia.

Neubauer and colleagues (Chap. 25) present a schema for considering possible mechanisms of decreased respiration during hypoxia. The first is related to the vasodilatory effect of hypoxia on medullary blood vessels, leading to increased blood flow, local reduction of medullary extracellular fluid (ECF) P_{CO_2}, development of ECF alkalosis, and consequently somewhat less stimulation of the chemoreceptors. This mechanism applies during mild hypoxia, but with more severe hypoxia (e.g., 10% O_2) a metabolic acidosis supervenes, and thus the depression must occur by other mechanisms.

The second mechanism, which occurs with very severe hypoxia, involves a loss of high-energy phosphates. To support this mechanism, Hitzig (Chap. 26) presents nuclear magnetic resonance (NMR) studies showing that 2% O_2 breathing led to almost complete disappearance of phosphocreatine and ATP; after 5 min the process appeared to be irreversible.

The third mechanism involves moderately severe hypoxia, represented by breathing 8–10% O_2; here there is a marked but reversible depression of respiratory activity, even to the point of apnea, but there is no evidence from NMR studies that phosphocreatine/ATP ratios (a measure of energy charge on the cells) have changed (see Hitzig, Chap. 26). This is in keeping with the finding that an excitatory input is still capable of causing medullary neurons to fire (Richter and Acker, Chap. 27) and that hypercapnic stimulation can cause respiratory rhythm to reappear (Neubauer et al., Chap. 25). The mechanisms involved in the respiratory depression of this type include (a) increased production, during hypoxia, of inhibitory neurochemicals such as GABA (Kazemi et al., Chap. 24), adenosine, and the opioid peptides; (b) depletion of excitatory amines; (c) the effects of changes in the extra-cellular ionic environment on neuronal function (Richter and Acker, Chap. 27); and (d) the effects of lactic acid (Neubauer et al., Chap. 25). The evidence presented supports the possibility that all of these are potential mechanisms, but no specific one can, at the present time, be considered dominant.

These chapters show that the respiratory depression that occurs during moderately severe hypoxia cannot be considered as due to a simple loss of energy substrates, such as occurs with anoxia or ischemia. It has been suggested that the third type of depression is an adaptive mechanism that protects neurons from damage during hypoxia by reducing neuronal activity.

In addition to the direct effect of acute hypoxia on the brain-stem mechanisms evidence for long-lasting post-hypoxic central inhibition and facilitation of respiration are discussed by Gallman and Millhorn.

Taken together these chapters clearly demonstrate that hypoxia elicits multiple effects on the central nervous systems. Some of these effects influence respiratory neuron activities with varying time-courses. The mechanisms and the precise site of these effects are unknown.

24

Role of Medullary Glutamate in the Hypoxic Ventilatory Response

H. KAZEMI, C.-H. CHIANG, AND B. HOOP

Recent evidence suggests that neurotransmitters in the brain have modulating effects on the activity of central respiratory neurons. Two amino acid neurotransmitters, γ-aminobutyric acid (GABA) and glutamic acid, have opposing effects on the membrane potential of individual medullary respiratory neurons, with GABA being an inhibitory neurotransmitter and glutamate an excitatory one (20). Glutamate is assumed to be released by primary afferent fibers (5). There is a significant concentration of glutamate-sensitive receptors on medullary respiratory neurons (16) and centrally applied glutamate increases ventilation primarily by increasing tidal volume and inspiratory force (3).

The glutamate content of the brain is also altered during hypoxia and hypercapnia (4,17,19,23). Hypoxia increases ventilation, and this increase is dependent on stimulation of peripheral chemoreceptors. The present study addresses the question of the relationship between hypoxia and brain amino acid neurotransmitters in anesthetized dogs with intact or denervated peripheral chemoreceptors and suggests a possible role for medullary glutamate in the ventilatory response to hypoxia.

METHODS

Mongrel dogs weighing 13–25 kg were anesthetized with intravenous sodium pentobarbital, 30 mg/kg initially and 4.5 mg/kg every 2 h during the experiment. Ventilation was maintained through an endotracheal tube by a constant volume respirator (Harvard Apparatus Company, Dover, MA). Tidal volume and frequency of the respirator were adjusted to maintain P_aCO_2 in the 35- to 38-mmHg range. A polyethylene catheter was inserted in the femoral artery, and arterial blood pressure was monitored oscillographically through a Statham transducer. A femoral vein was also cannulated. The rectal temperature was monitored continuously and was maintained at 38°C with a thermostatted blanket.

The study consisted of 33 dogs which were divided into two groups:

Group I animals (18 dogs) with intact peripheral chemoreceptors were ventilated on room air under normocapnic conditions. Five of these dogs were ventilated on room air for another hour and served as control animals in this group. The other 13 dogs were ventilated on 7% O_2 in N_2 for 1 h and periodic measurements were made as described below.

Group II animals (15 dogs) were prepared as in group I and ventilated on room air. They underwent bilateral carotid body denervation and cervical vagotomy (see below). After chemodenervation, 5 of the dogs were ventilated on room air under normocapnic conditions for 1 h. The other 10 dogs were ventilated on 7% O_2 in N_2 for 1 h.

Chemodenervation

Bilateral cervical vagotomy and carotid body denervation were performed following a midline incision in the anterior neck. The cervical vagosympathetic nerve trunk was exteriorized on each side and cut at the level of thyroid cartilage. After the common carotid artery and carotid sinus were identified on each side of the neck, the adventitia was completely stripped away from common, internal, and external carotid arteries, and their branches in a region 2 cm above and below the bifurcation of the carotid artery and all nerve connections were severed. To test the adequacy of the peripheral chemodenervation, we measured the ventilatory response to transient hypoxia. We removed the animals from the ventilator and recorded respiration on a spirometer filled with room air. Then we switched the spirometer gas to nitrogen and recorded four to seven consecutive breaths. The anoxic challenge was done before and after chemodenervation. Chemodenervation was judged adequate when there was no ventilatory response to transient hypoxia. This was the case in every animal included in group II.

Both groups of animals, intact and chemodenervated, were then placed prone on the operating table and the head was placed in a stereotaxic instrument. Muscles over the skull and the back of the neck were dissected away. A polyethylene catheter was placed in the sagittal sinus with the tip of the catheter directed caudally. A No. 18 spinal needle was inserted into cisterna magna. Once the animals were prepared in this manner and ventilated mechanically, they were then paralyzed by intravenous injection of 200 mg succinylcholine.

Measurements

After the animals had been prepared and paralyzed, each experimental period of 1 h was begun. We obtained 3-ml arterial and sagittal sinus blood samples in heparinized syringes at 0 time and at 30 and 60 min of the experimental period. Simultaneously with the blood samples, 1-ml cisternal cerebrospinal fluid (CSF) samples were obtained anaerobically from the spinal needle through a three-way stopcock into dry 1-ml syringes. The dead space of the syringe and stopcock was flushed with

CSF just before sampling. CSF samples contaminated with blood or air bubbles were discarded. pH, Pco_2, and Po_2 of arterial blood, sagittal sinus blood, and CSF were immediately measured by appropriate electrodes (Instrumentation Laboratory Systems 1303, Lexington, MA) at 38°C. Bicarbonate contents of blood and CSF samples were calculated from the Henderson–Hasselbach equation. Arterial blood pressure, body temperature, and heart rate were recorded at the same time periods. Lactate was measured by the enzymatic technique in all blood and CSF samples.

At the end of each experiment, the brain was exposed by removing the cranial vault. With a scalpel, the dura mater was cut open at the level of cisterna magna. Then the whole brain, including medulla oblongata, was removed rapidly and immediately frozen in liquid N_2. The average time between incising the brain and immersion into liquid N_2 was 5 s. The frozen brain was then dissected. The cortex of the anterior sigmoid gyrus (equivalent to the motor area of human brain) and the medulla were separated. These segments of the brain were weighed and deproteinized rapidly in 10 volumes of chilled 8% perchloric acid per gram of brain with a tissue homogenizer. The amino acid content of cortex and medulla were then determined by ion-exchange column chromatography (Model 119CL Amino Acid Analyzer; Beckman Instruments, Wakefield, MA).

Analysis of variance (ANOVA) was used for testing the null hypothesis—that is, whether or not mean values were the same in all groups. Mean values that differed between groups were further examined for correlations with linear regression analysis. A level of confidence of 99% was chosen for the correlation coefficient. ANOVA was used for statistical analysis of brain amino acid content.

RESULTS

During the conduct of these experiments, it became apparent that the pattern of change in brain amino acid content during hypoxia differs, depending on whether there is an increase in CSF and blood lactate. Therefore, data from animals in groups I and II are presented separately in three subgroups: (a) control, (b) hypoxia without lactate increase, and (c) hypoxia with lactate increase. The criterion used to assign hypoxic animals to category (c) required that arterial lactate concentration be ≥ 1 SD greater than the mean arterial lactate concentration of the corresponding normoxic group. In all but one case, lactate concentrations increased by *several* standard deviations, and there was a corresponding increase in nearly every CSF lactate value.

Blood and CSF Po_2, and lactate content for group I (intact chemoreceptors) and group II (chemodenervated animals) are given in Table 24.1. In the group I controls (animals breathing room air), there were no time-dependent changes in any of these parameters. In group I dogs breathing the hypoxic gas mixture at constant $\dot{V}_E$ without an increase in lactate, the mean P_aO_2 fell from 119 ± 8.49 mmHg to 30.57 ± 3.05 mmHg after 60 min of hypoxia, and the sagittal sinus Po_2 fell from 38.43 ± 8.20 to 21.21 ± 2.94 mmHg. There were no significant changes in Pco_2, pH, or $[HCO_3^-]$ in these animals (data not shown).

Table 24.1 PO_2 and Lactate During Hypoxia

	Control				No lactate change				Lactate increase			
	0 min		60 min		0 min		60 min		0 min		60 min	
	PO_2	Lact.	PO_2	Lact.	PO_2	Lact.	PO_2	Lact.	PO_2	Lact.	PO_2	Lact.
Group I[a]	(n = 5)				(n = 7)				(n = 6)			
Arterial	111.6 ±3.06	0.48 ±0.17	113 ±2.41	0.46 ±0.18	119 ±8.49	0.59 ±0.14	30.6* ±3.05	0.62 ±0.23	108.2 ±5.1	0.69 ±0.20	25.2* ±2.5	2.64* ±0.43
Sag. sinus	41.7 ±1.75	0.52 ±0.17	41.7 ±1.43	0.49 ±0.13	38.4 ±8.2	0.61 ±0.07	21.2* ±2.94	0.74 ±0.23	41.8 ±2.98	0.74* ±0.13	18.0* ±1.30	2.69* ±0.60
CSF	—	1.10 ±0.15	—	1.15 ±0.33	—	1.20 ±1.15	—	1.45 ±0.14	—	1.07 ±0.32	—	2.38* ±0.54
Group II[b]	(n = 5)				(n = 5)				(n = 5)			
Arterial	102.8 ±6.94	0.91 ±0.22	89.0 ±14.67	0.99 ±0.40	108.4 ±10.02	0.63 ±0.12	46.6* ±1.33	0.74 ±0.09	109 ±6.24	1.38 ±0.53	33.0* ±2.92	3.49* ±1.4
Sag. sinus	45.6 ±2.35	1.22 ±0.39	42 ±4.34	0.98 ±0.40	44.4 ±0.40	0.82 ±0.20	32.80* ±1.36	1.11 ±0.29	47.7 ±5.11	1.26 ±0.56	21.0* ±2.27	3.28* ±1.5
CSF	—	0.96 ±0.07	—	1.32 ±0.14	—	1.13 ±0.21	—	1.52 ±0.34	—	1.62 ±0.57	—	3.62* ±0.91

Note: Group I = intact; group II = peripherally chemodenervated; n = number of dogs in each group. Values are expressed as means $\pm$ SEM. Units for PO_2, mmHg; for lactate, mmol/l.
*Significantly different from 0-min value at $p < .01$.

In those intact animals in whom lactate increased during hypoxia in both blood and CSF, the mean P_aO_2 fell to 25.17 ± 2.5 mmHg at 60 min of hypoxia, a value significantly different ($p < .05$) from the P_aO_2 in intact animals at 60 min of hypoxia in whom lactate did not increase (Table 24.1). There were no significant changes in blood or CSF Pco_2, pH, or [HCO_3^-].

In the chemodenervated animals in the control group breathing room air (group II controls), no significant changes in oxygenation, acid–base balance, or lactate occurred during the 1-h experimental period (Table 24.1). In the chemodenervated animals breathing the hypoxic gas mixture in whom lactate did not increase, the mean P_aO_2 fell from 108.4 ± 10.02 to 46.60 ± 1.33 after 60 min of hypoxia. No changes in blood or CSF acid–base balance or lactate occurred. In the chemodenervated animals in which blood and CSF lactate increased during hypoxia (Table 24.1), the mean P_aO_2 fell from 109.0 ± 6.24 to 33.0 ± 2.92 mmHg at 60 min of hypoxia. There were no significant changes in blood and CSF Pco_2, pH, or [HCO_3^-].

In the cortex, the mean glutamate concentration (Fig. 24.1) was elevated in intact animals only when there was no blood lactate increase (ANOVA, $d.f.$: 5.30; $F = 5.36$, $p < .005$). There was no such glutamate increase in denervated animals. In the medulla, mean glutamate was also elevated in intact animals with no lactate increase ($F = 6.51$, $p < .05$). There was a similar but not significant trend in medullary glutamine ($F = 1.41$, $p = 0.25$; Fig. 24.2). GABA increased in the medulla significantly in the chemodenervated animals during hypoxia only with lactate increase (Fig. 24.3) and in the cortex in the intact animals with hypoxia and lactate increase. The rise in medullary GABA correlated significantly with sagittal sinus Po_2 in the chemodenervated animals.

DISCUSSION

Several previous studies of the amino acid content of whole brain or brain cortex during hypoxia (5% O_2) where hypocapnia was also present have shown increases in the content of GABA and alanine in mouse, rat, guinea pig, and dog (17,19,24). Because CO_2 fixation in the brain alters the content of some of the CNS amino acids (23), one needs to separate the effects of hypoxia from those of hypocapnia.

The present study was conducted in anesthetized, mechanically ventilated dogs, breathing 7% O_2 at constant $\dot{V}_E$ whose P_aCO_2 was kept normal. Once the data on brain amino acids were analyzed, it became apparent that changes in brain amino acid levels were different when lactate in blood and CSF had increased during hypoxia as compared to when no increase in lactate had occurred. Because the lactate increase in the CSF reflects a concurrent increase in brain lactate but not that in the plasma (12,14), it may therefore be assumed that increases in brain lactate affect concentration of certain amino acids.

For the intact dogs during hypoxia (mean $P_aO_2 = 30.57 \pm 3.05$ mmHg) without a lactate increase, glutamate increased significantly in both cortex and medulla, but in more severe hypoxic conditions (mean $P_aO_2 = 25.17 \pm 2.55$ mmHg) with lactate increase, glutamate remained unchanged in cortex and medulla (Fig. 24.1).

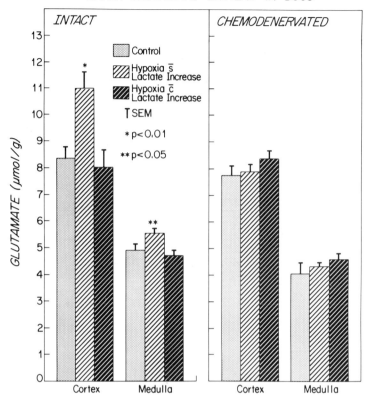

Fig. 24.1 Glutamate content of cerebral cortex and medulla in the dog after 1 h of hypoxia (7% O_2 in O_2 at constant $\dot{V}$E) in two groups of animals, with intact peripheral chemoreceptors and after peripheral chemodenervation. Control animals breathed room air. Each hypoxic group is further subdivided, based on whether there was increased lactate in the CSF or not. Mean values in at least five dogs for each subgroup.

Glucose and glutamine are the two potential precursors of glutamate (8). Glutamate can be synthesized by hydrolysis of glutamine, a reaction catalyzed by the enzyme glutaminase, or it can be synthesized from glucose by oxidative metabolism and transamination of the α-ketoglutarate. Bradford and Ward (1) showed that nerve terminals contain large quantities of glutaminase and suggested that this enzyme plays the major role in the production of the neurotransmitter glutamate. Cotman and co-workers (8,9) and Tapia (18) showed that about two-thirds of the glutamate was produced from glutamine and about one-third from glucose, and in our studies there was a linear relationship between the brain content of glutamine and glutamate.

In hypoxia in the intact control group of animals, glutamate and glutamine contents were significantly higher in the cortex than in the medulla. These differences may be due to variations in metabolic rate with the neuron packing density

BRAIN GLUTAMINE CONTENT IN DOGS

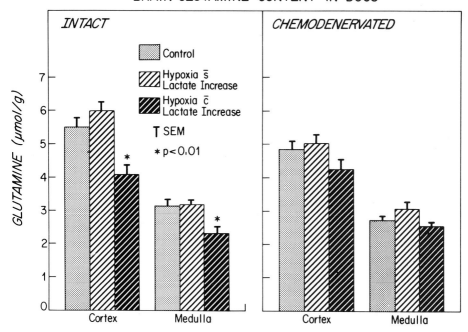

Fig. 24.2 Glutamine content of cerebral cortex and medulla in the dog after 1 h of hypoxia. The same animals as in Fig. 24.1.

Fig. 24.3 GABA content of cerebral cortex and medulla in the dog after 1 h of hypoxia. The same animals as in Fig. 24.1.

BRAIN GABA CONTENT IN DOGS

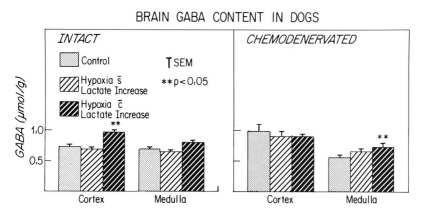

(glia/neuron indices) (21), or to different functional activities in cortex and medulla.

Studies looking at the effects of hypoxia ($F_{I_{O_2}}$ = 0.11–0.09) on the function of the human brain have shown lethargy, euphoria, irritability, hallucination, impaired critical judgment, and muscular incoordination (7). Our results suggest that during low O_2 breathing, the increase in the excitatory neurotransmitter glutamate in the brain cortex may be responsible for behavioral changes (irritability and euphoria), and increased glutamate in medulla may be responsible for the increases in ventilation and blood pressure. After peripheral chemodenervation, brain glutamate failed to increase during hypoxia. This lack of increase in glutamate may account for the absence of a ventilatory response to hypoxia after chemodenervation.

Depression of ventilation by hypoxia has been repeatedly demonstrated in chemodenervated and intact animals (2,6). Weiskopf and Gabel (22) found evidence for the depressant effect of hypoxia in awake human subjects. There is no real clue to the mechanism of the depressant effect of hypoxia. Hypoxia increases cerebral blood flow (11), but the increased blood flow may not be able to compensate for the low O_2 content of blood in severe hypoxia, and thus O_2 delivery to brain tissue is reduced. Whether GABA plays a role in the ventilatory depression of hypoxia is unknown. In our studies, there was a negative correlation between medullary GABA content and sagittal sinus P_{O_2} in the chemodenervated animals only. Other studies have shown that centrally applied GABA depresses ventilation (10,13,25), and it is possible that the ventilatory depression with severe hypoxia in chemodenervated animals could be related to the increase in medullary GABA.

The increase in GABA during hypoxia is probably related to the availability of α-ketoglutarate, since the latter is important in the degradation of GABA and synthesis of glutamate. During severe hypoxia or anoxia, the level of α-ketoglutarate declines rapidly since the Krebs cycle intermediates depend on aerobic metabolism. With a reduction in α-ketoglutarate, GABA cannot be degraded, but it can still be formed from glutamate because glutamic acid decarboxylase (GAD), the enzyme necessary for conversion of glutamate to GABA, is an anaerobic enzyme and allows for GABA formation to proceed during hypoxia (15).

Based on our studies on brain amino acid changes during hypoxia and observations by others on the ventilatory response to hypoxia, a speculative hypothesis about the central mechanisms of ventilatory and circulatory stimulation and possible depression to hypoxia may be offered. In hypoxia, oxygen deprivation stimulates peripheral circulatory and respiratory chemoreceptors. The afferent nerve fibers carry the chemoreceptor impulses to respiratory and circulatory centers, causing release of the excitatory neurotransmitter glutamic acid, which stimulates respiratory and circulatory neurons, resulting in increased ventilation and blood pressure. However, in severe hypoxia, the cerebral metabolic pathway becomes anaerobic, increasing the inhibitory neurotransmitter GABA, which then results in decreased ventilation and blood pressure. With peripheral chemodenervation, afferent impulses do not reach the respiratory and circulatory centers; therefore, there is no glutamate release and no increase in ventilation or blood pressure. The depression of ventilation with severe hypoxia, particularly in the chemodenervated animals, may be related to the medullary GABA increase. This hypothesis would not exclude the possibility that brain amino acid changes could be due in part to changes in cerebral blood flow or pattern of distribution of cerebral perfusion during hypoxia with intact or denervated peripheral chemoreceptors.

ACKNOWLEDGMENTS

This work was supported in part by NIH grants HL-29493 and HL-29629. C.-H. Chiang participated in this effort while on a leave of absence from the Pulmonary Service, Tri-Service General Hospital, Taipei, Taiwan; he was supported by a fellowship from the Government of the Republic of China (Taiwan).

REFERENCES

1. Bradford, H. F., and H. K. Ward. On glutaminase activity in mammalian synaptosomes. *Brain Res. 110:* 115–125, 1976.
2. Cherniack, N. S., S. G. Kelson, and S. Lahiri. The effects of hypoxia and hypercapnia on central nervous system output. In: *Respiratory Adaptations, Capillary Exchange and Reflex Mechanism,* ed. A. S. Paintal and P. Gill-Kumar. Delhi: Vallabhbhai Patel Chest Institute, 1977, pp. 312–325.
3. Chiang, C.-H., P. Pappagianopoulos, B. Hoop, and H. Kazemi. Central cardiorespiratory effects of glutamate in dogs. *J. Appl. Physiol. 60:* 2056–2062, 1986.
4. Duffy, T. E., S. R. Nelson, and O. H. Lo. Cerebral carbohydrate metabolism during acute hypoxia and recovery. *J. Neurochem. 19:* 959–977, 1972.
5. Fagg, G. E., and A. C. Foster. Amino acid neurotransmitters and their pathways in the mammalian central nervous system. *Neuroscience 9:* 701–709, 1983.
6. Gemmil, C. L., and D. L. Reeves. The effect of anoxemia in normal dogs before and after denervation of carotid sinuses. *Am. J. Physiol. 105:* 487–495, 1933.
7. Gibson, G. E., W. Pulsinelli, J. P. Blass, and T. E. Duffy. Brain dysfunction in mild to moderate hypoxia. *Am. J. Med. 70:* 1247–1254, 1981.
8. Hamberger, A. C., G. H. Chiang, E. S. Nylen, S. W. Scheff, and C. W. Cotman. Glutamate as a CNS transmitter: I. Evaluation of glucose and glutamine as precursors for the synthesis of preferentially released glutamate. *Brain Res. 168:* 513–530, 1979.
9. Hamberger, A. C., G. H. Chiang, E. Sandoval, and C. W. Cotman. Glutamate as a CNS transmitter: II. Regulation of syntheses in the releasable pool. *Brain Res. 168:* 531–541, 1979.
10. Hedner, J., P. Hedner, P. Wessberg, and J. Jonason. An analysis of the mechanism by which γ-aminobutyric acid depresses ventilation in the rat. *J. Appl. Physiol. 56:* 849–856, 1984.
11. Johannsson, H., and B. K. Siesjo. Cerebral blood flow and oxygen consumption in the rat in hypoxic hypoxia. *Acta Physiol. Scand. 93:* 269–276, 1984.
12. Kazemi, H., L. M. Valenca, and D. C. Shannon. Brain and cerebrospinal fluid lactate concentration in respiratory acidosis and alkalosis. *Respir. Physiol. 6:* 178–186, 1969.
13. Kneussl, M., P. Pappagianopoulos, B. Hoop, and H. Kazemi. Reversible depression of ventilation and cardiovascular function by ventriculocisternal perfusion with γ-aminobutyric acid in dogs. *Am. Rev. Respir. Dis. 133:* 1024–1028, 1986.
14. Leusen, I., E. Lacroix, and G. Demeester. Lactate and pyruvate in the brain of rats during changes in acid–base balance. *Arch. Int. Physiol. Biochem. 75:* 310–324, 1967.
15. McGeer, P. L., and E. G. McGeer. Amino acid neurotransmitters. In: *Basic Neurochemistry,* ed. C. J. Siegel, R. W. Albers, R. Katzman, and B. W. Agranoff. Boston: Little, Brown, 1981, pp. 233–252.

16. Monaghan, D. T., and C. W. Cotman. Distribution of N-methyl-D-aspartate-sensitive L-[^{3}H]glutamate-binding sites in rat brain. *J. Neurosci. 5:* 2909–2919, 1985.
17. Norberg, K., and B. K. Siesjo. Cerebral metabolism in hypoxic hypoxia: II. Citric acid cycle intermediates and associated amino acids. *Brain Res. 86:* 45–54, 1975.
18. Tapia, R. Glutamine metabolism in brain. In: *Glutamine: Metabolism, Enzymology and Regulation,* ed. J. Mora and R. Palacio. New York: Academic Press, 1980, pp. 285–297.
19. Tews, J. K., S. H. Carter, P. D. Roa, and W. E. Stone. Free amino acids and related compounds in dog brain: postmortem and anoxic changes, effects of ammonium chloride infusion, and levels during seizures induced by picrotoxin and by pentylenetrazol. *J. Neurochem. 10:* 641–653, 1963.
20. Toleikis, J. R., and D. T. Frazier. Effects of L-glutamate and GABA on the response of expiratory neurons to mechanical loads. *J. Neurosci. Res. 7:* 443–452, 1982.
21. Tower, D. B., and O. M. Young. The activities of butyryl-cholinesterase and carbonic anhydrase, the rate of anaerobic glycolysis, and the question of a constant density of glial cells in cerebral cortex of various mammalian species from mouse to whale. *J. Nuerochem. 20:* 269–278, 1973.
22. Weiskopf, R. B., and R. A. Gabel. Depression of ventilation during hypoxia in man. *J. Appl. Physiol. 39:* 911–915, 1975.
23. Weyne, J., F. Van Leuven, H. Kazemi, and I. Leusen. Selected brain amino acids and ammonium during chronic hypercapnia in conscious rats. *J. Appl. Physiol. 44:* 333–339, 1978.
24. Wood, J. D., W. J. Watson, and A. J. Ducker. The effect of hypoxia on brain γ-aminobutyric acid levels. *J. Neurochem. 15:* 603–608, 1968.
25. Yamada, K. A., P. Hamosh, and R. A. Gillis. Respiratory depression produced by activation of GABA receptors in hindbrain of cat. *J. Appl. Physiol. 51:* 1278–1286, 1981.

25

Modulation of Respiratory Output by Brain Hypoxia

J. A. NEUBAUER, J. E. MELTON, AND N. H. EDELMAN

Although it has long been known that systemic hypoxia in the absence of peripheral chemoreceptor stimulation causes respiratory depression, the precise nature of this phenomenon has remained elusive from both descriptive and mechanistic points of view. The physiological relevance of hypoxic depression of breathing can be found in both unanesthetized newborn and adult mammals. In the newborn, the respiratory response to hypoxia is unsustained, despite a sustained stimulation of the peripheral chemoreceptors (1,23). Thus, central hypoxic depression of respiration is able to dominate the peripheral response to hypoxia within minutes, giving the response a biphasic character. Although not as pronounced as the newborn's response, and having slower dynamics, there appears to be a remnant of this phenomenon in the adult. In unanesthetized adult animals, the initial increase in ventilation shows a significant roll-off after 15–30 min of continued hypoxia (8,13,29). Although some of the response may be attributable to peripheral effects such as reduction in systemic metabolic rate and reduction of mechanical output of respiratory muscles, there is convincing evidence that the major locus of the hypoxic effect is within the central nervous system.

At least three general mechanisms have been proposed to explain hypoxic depression. First, it has been suggested that the vasodilatory effect of hypoxia on brain blood vessels may cause hyperperfusion of the medullary chemoreceptors relative to their metabolism, resulting in an alkaline shift of pH and less stimulation. Evidence for this effect exists (21); however, we have shown that the alkalosis at the surface of the ventral medulla is generally transient, occurring only during mild hypoxia. With progressive brain hypoxia, it is rapidly replaced by an intense acidosis as the degree of hypoxia becomes more severe. We have called the depression of respiration associated with ventral medullary alkalosis *type I* hypoxic depression. The spectrum of its physiological significance is uncertain; however, we believe that it probably contributes to hypoxic depression of respiration during

REM sleep (24). At the other extreme, there must be a point at which oxygen delivery is insufficient to maintain aerobic metabolism and cell integrity. We have termed this *type III* hypoxic depression. *Type II* hypoxic depression is the intervening phase; it is associated with brain acidosis and greater respiratory depression than is type I, but occurs with levels of brain hypoxia not ordinarily associated with depletion of high-energy phosphates.

It is the mechanism responsible for type II hypoxic depression which we are currently pursuing. Since we have shown that the respiratory depression resulting from brain hypoxia is specific and not due to a generalized metabolic failure of respiratory neurons (17), we have focused on mechanisms that can promote hyperpolarization of respiratory neurons without impairing an excitatory response to an intense stimulus. A relative hyperpolarization could be achieved by an alteration in the balance between inhibitory and excitatory neuroeffectors.

There are several neuroeffector candidates that have been shown either directly or indirectly to change with brain hypoxia. The synthesis and release of several excitatory neurotransmitters—acetylcholine, adrenergic amines, glutamate, and aspartate—decrease during hypoxia (2,6,7,9,16). In contrast, there is a general increase in the concentrations of the neuronal depressants—opioids, adenosine, GABA, alanine, and lactic acid (7,9,12,30,31). In an effort to identify which inhibitory neuroeffectors are responsbile for hypoxic depression of respiratory output, we have determined the effect of a number of selective antagonists in our cat model of progressive brain hypoxia produced by inhalation of carbon monoxide.

METHODS

General Preparation

Adult cats (3.5–5.0 kg) were preanesthetized with ketamine HCl (2.2 mg/kg, i.m.) and acepromazine (1.1 mg/kg, i.m.) and then anesthetized with α-chloralose (40 mg/kg, i.v.). Rectal temperature was monitored and maintained at 38°C throughout the experiment. Venous and arterial catheters were inserted for recording arterial blood pressure (Statham 23Db pressure transducer), sampling arterial blood, and administering drugs. Blood gas tensions (P_{O_2} and P_{CO_2}) and pH were determined electrometrically at 38°C (Radiometer, Cleveland, OH). Arterial oxygen content (Lexicon) and carboxyhemoglobin and hemoglobin levels (IL182 Co-oximeter, specifically modified for cat blood, Instrumentation Laboratory, Lexington, MA) also were determined for each blood sample. The trachea was cannulated with an endotracheal tube (size No. 1, Shiley).

The midline structures superior to the tracheostomy were tied, cut, and reflected rostrally for exposure of the carotid sinus nerves and temporalis bone. The carotid sinus nerves were identified and sectioned bilaterally. Vagotomy was performed in all cats, except those in the naloxone series. The ventral surface of the medulla was exposed by removing a portion of the basioccipital bone and incising the dura and arachnoid membranes at the level of the roots of the twelfth cranial nerve. A flexible 1-mm-diameter, rounded, H^+-sensitive glass electrode and Ag/AgCl reference electrode (Microelectrodes, Londonderry, NH) were carefully positioned on the surface of the ventral medulla. The brain surface and electrodes were protected from heat and CO_2 loss by either trapping a small pool of CSF (1.5–2.0 mm) with a soft agar scal (group I) or by creating a deep (1.5–2.0 cm) pool of CSF above the brain surface (group II). Changes in H^+ activity were measured by using a digital display pH meter (Beckman Φ 71) with isolated input, and the signal was amplified and recorded. Because calibration of the pH electrodes was performed in vitro using two phosphate buffer solutions (6.865 and 7.410, Radiometer), all pH data are reported as changes from baseline. The responsiveness of the pH system was checked in vivo prior to every study by recording the delay and magnitude of the decrease in ventral medullary surface pH to an abrupt increase in end-tidal CO_2. The criteria for acceptance necessitated that the pH change within 5–15 s after a change in $P_{ET}CO_2$ with a magnitude of 0.003–0.007/mmHg end-tidal CO_2. $P_{ET}CO_2$ was generally increased 14–28 mmHg.

Respiratory output was assessed by measuring either the inspiratory flow with a Fleisch 00 pneumotachograph and a Validyne differential pressure transducer in spontaneously breathing cats (naloxone series), or the phrenic neurogram in paralyzed (gallamine HCl, 2 mg/kg/h, i.v.), mechanically ventilated cats. The phrenic nerve was isolated at the C4–5 level, desheathed, placed on bipolar gold electrodes, and bathed in mineral oil. The raw neurogram signal was amplified, filtered with a band pass of 0.1 to 10 kHz (differential amplifier, CWE, Inc.), full-wave rectified, and integrated with a time constant of 100 ms (moving-averaged, third-order Paynter filter; CWE, Inc.). The raw phrenic neurogram and moving average signals were continuously recorded, and the signal was A–D converted (Data Transformations) and analyzed breath by breath by an IBM-XT computer. End-tidal CO_2 was monitored (Godard Capnograph), recorded, and maintained constant in mechanically ventilated cats by servo-adjustment of the ventilatory frequency.

In order to keep the mean arterial blood pressure constant, the abdominal aorta was cannulated just proximal to the bifurcation of the femoral arteries and the cannula connected to a low impedance–high capacitance reservoir of an isotonic mannitol–saline solution.

Experimental Protocol

The respiratory and ventral medullary pH responses to progressive brain hypoxia were compared before and after pretreatment with selective antagonists of the specific inhibitory neuroeffectors. Progressive brain hypoxia was produced with inhalation of 0.5–1.0% CO, 40% O_2 (balance N_2). After a stable 5-min baseline was established while the animal breathed 40% O_2 (balance N_2), a control response to progressive carboxyhemoglobin was obtained. Ventral medullary pH, respiratory output, end-tidal CO_2, and arterial blood pressure were continuously recorded. Arterial blood was sampled every few minutes and at the end of CO exposure. Inhalation of CO was continued until respiratory output was reduced to at least 40% of baseline. Subsequent inhalation of 100% O_2 (approximately 45 min), was used to reduce the arterial COHb levels to <10%. The response to progressive carboxyhemoglobinemia was repeated after administration of specific antagonists using the same protocol.

Role of Endogenous Opioids in Hypoxic Depression of Respiration: Naloxone

The ventilatory and ventral medullary pH responses to progressive brain hypoxia were determined in spontaneously breathing cats using 1% CO, 40% O_2 (balance N_2). After a control response was obtained, naloxone HCl (0.1 mg/kg) was administered intravenously. A new stable baseline minute ventilation was generally reached after 5 min, at which point the second response to progressive hypoxia was determined.

Role of Adenosine in Hypoxic Depression of Respiration: Theophylline

The phrenic neurogram and ventral medullary pH responses to progressive brain hypoxia (0.5% CO, 40% O_2, balance N_2) were determined in paralyzed, mechanically ventilated cats while end-tidal CO_2 and mean arterial blood pressure were kept constant. Responses were determined before and after pretreatment with the adenosine antagonist theophylline. Theophylline (20 mg/kg) was administered by an intravenous infusion over 30–40 min. Thirty minutes after completion of the dose infusion, a second response to progressive CO hypoxia was determined.

Role of Lactic Acidosis in Hypoxic Depression of Respiration: Sodium Dichloroacetate

The ventral medullary pH and phrenic neurogram responses to progressive brain hypoxia (0.5% CO, 40% O_2, balance N_2) were determined before and 15 min after administration of sodium dilchoroacetate (500 mg/kg). Sodium dichloroacetate was prepared by neutralizing a solution of dichloroacetic acid in distilled water with NaOH.

Role of GABA in Hypoxic Depression of Respiration: Bicuculline

The effect of brain hypoxia on the dose–response curve of minute phrenic activity to the GABA antagonist bicuculline was assessed by determining dose–response curves with and without brain hypoxia. Dose–response curves were determined by recording the phrenic neurogram response to cumulative doses of bicuculline (0.01 mg/kg/min, i.v.). A control dose–response was determined while ventilating the cat on 40% O_2. The effect of brain hypoxia on the dose–response curve was assessed after first depressing phrenic nerve activity with inhalation of 0.5% CO, 40% O_2 (balance N_2), then maintaining that level of hypoxemia by a rebreathing circuit with a CO_2 scrubber, and determining the phrenic neurogram response to cumulative doses of bicuculline using the same protocol as for the control response.

RESULTS AND DISCUSSION

Role of Endogenous Opioids in Hypoxic Depression: Naloxone

Since it had been shown that the apnea of neonatal asphyxia could be reversed by using the opioid antagonist naloxone (3,4), we assessed whether endogenous opioids played a role in our model of hypoxic depression. Although we could show

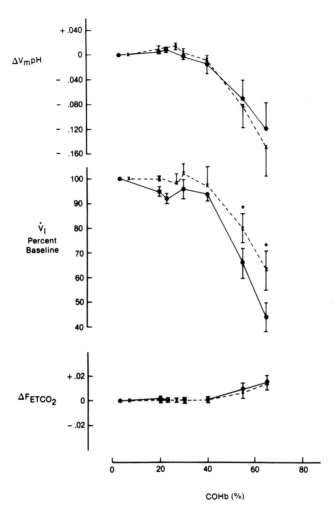

Fig. 25.1 Ventilatory and ventral medullary surface pH (V_mpH) reponses to progressive car-boxyhemoglobinemia before (●————●) and after naloxone (x---x). Changes (means ± SE) in V_mpH, minute ventilation ($\dot{V}_I$), and end-tidal fractional concentration of CO_2 ($F_{ET}CO_2$) are plotted against percent arterial carboxyhemoglobin (COHb). Asterisks denote a signifi-cant ($p < .05$) difference in the response after naloxone.

that opioids mediate a portion of the depression of ventilation, blocking their effect did not eliminate the respiratory depression to acute brain hypoxia (20). The ven-tilatory and ventral medullary pH responses to progressive carboxyhemoglobine-mia before and after naloxone are shown in Fig. 25.1. Prior to naloxone, increasing the COHb to 55% was associated with a substantial ventral medullary surface aci-dosis (i.e., the ventral medullary pH decreased by 0.071 ± 0.032 pH units) and a significant reduction in minute ventilation (66 ± 6% of baseline) due to significant declines in both frequency and tidal volume. Administration of naloxone did not alter the basic characteristics of the surface pH profile during progressive brain hypoxia; however, there was a smaller, but significantly less, reduction in ventilation. After naloxone, although the progressive acidosis of brain hypoxia (i.e., a decline in ventral medullary pH of 0.082 ± 0.036 pH units at 55% COHb) was still associated with a progressive decline in ventilation, there was less depression at any given level of carboxyhemoglobinemia. Thus, when COHb was increased to 55%, minute ventilation was reduced to only $81 \pm 9\%$ of baseline, which was significantly less than the reduction to 66% seen prior to naloxone.

When we examined the naloxone effect on hypoxic depression in terms of the tidal volume and frequency components, we found that the naloxone effect was not due to a difference in the frequency response but rather to a progressive increase in tidal volume during progressive carboxyhemoglobinemia.

Because central acidotic stimulation of ventilation is usually manifested as an increase in tidal volume, the ability of naloxone to uncover an increase in tidal volume with progressive brain hypoxia suggested that there might be a reestablishment of an acid stimulation of central chemosensitive cells by the metabolic acidosis of brain hypoxia although this effect of acid stimulation is quite small. In fact, when a linear regression analysis of change in tidal volume versus change in ventral medullary surface pH was performed, it was found that before naloxone there was virtually no tidal volume response to medullary acidosis whereas after naloxone there was a significantly greater ($p < .02$) response to the metabolic acidosis of brain hypoxia ($\Delta V_1 = -60.3$ ml/pH unit of -0.00976, $r = -0.937$). This was within the range of ventilatory responses to "metabolic" acidosis that have been previously reported (25,27). These observations suggest that administration of naloxone restored the ventilatory response to metabolic acidosis, which had been blunted by endogenous opioids during the production of progressive brain hypoxia.

Role of Adenosine in Hypoxic Depression: Theophylline

A potential role for the inhibitory neuroeffector adenosine was suggested by Millhorn and associates (18), who showed that the adenosine antagonist theophylline eliminated the post-hypoxic depression of respiratory output in anesthetized cats. Thus, to assess the role of adenosine on the progressive depression of respiration during hypoxia, we determined the effect of theophylline on hypoxic depression of respiration in our model (22).

The effect of theophylline on the minute phrenic nerve response to reductions in arterial oxygen content by progressive carboxyhemoglobinemia is shown in Fig. 25.2 for a representative animal. Similar to the naloxone studies, pretreatment with theophylline produced only a minor attenuation of the hypoxic depression of minute phrenic nerve activity and did not significantly alter the course of hypoxic depression. In the mean data for the group, it was found that prior to theophylline administration, a 50% reduction in arterial oxygen content was associated with $34 \pm 12\%$ reduction in phrenic nerve activity, whereas after theophylline, equivalent reductions in arterial oxygen content diminished phrenic nerve activity by $18 \pm 8\%$. The difference in the responses with or without pretreatment with theophylline was due to an attenuation of the depression of peak phrenic nerve activity after antagonizing adenosine. Thus, although there is indirect evidence suggesting that adenosine may play a major role in the depression of respiration with brain

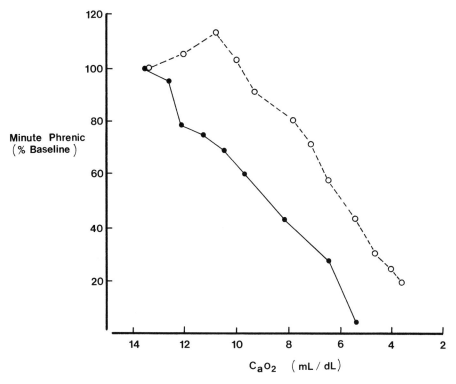

Fig. 25.2 Minute phrenic nerve response to progressive reductions in arterial oxygen content (C_aO_2) produced by inhalation of 0.5% CO in 40% O_2 before (●———●) and after (○---○) theophylline in a single cat.

hypoxia (18,30), this direct testing of adenosine's contribution to hypoxic depression reveals only a minor role.

Role of Lactic Acidosis in Hypoxic Depression: Sodium Dichloroacetate

In a third group of studies, we considered the lactic acidosis associated with brain tissue hypoxia. Although we generally think of acidosis as a respiratory stimulant, this stimulation is a unique characteristic of a small population of chemosensitive cells located near the surface of the ventral medulla. In contrast to this stimulatory effect, most CNS neurons respond to acidosis with a hyperpolarization and diminished acitivity (10,14,15,19). Because the acidosis of brain hypoxia is primarily due to the production of lactate, we could determine the role of lactic acid in hypoxic depression by preventing lactic acid formation with the use of sodium dichloroacetate (DCA) in our model of progressive CO hypoxia. DCA prevents lactate formation by enhancing the activity of pyruvate dehydrogenase through inhibition of the kinase responsible for inactivating the active form of the enzyme (5). Systemic administration of DCA was able to prevent the ventral medullary acidosis associated with progressive reductions in arterial oxygen content and dramatically pre-

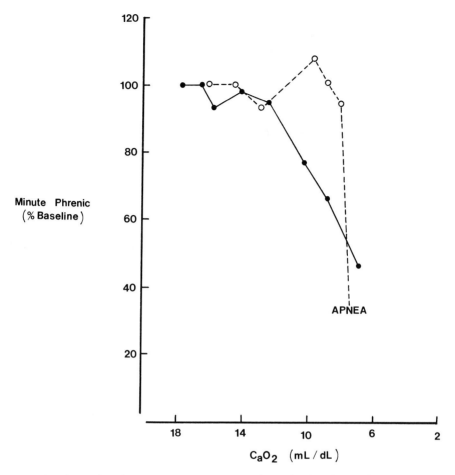

Fig. 25.3 Minute phrenic nerve response to progressive reductions in arterial oxygen content produced by inhalation of 0.5% CO in 40% O_2 before (●————●) and after (○---○) sodium dichloroacetate (DCA) in a single cat.

vented any significant depression of phrenic nerve activity until the hypoxemia became very severe, whereupon further CO-hypoxemia produced a precipitous decline in phrenic activity (Fig. 25.3). Thus, the progressive and graded brain lactic acidosis may contribute to a significant portion of the progressive decline in respiratory output with progressive CO hypoxia (26). Although intracellular acidosis may play a direct role in depression of respiratory neuronal activity by directly affecting membrane potentials, a more likely explanation is that intracellular acidosis contributes to membrane hyperpolarization by promoting the production of a potent inhibitory neurotransmitter (e.g., GABA).

Role of GABA in Hypoxic Depression of Respiration: Bicuculline

The rate of synthesis of GABA is sensitive to the effects of reductions in oxygen availability and increases in intracellular acidity. Reductions in oxygen diminish the degradation of GABA by reducing the concentration of α-ketoglutarate via the TCA cycle which is necessary for the transamination of GABA. In addition, an increase in the intracellular acidity favors the production of GABA (32) because the optimal pH values for the two key enzymes are 7.0 for glutamic acid decarboxylase (which catalyzes synthesis of GABA from glutamic acid) and 8.0 for GABA transaminase (which catalyzes the degradation of GABA). Thus, the fourth inhibitory neurotransmitter that was assessed for a contributory role in the hypoxic depression of respiration in our model of progressive brain hypoxia was GABA.

The effect of brain hypoxia on the dose–response curves of minute phrenic nerve activity versus the GABA antagonist bicuculline is shown in Fig. 25.4. In the absence of hypoxia, only small doses of bicuculline were necessary to stimulate phrenic output maximally at subseizure levels, indicating that in the anesthetized cat, GABA was at concentrations that contribute a tonic inhibitory influence on phrenic nerve activity. In the presence of brain hypoxia and significant respiratory depression, the dose–response curve is shifted toward higher doses, reflecting the ability of brain hypoxia to increase the concentrations of brain GABA. However, what is most important in this dose–response curve is that the maximum level of the phrenic nerve response is the same with and without brain hypoxia, suggesting

Fig. 25.4 Effect of brain hypoxia, produced by reducing arterial content with 0.5% CO in 40% O_2, on the dose–response curves of minute phrenic nerve activity versus the GABA antagonist bicuculline in a single cat.

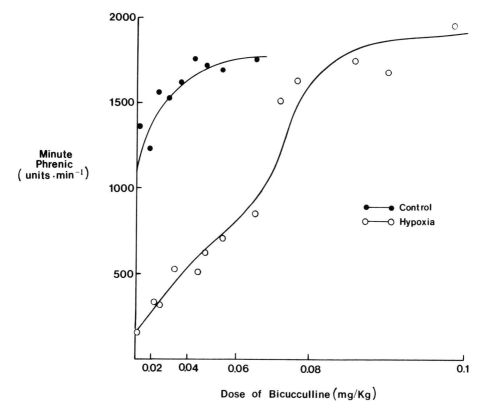

that there is true competitive inhibition. Thus, reversing the inhibitory influence of GABA during brain hypoxia restored phrenic activity to maximum stimulation. We believe that these results suggest that GABA may be the principal inhibitory neurotransmitter mediating respiratory depression during type II hypoxic depression, and that the levels of GABA may be regulated via cellular acidosis.

The effect of brain hypoxia on cellular metabolism to favor production of inhibitory neuroeffectors is an adaptive mechanism that provides the brain with relative resistance to permanent cellular damage by diminishing the external work of neuronal activity. This depression of respiratory neurons is specific for brain hypoxia since it does not prevent the neuronal circuitry from responding to other stimuli, such as hypercapnia (17). Thus, it is a depression manifested as an increased threshold for respiratory stimuli without an alteration of intrinsic responsiveness, as would occur with hyperpolarization of all respiratory neuronal pools.

If we postulate that central hypoxic depression is a protective mechanism, then it is reasonable to suggest that it may be a conserved function whose general mechanisms are used more prominently by lower animals that have evolved a tolerance for hypoxic environments. The specific strategies that assist hypoxia-tolerant animals in maintaining cellular integrity when oxygen becomes a limited substrate have been enumerated in a recent review (11). Animals that can be classified as hypoxia-tolerant are generally able to prevent accumulation of lactic acidosis with a reverse Pasteur effect; their membranes tend to be less permeable to ions; they decrease their metabolism so that ATP utilization is regulated to synthesis; and they are better able to maintain stable membranes with stable ion gradients.

It seems clear that the key to surviving the detrimental effects of hypoxia is having the ability to maintain the integrity of membrane and ionic gradients. Although mammals appear to lack the special qualities that endow, for example, turtles with their extraordinary tolerance to hypoxia (28), the mammalian nervous system can minimize the effect of hypoxia at the cellular level. Specifically, cellular metabolic mechanisms that promote membrane hyperpolarization reduce the basal activity and thereby reduce the metabolic drain of membrane ion pumps. Thus, this adaptation to hypoxia might subserve a protective function by limitation of motor activity as well as conservation of high-energy substrates within neuronal cells. In addition, because neuronal firing stresses ionic pumps, reducing discharge rate could provide a means for delaying the loss of cellular integrity.

REFERENCES

1. Blanco, C. E., M. A. Hanson, P. Johnson, and H. Rigatto. The pattern of breathing of kittens during hypoxia. *Pediatr. Res. 15:* 652, 1981.
2. Brown, R. M., S. R. Snider, and A. Carlsson. Changes in biogenic amine synthesis and turnover induced by hypoxia and/or foot shock stress. II. The central nervous system. *J. Neurol. Trans. 35:* 293–305, 1974.
3. Chernick, V., and R. J. Craig. Naloxone reverses neonatal depression caused by fetal asphyxia. *Science 216:* 1252–1253, 1982.
4. Chernick, V., D. L. Madansky, and E. E. Lawson. Naloxone decreases the duration of primary apnea with neonatal asphyxia. *Pediatr. Res. 14:* 357–359, 1980.

5. Crabb, D. W., E. A. Yount, and R. A. Harris. The metabolic effects of dichloroacetate. *Metabolism 30:* 1024–1039, 1981.
6. Davis, J. N., and A. Carlsson. Effect of hypoxia on monoamine synthesis levels and metabolism in rat brain. *J. Neurochem. 21:* 783–790, 1973.
7. Duffy, T. E., S. R. Nelson, and O. H. Lowry. Cerebral carbohydrate metabolism during acute hypoxia and recovery. *J. Neurochem. 19:* 959–977, 1972.
8. Easton, P. A., L. J. Slykerman, and N. R. Anthonisen. Ventilatory response to sustained hypoxia in normal adults. *J. Appl. Physiol. 61:* 906–911, 1986.
9. Erecinska, M., D. Nelson, D. F. Wilson, and I. A. Silver. Neurotransmitter amino acids in the CNS. I. Regional changes in amino acid levels in rat brain during ischemia and reperfusion. *Brain Res. 304:* 9–22, 1984.
10. Gill, P. K., and M. Kuno. Properties of phrenic motoneurones. *J. Physiol.* (Lond.) *168:* 258–273, 1963.
11. Hochachka, P. W. Defense strategies against hypoxia and hypothermia. *Science 231:* 234–241, 1986.
12. Iversen, K., T. Hedner, and P. Lundborg. GABA concentrations and turnover in neonatal rat brain during asphyxia and recovery. *Acta Physiol. Scand. 118:* 91–94, 1983.
13. Kagawa, S., M. J. Stafford, T. B. Waggener, and J. W. Severinghaus. No effect of naloxone on hypoxia-induced ventilatory depression in adults. *J. Appl. Physiol. 52:* 1030–1034, 1982.
14. Krynjevic, K., M. Randic, and B. K. Siesjo. Cortical CO_2 tension and neuronal excitability. *J. Physiol.* (Lond.) *176:* 105–122, 1965.
15. Marino, P. L., and T. W. Lamb. Effects of CO_2 and extracellular H^+ iontophoresis on single cell activity in the cat brainstem. *J. Appl. Physiol. 38:* 688–695, 1975.
16. McNamara, M. C., J. L. Gingras-Leatherman, and E. E. Lawson. Effect of hypoxia on brainstem concentration of biogenic amines in postnatal rabbits. *Dev. Brain Res. 25:* 253–258, 1986.
17. Melton, J. E., J. A. Neubauer, and N. H. Edelman. CO_2 sensitivity of the cat phrenic neurogram during hypoxic respiratory depression *Appl. Physiol. 65:* 736–743, 1988.
18. Millhorn, D. E., F. L. Eldridge, J. P. Kiley, and T. G. Waldrop. Prolonged inhibition of respiration following acute hypoxia in glomectomized cats. *Respir. Physiol. 57:* 331–340, 1984.
19. Mitchell, R. A., and D. A. Herbert. The effect of carbon dioxide on the membrane potential of medullary respiratory neurons. *Brain Res. 75:* 345–349, 1974.
20. Neubauer, J. A., M. A. Posner, T. V. Santiago, and N. H. Edelman. Naloxone reduces the ventilatory depression of brain hypoxia. *J. Appl. Physiol. 63:* 699–706, 1987.
21. Neubauer, J. A., T. V. Santiago, M. A. Posner, and N. H. Edelman. Ventral medullary pH and ventilatory responses to hyperperfusion and hypoxia. *J. Appl. Physiol. 58:* 1659–1668, 1985.
22. Nissely, F. P., J. E. Melton, J. A. Neubauer, and N. H. Edelman. Effect of adenosine antagonism on phrenic nerve output during brain hypoxia [Abstract]. *Fed. Proc. 45:* 1046, 1986.
23. Rigatto, H. Control of ventilation in the newborn. *Annu. Rev. Physiol. 46:* 661–674, 1984.
24. Santiago, T. V., J. A. Neubauer, and N. H. Edelman. Correlation between ventilation and brain blood flow during hypoxic sleep. *J. Appl. Physiol. 60:* 295–298, 1986.
25. Shams, H. Differential effects of CO_2 and H^+ as central stimuli of respiration in the cat. *J. Appl. Physiol. 58:* 357–364, 1985.
26. Simone, A., J. A. Nuebauer, J. E. Melton, and N. H. Edelman. Role of brain lactic acidosis in hypoxic depression of respiration *Appl. Physiol.* (in press).

27. Teppema, L. J., P.W.J.A. Barts, H. T. Folgering, and J. A. Evers. Effects of respiratory and (isocapnic) metabolic arterial acid–base disturbances on medullary extracellular fluid pH and ventilation in cats. *Respir. Physiol. 53:* 379–395, 1983.

28. Ultsch, G. R., and D. C. Jackson. Long-term submergence at 3°C of the turtle, *Chrysemys picta bellii,* in normoxic and severely hypoxic water. *J. Exp. Biol. 96:* 11–28, 1982.

29. Weil, J. V., and C. W. Zwillich. Assessment of ventilatory response to hypoxia: Methods and interpretation. *Chest 70* (Suppl.): 124–128, 1976.

30. Winn, H. R., R. Rubio, and R. M. Berne. Brain adenosine concentration during hypoxia in rat. *Am. J. Physiol. 241:* H235–H242, 1981.

31. Wood, J. D., W. J. Watson, and A. J. Ducker. The effect of hypoxia on brain γ-amino-butyric acid levels. *J. Neurochem. 15:* 603–608, 1968.

32. Wu, J.-Y. Purification, characterization and kinetic studies of GAD and GABA-7 from mouse brain. In: *GABA in Nervous System Function,* ed. E. Roberts, T. N. Chase, and D. B. Tower. New York: Raven Press, 1976, pp. 7–55.

26

Effects of Hypoxia on Brain Cell Acid–Base and High-Energy Phosphate Regulation by ^{31}P-NMR Spectroscopy

B. M. HITZIG

Adequate delivery of O_2 is important to proper central nervous sytem (CNS) function. The relationship between the partial pressure of O_2 in the breathing medium and CNS metabolism is often complicated by differences in the animal's ability to deliver O_2, as well as selective metabolic advantages enjoyed by specialized animals (e.g., diving animals). Semiaquatic, fresh-water turtles display a remarkable ability to tolerate prolonged, severe hypoxemia. They can remain submerged from hours to months (9,10,13,15,21), depending upon body temperature, and emerge from the water in good condition. This tolerance is thought to be due to the presence of "diving reflexes" and the ability of this animal to maintain its vital functions through anaerobic metabolism for the duration of the dive (1,20).

We have demonstrated that turtles possess sensitive mechanisms of central chemical control of ventilation (6). Hitzig (7) has shown that central chemosensors of turtles and goats function similarly, and that the sensitivity of relative ventilation to changes in acid–base status of brain extracellular fluids is the same in both animals. Turtles can therefore be used to study the effects of prolonged O_2 deprivation on central chemical control of ventilation, a basic and vital function of the CNS, the state of which can be considered representative of the viability of other life-sustaining CNS functions.

The ability of the CNS to perform a particular integrative function during stress is dependent upon how well the neurons of the brain adapt to that stress. Hypoxia at the cellular level presents neurons with two related but distinctly different problems: First, they are subjected to acid–base stress caused by the accumulation of lactic (fixed) acid, the end product of anaerobic glycolysis. Second, because of the lack of O_2, brain cells suffer a loss of reducing equivalents and therefore must cope with the resulting decreased ability to generate high-energy phosphate compounds through oxidative phosphorylation.

^{31}P-nuclear magnetic resonance spectroscopy (NMR) allows us to examine CNS adaptations to each of these stresses individually. By using this technique, investigators may relate specific adaptations of one important regulated variable— for example, brain cell pH—to changes in high-energy phosphate regulation (11). ^{31}P-NMR coupled with surface-coil technology permits noninvasive, nondestructive, simultaneous measurements of brain intracellular pH (pH$_i$), and the levels of important compounds involved in high-energy phosphate metabolism. Relative levels of brain cell phosphocreatine (PCr), ATP, inorganic phosphate (P$_i$), and glycolytic intermediates can be obtained in unanesthetized animals. Serial measurements can be made in a time frame that allows the investigation of both steady- and non-steady-state phenomena (2,5,11).

In this chapter, we examine specific functions of the CNS during hypoxia on both an organ system and cellular level. The effects of O$_2$ deprivation on the integrative responses involved in central chemical control of ventilation in an animal model well-adapted to this stress will be discussed. Four groups (n = 6) of semiaquatic turtles *(Chrysemys scripta elegans)* were subjected to one of three experimental stresses related to the severe O$_2$ deprivation seen in apneic diving, and the central component of their ventilatory responses were measured. Additionally, endogenous levels of brain amino acid neurotransmitters known to be involved in the regulation of central control of ventilation were measured in similar groups of animals exposed to the same stresses. The results of these studies will enable us to gain additional insight into how the integrative mechanisms of the CNS, associated with central chemical control of ventilation, function during severe hypoxia.

^{31}P-NMR studies of the brain of conscious mice subjected to moderate to severe hypoxia are also discussed, and brain cell regulatory mechanisms associated with various levels of hypoxia are delineated. We measured brain pH$_i$ and the relative levels of high-energy phosphate compounds during experimentally induced moderate to severe hypoxia, and in acid–base stress that is associated with hypoxia.

METHODS

Turtle Ventilation Experiments

Adult turtles *(C. scripta elegans)* of either sex, weighing 1–2 kg, were obtained commercially. Chronic arterial catheters were implanted using the method developed by Jackson et al. (14). Arterial blood and cerebrospinal fluid (CSF) gas and pH measurements were made at appropriate times during the experiment. CSF was obtained from conscious animals using the method developed by Hitzig and Nattie (10). Ventilatory measurements were made using the buoyancy method originated by Jackson (12) which allows for the strict control of the animal's breathing mixture. Tidal volume (ml/breath), mean expired minute volume (ml [BTPS]*/kg/min, and respiratory frequency (breaths/min) were obtained.

---

*BTPS: body temperature, pressure, saturation.

All experiments were performed at 20°C. Control ventilatory measurements were made, and then the animals ($n = 6$) were subjected to 2 h of breathing one of four gas mixtures: 8% CO_2 in air (hypercapnia); 98% N_2–2% CO_2 (anoxia); 8% CO_2–92% N_2 (anoxia plus hypercapnia, a simulated dive); or air (controls). Ventilatory measurements were made every 30 min during the 2 h of breathing the experimental gases. Arterial blood gas and pH measurements were made immediately before and after the 2-h experimental breathing period. CSF total CO_2 was measured immediately after the 2-h experimental breathing period. CSF P_{CO_2} was estimated by adding 2 torr to the P_aCO_2 value. CSF pH was estimated by using the measured value for CSF total CO_2, the estimated CSF P_{CO_2}., and the Henderson–Hasselbach equation. This was necessitated by the small size of the CSF sample. Subsequent work in which CSF pH was directly measured in each of the experimental treatments confirmed that the estimated CSF pH values never differed from the measured values by more than 0.03 pH units (10).

Brain Amino Acid Measurements

The same experimental paradigm was used in this study as above, except that no ventilatory, arterial blood, or CSF measurements were made after turtles breathed the experimental gas mixtures for 2 h. Additionally, a group of turtles ($n = 6$) forced to dive in 20°C water for 2 h were added to the four groups of animals mentioned above. At the end of the 2-h experimental period, the animals were immediately decapitated (by guillotine), and the heads were instantly frozen in liquid N_2. The frozen medulla and midbrain were removed and the wet weights determined. One milliliter of cold perchloric acid (8% [w/v] in H_2O) was added for each 100 mg of brain tissue, and the mixture was uniformly homogenized in a blender at 3°C. γ-Aminobutyric acid (GABA), taurine, glycine, glutamic acid, and glutamine were measured chromatographically for each brain tissue sample by means of a cation-exchange column amino acid analyzer as reported previously (9).

Brain NMR Experiments

Unanesthetized outbred Swiss–Webster type CD-1 mice of either sex weighing 30–35 g were used in these experiments. We used a Bruker HX-270 Fourier-transform spectrometer with a 6.4-Tesla magnet. At the time of the experiment, the animals were placed in a specially designed probe in which the head was firmly held in position. The ³¹P-NMR signals from the animal's brain were monitored with a three-turn surface coil. The signal-to-noise ratio was high enough to obtain useful spectra within 2 min. A standard pulse sequence ($90–t–90– \ldots$) was used with a 2.5-s interpulse delay. The ratios of the concentrations of the high-energy phosphate compounds phosphocreatine and adenosine triphosphate (PCr/ATP) were determined by comparison of the signal-averaged resonance areas in each spectrum. These ratios are good indicators of the energy state of the cells being measured (2,5,11). A decrease in the PCr/ATP ratio signifies an increase in buffering of ATP by PCr and could mean an increase in brain cell ATP utilization, or a decrease in ATP production.

Brain pH_i was measured by comparison of the chemical shift of the P_i peak with previously determined calibration curves after the method of Moon and Richards (19). Comparison of the spectra taken in anesthetized mice before and after surgical removal of all the skin and muscles of the head confirmed that our signal originated from brain and not the muscle tissue of the head. The breathing mixture was strictly controlled by passing the gas from premixed pressurized cylinders through a tube into the bottom of the sealed probe.

The animals were given air to breathe, and control measurements were made for 30 min, with spectra being taken every 5 min. Hypoxic gas mixtures of 15%, 12%, 10%, 8%, 7%, 5%, and 2% O_2 in N_2 were administered for 20 min, and spectra were gathered every 5 min. Another group of animals ($n = 6$) were given a mixture of 10% CO_2/21% O_2 in N_2 to breathe for 40 min in order to assess the effects of acid–base stress alone on the above variables.

Statistical comparisons of the data taken from the various related experimental groups were made using analysis of variance (F-test) and unpaired Student's t-tests where applicable, as determined by the F-test.

RESULTS

Ventilation Experiments

At 30 min, there were large increases in both respiratory frequency (f) and tidal volume (V_T). From 30 to 120 min, the differences in V_T among the three experimental groups were not statistically significant. The data for normalized f (experimental value/control value) showed major differences among the groups (Fig. 26.1). The three experimental treatments resulted in an increase in f of approximately 2.5 fold within the first 30 min. During the next 30 min, f in the anoxic group decreased to 1.4 times the control—a statistically significant difference ($p <$ .01) from f values of the other two experimental groups. The f values increased slightly in hypercapnia, and remained at 2.5 times control levels in anoxia plus hypercapnia. Normalized f continued to rise to 3.1 times control values for the hypercapnic group during the final hour. The frequency decreased slightly (from 2.55 to 2.4) for anoxia plus hypercapnia from 60 to 90 min, and then decreased to 1.87 times the control in the final 30 min. The decreases were not statistically significant with increasing time, and the differences between the hypercapnic and the anoxic plus hypercapnic groups were not statistically significant for the entire experiment, according to the F-test. In sharp contrast to the other two groups, f in anoxia fell precipitously after 30 min to a point where it was not statistically different from control values at 60 min, and remained there for the duration of the experiment.

The experimental treatments produced a marked acidosis after 120 min in both arterial blood and CSF. The acidoses was most severe in the CSF, and estimated CSF pH was lowest in anoxia plus hypercapnia (Fig. 26.1).

Brain Amino Acid Experiments

In each experimental treatment where anoxia was present, mean brain tissue GABA levels (midbrain and medulla) were significantly elevated above controls ($p < .01$). Figure 26.2 reveals that this increase ranged from 47% (from 1.91 to 2.80

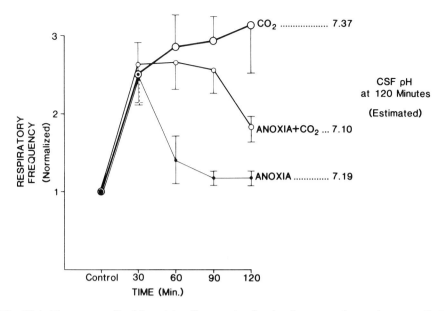

Fig. 26.1 Mean normalized breathing frequencies for the three experimental groups. Each data point represents the mean $\pm$ SE of all the values obtained for each animal divided by its own control. Note that the levels of respiratory frequency do not correlate with estimated CSF pH (10).

Fig. 26.2 Comparison of normalized brain tissue free GABA and taurine concentrations (μmol/g of brain wet wt) for the four experimental groups (9). Note that GABA levels are elevated in all treatments involving anoxia, whereas taurine levels vary with the experimental condition (see text).

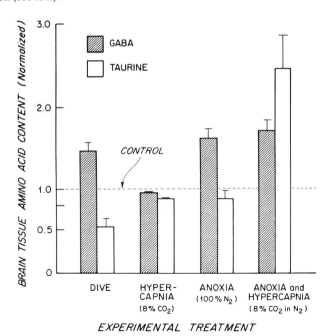

μmol/g brain tissue) during forced diving, to 72% (from 1.91 to 3.2 μmol/g brain tissue) during anoxia plus hypercapnia. Mean brain tissue taurine levels during diving were significantly decreased ($p < .05$) by 44% (from 1.91 to 1.80 μmol/g brain tissue). Interestingly, anoxia plus hypercapnia (simulated dive) resulted in a significant increase in brain tissue taurine ($p < .01$) of 113% (from 1.91 to 4.08 μmol/g brain tissue), whereas anoxia alone resulted in no significant change. Hypercapnia alone resulted in no significant changes in either GABA or taurine. There were no significant changes in glutamic acid, glutamine, or glycine after 2 h of any of the experimental protocols.

Brain NMR Experiments

Decreasing the inspired P_{O_2} to 8% had no effect upon PCr/ATP ratios (1.71 ± 0.09) in the six animals tested. Five minutes of breathing 7% O_2 resulted in a decrease in the PCr/ATP ratio to 1.44 (± 0.11), and the area under the phosphatidyl-N-methylethanolamine (PME) peaks increased an average of 14%. Intracellular pH remained constant (see Fig. 26.3 for an example). Five minutes of breathing 2% O_2 in N_2 (severe hypoxia) resulted in almost a complete loss of PCr and ATP with a large increase in P_i (Fig. 26.3). Under these conditions, brain cell pH became very acid (6.42 ± 0.07 units). Imposition of acid–base stress alone (breathing 10% CO_2, 21% O_2 in N_2) resulted in no change in the PCr/ATP ratios or in pH_i.

DISCUSSION

The purpose of this series of experiments was to examine CNS function during hypoxia on both the organ system and the cellular levels. On an organ system level, there may be integrated regulatory mechanisms which, under activation by hypoxia, modify the output of the system by altering the response of individual cells, or groups of cells. Inadequate delivery of oxygen, resulting from hypoxia, affects the ability of brain cells to produce the high-energy phosphates necessary to keep them alive and functioning.

Ventilatory Experiments

The semiaquatic turtle *Chrysemys scripta elegans* has been shown to possess sensitive mechanisms of central chemical control of ventilation (6,7). Perfusion of the brain ventricular system with mock CSF containing various concentrations of fixed acid resulted in large and predictable alterations in ventilation. Hitzig (7) demonstrated that the sensitivity of relative ventilation to alterations in the acid–base status of brain extracellular fluid (ECF) is the same in turtles and goats; therefore, turtles are a good experimental model for the study of central chemical ventilatory drive. Central control of ventilation is a basic and important function of the CNS, and studying how hypoxia affects this system is important in understanding the overall CNS response to this stress.

Hitzig et al. (8) observed that the ventilatory response of these animals to

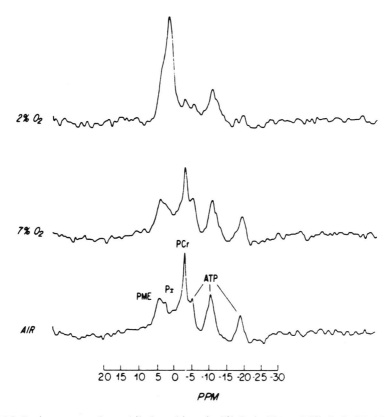

Fig. 26.3 Brain spectra taken while breathing air, 7% O_2 in N_2, and 2% O_2 in N_2. Note that the phosphatidyl-N-methylethanolamine (PME) and P_i peaks increased and the PCr peak decreased while ATP remained constant, with 7% O_2 breathing. With 2% O_2 breathing, the increase in the P_i peak was maximized, while there was a dramatic decrease in PCr and ATP. These changes were observed within 5 min. after breathing of the gas mixtures was initiated.

changes in the acid–base status of brain ECF consisted of alterations in f. Tidal volume changes were completely independent of acid–base changes in brain ECF. They concluded that central chemical control of ventilation involved alterations in respiratory frequency only, and that tidal volume changes were stimulated by receptors outside the blood–brain barrier. This finding was supported by the work of Milsom and Jones (18). Changes in f, therefore, reflect changes in central chemical ventilatory drive. This relationship allowed us to study the central effects of the various experimental stresses by measuring changes in f.

Semiaquatic turtles can maintain prolonged apneic dives lasting from several hours to many months, depending upon body temperature (9,10,13,15,21). Jackson and Silverblatt (15) found that these animals could tolerate 2- to 4-h dives (at 24°C) despite severe metabolic (arterial blood [lactic acid] = 29 meq/l), and respiratory acidosis (P_{CO_2} = 100 torr). Clark and Miller (3) demonstrated that 3 h of N_2 breathing resulted in a 0.5-unit decrease in brain pH_i, with brain tissue lactic acid concentrations of 29 meq/l. The ability to tolerate prolonged dives is seemingly incongruous with highly developed mechanisms of central chemical control of ventilation. The drive to breathe in most mammals (with proven central chemical control of ventilation) would force termination of a voluntary dive within minutes. Even diving mammals and birds are severely limited in their ability to maintain a prolonged apneic dive when compared with turtles. Clearly, diving turtles must possess an effective means of attenuating their ventilatory drive.

In the first series of experiments, turtles were subjected to 2 h of one of three experimental stresses (hypercapnia, anoxia, or anoxia plus hypercapnia), and their ventilatory responses and blood and CSF acid–base variables measured. These experiments produced large alterations in the pH of arterial blood and CSF. The acidosis in arterial blood was generally less severe than in CSF (0.2–0.29 pH units for blood vs. 0.23–0.5 pH units for CSF). This finding may result from the fact that CSF is a dilute salt solution with very little weak acid buffer (protein).

As stated above, changes in f reflect the central ventilatory response to the experimental stresses. During the initial 30 min of the experiments, f was elevated to the same level in each of the three experimental treatments; however, by 60 min, f was significantly higher in the two groups in which CO_2 was present in the breathing mixture (Fig. 26.1). At 120 min, it can be seen that f does not correlate with CSF pH measurements; that is, there was no discernible relationship between increased f and decreased CSF pH, but increases in f did seem to match increases in inspired P_{CO_2}. This was true whether or not anoxia was also present. Increased endogenous CNS fixed acid (lactic acid) alone, although producing a much greater change in estimated CSF pH (7.19) than hypercapnia (7.37), did not cause sustainable dramatic increases in f. Similar findings were reported in cats (16). These results seem to suggest that CO_2 has a stimulatory effect on central chemical ventilatory drive independent of pH effects.

The differences in f observed in the anoxic group as compared to the hypercapnic group from 60 to 120 min could not be due to anoxic depression of ventilation caused by decreases in brain cell high-energy phosphates. Anoxia did not depress the central ventilatory response because the addition of CO_2 to the breathing mixture resulted in a significantly elevated f over that seen in anoxia alone. Additionally, Clark and Miller (3) noted small decreases in the ATP content of the brain cells of *Chrysemys* after 3 h of breathing N_2; brain tissue retained most of its ATP, whereas heart and liver did not. It is possible that the decrease in f seen at 120 min of anoxia plus hypercapnia as compared to 90 min signifies the beginning of anoxic depression since unlimited extension of anoxia must result in the death of the animal.

Brain Amino Acid Experiments

Presumably, central chemosensors function by relaying their information to a controller within the CNS, which in turn stimulates effectors to produce alterations in ventilation. Ventilatory drive could be modified at any point by a variety of endogenously produced substances to produce the observed changes. Theoretically, increased levels of CO_2 could modify the effects of these substances in some way, resulting in an increase in central ventilatory drive. To investigate this possibility, we measured changes in turtle brain amino acid neurotransmitters during the three experimental treatments mentioned above plus those seen during 2 h of actual diving.

Several amino acids that are found in the CNS in relatively high concentrations have been shown to be inhibitory neurotransmitters. These include γ-aminobutyric acid (GABA), glycine, and taurine. To date, GABA and taurine are known to decrease ventilation. Several investigators have shown that GABA depresses centrally mediated cardiorespiratory functions (22–24). Yamada et al. (24) demonstrated that injection of GABA into the cisternal CSF of cats produced a marked reduction in ventilation associated with a decrease in heart rate and blood pressure. Wessberg et al. (22) have shown that taurine, infused into the brain ventricles of rats, has a depressant effect on ventilation that is independent of GABA receptors. Perfusion of the brain ventricular system with mock CSF containing taurine depressed ventilation by decreasing inspiratory neural drive and also by depressing respiratory timing mechanisms. This work has not established any involvement of these substances in the physiological processes of central chemical control of ventilation. Increases in CNS endogenous production of these substances in response to appropriate acid–base stress, accompanied by predictable changes in ventilatory behavior, would be indicative of a physiological role.

These experiments were designed to test if increased endogenous production of these substances within the medulla and midbrain of the CNS is associated with inhibition of ventilation under conditions of physiological stress. Our results show that brainstem and medulla GABA concentrations increased significantly during every experimental stress involving anoxia, including diving (Fig. 26.2); therefore, GABA could be the substance reducing ventilatory drive during diving and anoxia. However, we found that brainstem and medullary GABA concentrations were elevated to their highest level during anoxia plus hypercapnia (simulated dive). This suggests that GABA is not the sole mediator of reduced ventilatory drive during diving. Increased GABA concentrations during anoxia are consistent with the known decrease in activity of the GABA-degrading enzymes seen under anaerobic conditions (17); therefore, increased brain GABA concentrations are not unexpected.

Brainstem and medullary taurine levels are significantly reduced during diving (from 1.91 to 1.08 μmol/g), whereas they are significantly elevated during anoxia plus hypercapnia (from 1.91 to 4.68 μmol/g). On the surface, these results seem to conflict with our data in turtles, since decreased rather than increased CNS taurine levels are associated with suppression of centrally mediated respiratory drive during diving; however, closer examination of the data reveals a possible hypothetical model that could explain these apparently divergent results.

The increases in brainstem and medullary GABA levels during anoxic states are controlled by the decrease in the degradation of GABA and probably not subject to negative feedback control; however, the changes in taurine levels may be regulated. Taurine could be acting as a GABA antagonist: It could indeed be inhibitory when acting alone, but its action could be to mitigate the effects of GABA when acting in concert. In this hypothetical model, taurine need not be excitatory; it could act to inhibit the output of GABA neurons, or have a direct antagonistic effect on GABA binding. The differences in taurine concentration between the actual and simulated dive (taurine decreases during apneic diving, but increases during anoxia plus hypercapnia) could be related to the fact that the animals are apneic during the real dive and breathing during the simulated dive. If taurine antagonizes the inhibitory effects of GABA on respiration, then the elevated levels of taurine during the simulated dive would allow the animal to increase its breathing despite large increases in brain GABA (which is not subject to regulation). The reductions in taurine during actual diving, while GABA levels are elevated, fit well with the hypothetical model since reduced taurine levels would allow GABA to exert a greater effect in inhibiting ventilation.

The observation that GABA levels are significantly increased in anoxia while taurine is unchanged from control levels also fits well with the model since f is significantly lower in anoxia alone than in any of the other experimental treatments (except diving). Both GABA and taurine levels are unchanged from controls during hypercapnia, thus not interfering with the stimulatory effect of hypercapnia on ventilation. This model is hypothetical, but the changes in medullary and midbrain taurine and GABA, which are associated with appropriate ventilatory changes during anoxia, suggest an active role for these substances in modulating centrally mediated ventilatory drive.

Brain ^{31}P-NMR in Hypoxia

Hypoxia can present brain cells with two separate but related stresses: (a) acid–base stress resulting from the accumulation of lactic acid, the end product of anaerobic glycolysis; and (b) reduction in the rate of oxidative phosphorylation if O_2 delivery is inadequate. ^{31}P-NMR spectroscopy can noninvasively and nondestructively measure variables associated with both stresses in an animal model (2,5,11). We have developed an NMR technique and RF coil configurations that allow us to make ^{31}P-NMR measurements on the brains of unanesthetized mice. This is important since it is well known that anesthesia (gas and barbiturate) reduces brain cell ATP levels (4). Additionally, barbiturate anesthesia has been shown to produce a metabolic acidosis in several species of experimental animals (4).

We induced moderate to severe hypoxia in six conscious animals. No changes in the spectra were observed until the O_2 content of the breathing mixture was reduced to 7%. This indicates that moderate hypoxia (down to 8% O_2) did not disrupt brain cell acid–base homeostasis or the relative levels of high-energy phosphates. However, 5 min of breathing 7% O_2 in N_2, resulted in a decrease in PCr with a 14% increase in PME, while ATP levels remained constant (see Fig. 26.3 for an example). The decrease in PCr caused the PCr/ATP ratio to decrease to 1.44 ($\pm$ 0.11), demonstrating that lowering inspired Po_2 to 7% results in decreases in the "energy charge" of brain cells. Brain pH_i remained constant, suggesting that there is pH compensation for increased levels of cellular lactic acid.

Five minutes of breathing 2% O_2 resulted in a marked decrease in PCr and ATP, with a concomitant increase in P_i (see Fig. 26.3 for an example). Brain pH_i became quite acidic (pH = 6.42) under these conditions. The increase in acid–base stress brought about by increased cellular levels of lactic acid, coupled with the severe reduction in aerobic production of ATP, combined to disrupt cellular mechanisms for maintenance of pH_i.

Respiratory acidosis was induced in six animals in order to ascertain if the reduction in PCr/ATP seen during severe hypoxia could have been due in part to the lactic acidosis. Exposing these animals to 40 min of breathing 10% CO_2 in a normoxic mixture resulted in no change in PCr/ATP or pH_i. These results demonstrate that decreases in pH_i alone do not produce changes in the energy state of the cell, suggesting that the loss of high-energy phosphates was due to the lack of O_2 and not contributed to by the lactic acid load. Additionally, they emphasize the ability of brain cells to regulate pH_i during acid–base stress.

In conclusion, these studies show that the CNS responds to hypoxia on both an organ system and a cellular level. Central ventilatory drive is modified during hypoxia, and the type and degree of modification depend upon the presence, or absence, of accompanying hypercapnia. Levels of amino acid neurotransmitters are altered during hypoxia, and these changes may be responsible for the modification of central ventilatory drive. Brain cells are resistant to moderate hypoxia and can compensate for the acid–base stress associated with hypoxia; they lose this ability as well as most of their high-energy phosphate compounds upon imposition of severe hypoxia.

ACKNOWLEDGMENTS

This work was supported by American Heart Association Grant-in-Aid 861030 and NIH Grant HL-29620. I wish to thank my co-workers Eric McFarland, Douglas C. Johnson, and Homayoun Kazemi, who participated in various aspects of these studies.

REFERENCES

1. Belkin, D. A. Anoxia tolerance in reptiles. *Science 139:* 492–493, 1963.
2. Chance, B., S. Eleff, J. S. Leigr, Jr., D. Sokolow, and A. Sapega. Mitochondrial regulation of phosphocreatine/inorganic phosphate ratios in exercising human muscle; a gated ³¹P NMR study. *Proc. Natl. Acad. Sci. U.S.A. 78:* 6714–6718, 1981.
3. Clark, V. M., and A. T. Miller, Jr. Studies on anaerobic metabolism in the fresh water turtle *(Pseudemys scripta elegans). Comp. Biochem. Physiol. 44:* 55–62, 1973.
4. Dempsey, J. A., and H. V. Forster. Mediation of ventilatory adaptations. *Physiol. Rev. 62:* 262–346, 1982.
5. Gadian, D. G. *Nuclear Magnetic Resonance and Its Applications to Living Systems.* Oxford: Clarendon Press, 1982, pp. 43–77.
6. Hitzig, B. M., and D. C. Jackson. Central chemical control of ventilation in the unanesthetized turtle. *Am. J. Physiol. 235 (Regulatory Integrative Comp. Physiol. 4):* R257–R264, 1978.
7. Hitzig, B. M. Temperature induced changes in turtle CSF pH and central control of ventilation. *Respir. Physiol. 49:* 205–222, 1982.
8. Hitzig, B. M., J. C. Allen, and D. C. Jackson. Central chemical control of ventilation and response of turtles to inspired CO_2. *Am. J. Physiol. 249 (Regulatory Integrative Comp. Physiol. 18):* R323–R328, 1985.
9. Hitzig, B. M., M. P. Kneussl, V. Shih, R. D. Brandstetter, and H. Kazemi. Brain amino acid concentrations during diving and acid–base stress in turtles. *J. Appl. Physiol. 58:* 1751–1754, 1985.
10. Hitzig, B. M., and E. E. Nattie. Acid–base stress and central chemical control of ventilation in turtles. *J. Appl. Physiol. 53:* 1365–1370, 1982.

11. Hitzig, B. M., J. W. Prichard, H. L. Canter, W. R. Ellington, J. S. Ingwall, C. T. Burt, S. I. Helman, and J. Koutcher. NMR spectroscopy as an investigative technique in physiology. *FASEB J. 1:* 22–31, 1987.

12. Jackson, D. C. The effects of temperature on ventilation in the turtle, *Pseudemys scripta elegans. Respir. Physiol. 12:* 131–140, 1971.

13. Jackson, D. C., and N. Heisler. Plasma ion balance of submerged anoxic turtles at 3°C: the role of calcium lactate formation. *Respir. Physiol. 49:* 159–174, 1982.

14. Jackson, D. C., S. E. Palmer, and W. L. Meadow. The effects of temperature and carbon dioxide breathing on ventilation and acid–base status of turtles. *Respir. Physiol. 20:* 131–146, 1974.

15. Jackson, D. C., and H. Silverblatt. Respiration and acid–base status of turtles following experimental dives. *Am. J. Physiol. 226:* 903–909, 1974.

16. Kiwull-Schöne, H., and P. Kiwull. Lack of ventilatory reaction to brain-stem acidosis induced by hypoxia [Abstract]. *Pflügers Arch. 391S:* 190, 1981.

17. McGeer, P. L., and E. G. McGeer. Amino acid neurotransmitters. In: *Basic Neurochemistry* (3rd ed.), ed. G. J. Siegel, R. W. Albers, B. W. Agranoff, and R. Katzman. Boston, MA: Little, Brown, 1981, p. 234.

18. Milsom, W. K., and D. R. Jones. Pulmonary receptor chemosensitivity and the ventilatory response to inhaled CO_2 in the turtle. *Respir. Physiol. 37:* 101–107, 1979.

19. Moon, R. B., and J. H. Richards. Determination of intracellular pH by ^{31}P magnetic resonance. *J. Biol. Chem. 248:* 7276–7278, 1973.

20. Robin, E. D., J. W. Vester, H. V. Murdaugh, Jr., and J. E. Millen. Prolonged anaerobiosis in a vertebrate: anaerobic metabolism in the freshwater turtle. *J. Cell. Comp. Physiol. 63:* 287–297, 1964.

21. Ultsch, G. R., and D. C. Jackson. Long-term submergence at 3°C of the turtle, *Chrysemys picta belli,* in normoxic and severely hypoxic water. I. survival, gas exchange, and acid–base status. *J. Exp. Biol. 96:* 11–28, 1982.

22. Wessberg, P., T. Hedner, J. Hedner, and J. Jonason. Effects of taurine and a taurine antagonist on some respiratory and cardiovascular parameters. *Life Sci. 33:* 1649–1655, 1983.

23. Yamada, K. A., R. Hamosh, and R. A. Gillis. Respiratory depression produced by activation of GABA receptors in hindbrain of cat. *J. Appl. Physiol. 51:* 1278–1286, 1981.

24. Yamada, K. A., W. P. Norman, P. Hamosh, and R. A. Gillis. Medullary ventral surface GABA receptors affect respiratory and cardiovascular function. *Brain Res. 248:* 71–78, 1982.

27

Respiratory Neuron Behavior During Medullary Hypoxia

D. W. RICHTER AND H. ACKER

Chemoreflexes are active during normocapnic, normoxic breathing (4,21) and become increasingly powerful during acute hypoxia and hypercapnia (26). The reflexes are, however, attenuated under chronic hypoxia and hypercapnia by endogenously released substances (5,6,12,34,35,37). Such decreased sensitivity may, in part, be responsible for ventilatory depression (11,24,25) and decreased excitability of respiratory structures within the brainstem, leading to primary apnea when respiratory neurons begin to fail to discharge rhythmically (17). This may be followed by blockade of synaptic interaction between different respiratory "centers" and hypoxic apnea (7,22).

To obtain more detailed information on the tolerance to hypoxia of the various mechanisms controlling the activity of medullary respiratory neurons, changes in tissue P_{O_2} and in the extracellular ion environment were determined in parallel with the spontaneous and stimulus-evoked discharge of medullary respiratory neurons during hypercapnia and hypoxia.

METHODS

Measurements were performed in 25 cats of either sex (body weight, 2–2.5 kg) which were anesthetized with sodium pentobarbitone (60 mg/kg), paralyzed with gallamine triethiodide (15 mg/kg) or pancuronium bromide (15 mg/kg), and artificially ventilated. Ventilation was adjusted to an end-tidal CO_2 concentration between 3% and 5%. Arterial P_{O_2}, P_{CO_2}, and pH were measured with O_2, CO_2, and pH electrodes in 0.5-ml blood samples drawn through a catheter in the femoral artery. The rectal temperature was maintained between 37 and 38°C by external heating.

267

The spinal cord was exposed by laminectomy for electrical stimulation at the C-3 level by use of bipolar stainless-steel electrodes. The vagus nerves were freed in the neck and stimulated with platinum hook electrodes. Phrenic nerve activity was recorded as a monitor of the central respiratory rhythm. Chemoreceptor afferents were kept intact.

The head was fixed in an antiflexed position, and the medulla exposed by occipital craniotomy. Medullary respiratory neurons were localized within the dorsal respiratory group (DRG)—that is, within an area 0–2 mm rostral to the obex, 1.5–2.5 mm lateral to the midline, and 1.5–2.5 mm ventral to the dorsal surface— or within the ventral respiratory group (VRG)—that is, within a region 0–2 mm rostral to the obex, 3–4 mm lateral to midline within a depth of 2.5–3.5 mm ventral to the dorsal surface.

Tissue oxygen tensions (P_{O_2}), activities of potassium (aK) and calcium (aCa) ions, and neuronal spike activity were measured within the DRG or VRG regions using either one compound electrode or two separate electrodes placed close to each other. The P_{O_2}, was measured with the polarographic method; the ion activities were determined with double- or three-barreled electrodes which were filled with potassium or calcium exchange resin (1,31). The reference barrel of the microelectrodes was filled with 150 mM NaCl solution.

Tissue P_{O_2}, changes in extracellular ion activities, and the neuronal discharge were measured during hyperoxic hypercapnia (6% CO_2 in 20% or 100% O_2), normocapnic hypoxia (10–15% O_2 in N_2), and asphyxia (ventilation stopped).

RESULTS

Within brainstem respiratory areas, the lowest levels of extracellular aK ranged from 3 to 3.6 mmol/l and those of aCa from 1.2 to 1.5 mmol/l. Superimposed on these levels were fluctuations of ion activities that occurred in synchrony with every burst discharge of medullary respiratory neurons. The amplitude of these fluctuations was 0.3–1.0 mmol/l for aK and 0.02–0.1 mmol/l for aCa. Tissue P_{O_2} remained constant at 60–80 torr when the animals were ventilated with oxygen-enriched air. The values measured for aK, aCa, and P_{O_2} were similar within the different areas (DRG, VRG) of respiratory neurons.

Superficial application of ouabain in a concentration of 0.4 mmol/l on the dorsal surface of the brainstem was followed by an increase in the mean level of aK by about 0.5 mmol/l within the region of DRG neurons without effect on the amplitude of the periodic fluctuations of aK.

Antidromic and synaptic activation of DRG and VRG respiratory neurons by repetitive spinal cord stimulation evoked an increase in aK of 0.5–1.0 mmol/l and a fall in aCa of 0.4–1.0 mmol/l. Similar changes in aK and aCa were measured when DRG neurons were synaptically activated by repetitive vagus nerve stimulation. Tissue P_{O_2} decreased by 10–40 torr (Fig. 27.1).

Hyperoxic hypercapnia led to an increase in mean level and amplitudes of periodic fluctuations of aK without significantly changing aCa or P_{O_2} within the region of both DRG and VRG neurons.

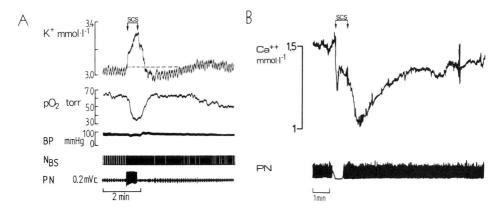

Fig. 27.1 Changes in extracellular potassium activity (K^+), calcium activity (Ca^{2+}), and tissue oxygen tension (P_{O_2}) during synaptic activation of medullary inspiratory neurons of the ventral group by repetitive spinal cord stimulation (100 Hz, 0.1 ms, 3 mA). PN, phrenic neurogram; N_{BS}, discharge of action potentials of inspiratory (bulbospinal) neurons: SCS, spinal cord stimulation.

Normocapnic hypoxia and asphyxia, however, evoked a fall in P_{O_2} to zero level within 2–3 min, and during this time, aK increased by 0.5–1.0 mmol/l. Calcium activity increased by 0.4–0.6 mmol/l, and in some cases this increase was preceded by a transient decrease of 0.1–0.4 mmol/l. The amplitudes of rhythmic aK fluctuations became larger initially, but then progressively decreased and finally disappeared. The aK level continued to increase as long as the hypoxia or asphyxia lasted (Fig. 27.2).

With the same time course as rhythmic aK fluctuations, peak discharge frequency of inspiratory neurons increased and then decreased whereas the duration of the burst discharge normally became longer. The rhythmic discharge of neurons was sometimes replaced by a tonic discharge which faded and finally ceased completely. Phrenic nerve activity also revealed an initial increase in peak inspiratory discharge and in burst frequency, but then decreased in amplitude. Rhythmic activity disappeared and only a weak tonic discharge component persisted for the next 1–2 min. This apnea was interrupted only by short bursts of gasplike discharges (Fig. 27.3).

When brainstem hypoxia persisted longer, the mean level of aK continued to increase above 4–5 mmol/l, although inspiratory neurons had stopped discharging and aK no longer revealed periodic fluctuations. During such early apneic situations, electrical stimulation of the spinal cord evoked additional transient increases in aK. Maximal aK levels of 11 mmol/l were measured during hypoxic tests lasting 5 min, and aK levels above 30–40 mmol/l were measured during lethal asphyxia.

Resumption of ventilation after 3–4 min of central apnea was followed by an increase in tissue P_{O_2} and a decrease in aK and aCa. Control levels were normally reached within 5 min. Under- and overswings, respectively, were normally seen in aK and P_{O_2}. In cases where hypoxia was of fairly long duration, aK remained elevated for longer than 5 min, although P_{O_2} had reached control levels. Rhythmic respiratory activity reappeared only if aK fell to control levels (and sometimes

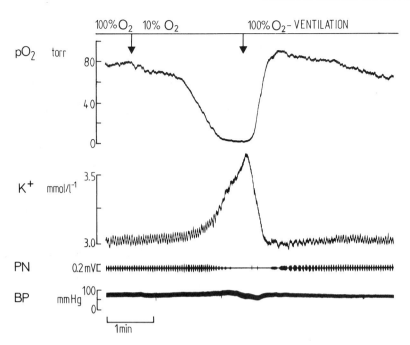

Fig. 27.2 Changes in tissue oxygen tension (P_{O_2}), extracellular potassium activity (K^+) in the ventral group of respiratory neurons, and phrenic nerve activity (PN) during ventilation of the animal with hypoxic gas (10% O_2 in 90% N_2). BP, arterial blood pressure.

below control). The pattern of central inspiratory activity, however, was changed in most cases in that for the first 2–3 min, burst discharges of inspiratory neurons were prolonged as a result of prolonged and increased postinspiratory activity. The amplitude of peak inspiratory activity, however, was normally reduced, as was the frequency of central respiratory activity (Fig. 27.3).

DISCUSSION

These experiments have shown that rhythmic respiratory activity within the brainstem evokes changes in the extracellular ionic environments of medullary respiratory neurons (31). The disturbances in the ionic environment of respiratory neurons are transient and seem to be effectively counterbalanced by active-transport mechanisms. These transport systems, however, are not protected by special hypoxia-tolerant properties and need an adequate energy supply. The changes in the ionic environment become larger and persistent when the energy supply is blocked either by ouabain or by lack of oxygen during hypoxia, when respiratory neurons are synaptically driven by afferent inputs from peripheral and central chemoreceptors and possibly other brain structures. The increase in aK indicates massive efflux of K^+ from the neurons which, as in other types of neurons, seems to be attributable to an increased (voltage-independent, possibly ATP-dependent) potas-

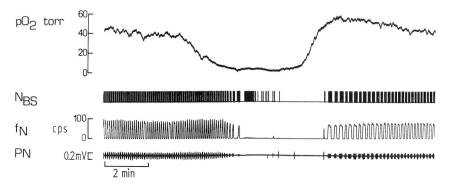

Fig. 27.3 Response of an inspiratory bulbospinal neuron and phrenic nerve discharge to hypoxia. Ventilation of the animal with 10% O_2 in 90% N_2 evoked a decrease of tissue oxygen tension (P_{O_2}) to zero level and an increase of the extracellular potassium activity (not illustrated) by 1 mmol/l above the control level of 3.1 mmol/l. The inspiratory neuron stopped discharging rhythmic bursts of action potentials (N_{BS}) and, for a short time (less than 2 min.), fired tonically before it ceased discharging. The phrenic nerve discharge (PN) stopped at the same time. Extracellular potassium activity decreased below control levels, and neuronal discharge and phrenic nerve discharge reappeared after the animal was reventilated with oxygen-enriched air. Note that the discharge frequency (f_N) of the inspiratory neuron and the phrenic nerve activity showed enhanced postinspiratory discharges.

sium conductance, resulting in membrane hyperpolarization at an early stage of hypoxia (15,18,19). Increased membrane conductance and hyperpolarization of respiratory neurons would explain the observed decrease in discharge frequency of inspiratory neurons even though excitatory synaptic drive from the chemoreceptors is still enhanced under hypoxia. Inhibitory synaptic inputs from other brain regions may initially contribute to this effect (12,24,37), but within a short time, GABA-ergic synaptic inhibition is probably abolished (15). Blockade of expiratory synaptic inhibition would explain the observed prolongation of the burst discharge in inspiratory neurons before the discharge becomes tonic.

The transient decrease in aCa that was seen at the beginning of hypoxia indicates an influx of Ca^{2+} into the respiratory neurons (2). Continuing influx of Ca^{2+} seems to be superimposed on a subsequent increase in aCa that may reflect release of Ca^{2+} from binding sites on the membranes during the development of brain acidosis. An additional effect on aCa may be induced by the changes in aK. Failure of active membrane transport mechanisms and a persistent increase in extracellular aK results initially in membrane hyperpolarization of respiratory neurons, which subsequently gives way to depolarization. This, in addition to accumulation of intracellular Ca^{2+} (Ca^{2+} influx, release from intracellular binding sites or stores, and blockade of the active Na–Ca exchange) and acidification of the outer and inner membrane surface, inactivates membrane currents that are essential to the repetitive discharge capacity of respiratory neurons (9,10,23,30)—that is, the low-threshold Ca-current, Na-currents, and voltage- and calcium-dependent K-currents (8,14,15,20,27,38,39). Inactivation of these currents would explain why inspiratory neurons stop discharging action potentials although synaptic activation is still increased. The central respiratory rhythm comes to complete arrest and stops in "primary apnea." This conclusion is consistent with the finding that only sharp and unpatterned, gasplike discharges were observed under this condition.

Conduction of afferent activity in nerve fibers of peripheral chemoreceptors and activation of other afferents converging on respiratory neurons seem to persist during this period of primary apnea because electrical stimulation of afferent inputs from the spinal cord evokes activation of the neurons and produces an additional increase in extracellular aK. Resumption of ventilation and energy supply to the respiratory network therefore stimulates active transport systems that normalize and transiently even decrease aK below control levels, and reestablishes the conditions necessary for normal synaptic interaction between respiratory neurons. The respiratory rhythm can start again, although its pattern seems to be changed. These changes in the central respiratory pattern may be explained by changes in the synaptic interaction between the respiratory neurons themselves, and in the afferent inputs from peripheral and central chemoreceptors and those from higher brain structures. In our experiments, peak inspiratory discharge and central inspiratory frequency were decreased during recovery, indicating that inhibitory afferent inputs dominate, as described by Millhorn and colleagues (24). Postinspiratory activities, however, seem to be enhanced, possibly as a result of direct activation of postinspiratory neurons by afferent chemoreceptor discharge or by activated pontine structures (30,32; see also Ballantyne et al., Chap. 33, this volume). Enhanced postinspiratory discharge of inspiratory neurons may result also from their persistent membrane depolarization and hyperexcitability (36) during periods when they are not readily controlled by synaptic inhibition (15,16).

Persistence of synaptic excitation under anaerobic conditions, however, could lead to neuronal damage (33) because neurons remain incapable of maintaining calcium and potassium homeostasis. Extracellular potassium activity continues to increase, and this in turn must lead to further depolarization of the neurons (19). High-threshold Ca conductances could be activated (38, see also refs. 9,10) and a largely uncontrollable influx of Ca^{2+} would develop. Increased cytosolic Ca^{2+} might then act as a cellular toxin (3,18) and further disrupt various intracellular functions (29). Proteases (28) and phospholipases (13) would be activated, precipitating membrane hydrolysis and consequent final disruption of plasma and mitochondrial membranes, thus leading to irreversible damage of respiratory neurons.

ACKNOWLEDGMENTS
     This work was supported by the DFG.

REFERENCES

1. Acker, H. The meaning of tissue Po_2 and local blood flow for the chemoreceptive process of the carotid body. *Fed. Proc. 39:* 2641–2647, 1980.
2. Acker, H., and D. W. Richter. Changes in potassium activity, calcium activity and oxygen tension in the extracellular space of inspiratory neurones within the NTS of cats. In: *Neurogenesis of Central Respiratory Rhythm,* ed. A. L. Bianchi and M. Denavit-Saubie. Lancaster: MTP Press, 1985, pp. 183–185.

3. Berridge, M. J., and R. F. Irvine. Inositol triphosphate, a novel second messenger in cellular signal transduction. *Nature 312:* 315–321, 1984.

4. Biscoe, T. J., and M. J. Purves. Observations on the rhythmic variation in the carotid body chemoreceptor activity which has the same period as respiration. *J. Physiol. (Lond.) 190:* 389–412, 1967.

5. Black, A.M.S., J. H. Comroe, Jr., and L. Jacobs. Species differences in carotid body response of cat and dog to dopamine and serotonin. *Am. J. Physiol. 223:* 1097–1102, 1972.

6. Black, A.M.S., D. I. McCloskey, and R. W. Torrance. The response of carotid body chemoreceptors in the cat to sudden changes of hypercapnic and hypoxic stimuli. *Respir. Physiol. 131:* 36–49, 1971.

7. Bystrzycka, E., B. S. Nail, and M. J. Purves. Central and peripheral neural respiratory activity in the mature sheep foetus and newborn lamb. *Respir. Physiol. 25:* 199–215, 1975.

8. Carbone, E., R. Fioravanti, G. Prestipino, and E. Wanke. Action of extracellular pH on Na^+ and K^+ membrane currents in the giant axon of *Loligo vulgaris. J Membr. Biol. 43:* 295–315, 1978.

9. Champagnat, J., T. Jacquin, and D. W. Richter. Voltage-dependent currents in neurones of the nuclei of the solitary tract of rat brainstem slices. *Pflügers Arch. 406:* 372–379, 1986.

10. Champagnat, J., D. W. Richter, T. Jacquin, and M. Denavit-Saubie. Voltage-dependent conductances in neurons of the ventrolateral nTS in rat brainstem slices. In: *Neurobiology of the Control of Breathing,* ed. C. von Euler and H. Lagercrantz. New York: Raven Press, 1987, pp. 217–221.

11. Cherniack, N. S., N. H. Edelman, and S. Lahiri. Hypoxia and hypercapnia as respiratory stimulants and depressants. *Respir. Physiol. 11:* 113–126, 1970.

12. Daly, J. W., R. F. Burns, and S. H. Snyder. Adenosine receptors in the central nervous system: relationship to the central actions of the methylxanthines. *Life Sci. 28:* 2083–2097, 1981.

13. Derksen, A., and P. Cohen. Patterns of fatty acid release from endogenous substrates by human platelet homogenates and membranes. *J. Biol. Chem. 250*(24): 9342–9347, 1975.

14. Drouin, H., and R. The. The effects of reducing extracellular pH on the membrane currents of the Ranvier node. *Pflügers Arch. 313:* 80–88, 1969.

15. Fujiwara, N., H. Higashi, K. Shimoji, and M. Yoshimura. Effects of hypoxia on rat hippocampal neurones in vitro. *J. Physiol. (Lond.) 384:* 131–151, 1987.

16. Groul, D. C., J. L. Barker, L.-Y.M. Huang, J. F. MacDonald, and T. G. Smith, Jr. Hydrogen ions have multiple effects on the excitability of cultured mammalian neurons. *Brain Res. 183:* 247–252, 1980.

17. Gutheroth, W. G., I. Kawabori, D. Breazeale, and G. McGough. Hypoxic apnea and gasping. *J. Clin. Invest. 56:* 1371–1377, 1975.

18. Hansen, A. J. Effect of anoxia on ion distribution in the brain. *Physiol. Rev. 65:* 101–148, 1985.

19. Hansen, A. J., J. Hounsgaard, and H. Jahnsen. Anoxia increases potassium conductance in hippocampal nerve cells. *Acta Physiol. Scan. 115:* 301–310, 1982.

20. Hille, B. Charges and potentials at the nerve surface: divalent ions and pH. *J. Gen. Physiol. 51:* 221–236, 1968.

21. Hornbein, T. F., Z. J. Griffo, and A. Roos. Quantitation of chemoreceptor activity: interrelation of hypoxia and hypercapnia. *J. Neurophysiol. 24:* 561–568, 1961.

22. Lawson, E. E., and B. T. Thach. Respiratory patterns during progressive asphyxia in newborn rabbits. *J. Appl. Physiol. 43:* 463–474, 1977.

23. Mifflin, S., and D. W. Richter. The effects of QX-314 on medullary respiratory neurones. *Brain Res. 420:* 22–31, 1987.

24. Millhorn, D. E., F. L. Eldridge, J. P. Kiley, and T. G. Waldrop. Prolonged inhibition of respiration following acute hypoxia in glomectomized cats. *Respir. Physiol. 57:* 331–340, 1984.

25. Morrill, C. G., J. R. Meyer, and J. V. Weil. Hypoxic ventilatory depression in dogs. *J. Appl. Physiol. 38:* 143–146, 1975.

26. Mulligan, E., and S. Lahiri. Separation of carotid body chemoreceptor responses to O_2 and CO_2 by oligomycin and by antimycin A. *Am. J. Physiol. 242:* C200–C206, 1982.

27. Neumcke, B., W. Schwarz, and R. Staempfli. Increased charge displacement in the membrane of myelinated nerve at reduced extracellular pH. *Biophys. J. 31:* 325–332, 1980.

28. Pant, H., and H. Gainer. Properties of a calcium-activated protease in squid axoplasm which selectively degrades neurofilament proteins. *J. Neurobiol. 11:* 1–12, 1980.

29. Rasmussen, H., and P. G. Barrett. Calcium messenger system: an integrated view. *Physiol. Rev. 64:* 938–984, 1984.

30. Richter, D. W., D. Ballantyne, and J. E. Remmers. How is respiratory rhythm generated? A model. *News Physiol. Sci. 1:* 109–112, 1986.

31. Richter, D. W., H. Camerer, and U. Sonnhof. Changes in extracellular potassium during the spontaneous activity of medullary respiratory neurones. *Pflügers Arch. 376:* 139–149, 1978.

32. Richter, D. W., J. Champagnat, and S. Mifflin. Membrane properties involved in respiratory rhythm generation. In: *Neurobiology of the Control of Breathing,* ed. C. von Euler and H. Lagercrantz. New York: Raven Press, 1987, pp. 141–147.

33. Rothman, S. M. Synaptic activity mediates death of hypoxic neurons. *Science 220:* 536–537, 1983.

34. Rubio, R., R. M. Berne, E. L. Bockman, and R. R. Curnish. Relationship between adenosine concentration and oxygen supply in rat brain. *Am. J. Physiol. 228:* 1896–1902, 1975.

35. Sampson, S. R. Mechanism of efferent inhibition of carotid body chemoreceptors in the cat. *Brain Res. 45:* 266–270, 1972.

36. Schiff, S. J., and G. G. Somjen. Hyperexcitability following moderate hypoxia in hippocampal tissue slices. *Brain Res. 337:* 337–340, 1985.

37. Snyder, S. H., J. J. Katims, Z. Annau, R. F. Burns, and J. W. Daly. Adenosine receptors and behavioral actions of methylxanthines. *Proc. Natl. Acad. Sci. U.S.A. 78:* 3260–3264, 1981.

38. Spitzer, N. C. Low pH selectively blocks calcium action potentials in amphibian neurons developing in culture. *Brain Res. 161:* 555–559, 1979.

39. Woodhull, A. M. Ion blockage of sodium channels in nerve. *J. Gen. Physiol. 61:* 687–708, 1973.

28

Long-Lasting Facilitation and Inhibition of Respiration Elicited by Hypoxia in Glomectomized Cats

E. A. GALLMAN AND D. E. MILLHORN

Hypoxia presented to peripheral chemoreceptors causes an increase in ventilation. In the absence of peripheral chemoreceptors, hypoxia acts centrally to produce respiratory depression (12). The central depressive effect of hypoxia upon respiratory output is not fully understood but may involve metabolic depression of central neurons (1), brain alkalosis due to increased cerebral blood flow (3), or release of adenosine (6,9).

This laboratory has recently performed studies in peripherally chemodenervated cats which indicate that, in addition to the direct effects noted above, acute hypoxia may induce a long-lasting centrally mediated inhibition of respiratory output (6). Further work has shown that, in addition to the long-lasting central inhibition, hypoxia may elicit a long-lasting centrally mediated facilitation of respiration. These responses are masked during the actual hypoxic episode by the immediate depression of respiration, but, because of their long-lasting nature, they can be seen during the post-hypoxic period. The long-lasting facilitation should not be confused with the prolonged stimulation of respiration previously reported by Millhorn et al. (7). The earlier report dealt with a mechanism activated by stimulation of peripheral chemoreceptors. This long-lasting mechanisms discussed here are activated by hypoxia in the absence of input from peripheral chemoreceptors.

METHODS

Studies were performed in anesthetized, paralyzed, ventilated, and peripheral chemo-denervated cats. End-tidal P_{CO_2} was servo-controlled at the desired level $\pm$

0.5 torr. Temperature was servo-controlled at $37° \pm 0.5°C$. Arterial blood pressure was monitored through a catheter placed in the femoral artery. Hypoxia was produced by ventilating for 10 min with reduced inspired oxygen ($F_IO_2 = 0.06–0.15$). At other times, cats were ventilated with 100% oxygen. Blood samples were drawn at the end of each 10-min hypoxic episode and analyzed to determine the actual degree of hypoxemia. Phrenic nerve activity was recorded as an index of the output of the central respiratory control network. Minute phrenic activity, the product of phrenic rate and peak phrenic activity, was used as a neural equivalent of minute ventilation.

In addition to studying cats with intact brains, we investigated the central hypoxic response of cats following two types of ablation. The first, termed *high decerebration,* was a transection of the neuraxis rostral to the superior colliculi, which left the mesencephalon intact. The second, termed *low decerebration,* was a midcollicular transection, whch extended to the rostral border of the ventral pons.

RESULTS AND DISCUSSION

Our studies in peripherally chemodenervated cats with intact brains confimed previous findings from this laboratory that a brief episode of severe hypoxia ($P_aO_2 <$ 25 torr) can lead to an extended period of respiratory inhibition. Figure 28.1A presents the response of one such cat. As can be seen, the minute phrenic activity remained below the control level for at least 60 min following the return to ventilation with 100% O_2. The mean arterial pressure was unchanged during the course of the experiment. End-tidal P_aCO_2 was controlled at 26 torr throughout the control period, the hypoxic episode, and the 60-min recovery period. The brisk phrenic response to a 2-torr increase in P_aCO_2 immediately following the 60-min recovery period attests to the continued viability of the central respiratory networks.

While attempting to determine the degree of hypoxia necessary to elicit the long-lasting inhibitory response, we discovered that mild hypoxia was followed, not by inhibition, but by a long-lasting facilitation. The response of one cat to a P_aO_2 of 38 torr is shown in Fig. 28.1B. The mean arterial pressure and P_aCO_2 were unchanged throughout the experiment. The respiratory response during hypoxia was phrenic apnea, but within 15 min following the return to ventilation with 100% oxygen, phrenic activity was above the control level. It continued to increase for the remainder of the 60-min recovery period. The averaged responses of cats to

---

$\longrightarrow$

Fig. 28.1 Response of cats with intact brains following hypoxia. (**A**) Effect on phrenic activity of 10 min of severe (25 torr) hypoxia. The cat breathed 100% O_2 during control and recovery. Phrenic activity remained inhibited for the 60-min recovery period. Response to a 2-torr increase in PCO_2 after 60 min shows the viability of the respiratory network. (**B**) Effect on phrenic activity of 10 min of mild (38 torr) hypoxia in another cat. The cat breathed 100% O_2 during control and recovery. Phrenic activity was above control level by 15 min of recovery and continued to increase. (**C**) Averaged responses of cats with intact brains following severe (20–25 torr), moderate (26–35 torr), and mild (36–65 torr) hypoxia. Means $\pm$ SEM.

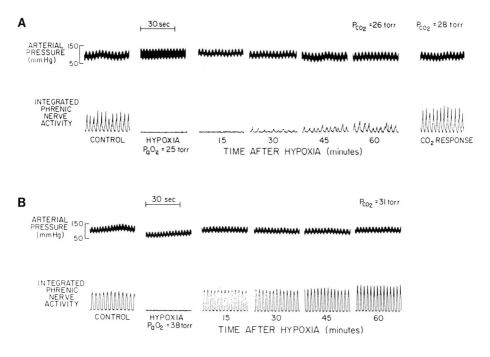

A

ARTERIAL PRESSURE (mmHg)

INTEGRATED PHRENIC NERVE ACTIVITY

30 sec

$P_{CO_2} = 26$ torr $P_{CO_2} = 28$ torr

CONTROL   HYPOXIA $P_aO_2 = 25$ torr   15   30   45   60 CO_2 RESPONSE

TIME AFTER HYPOXIA (minutes)

B

ARTERIAL PRESSURE (mmHg)

INTEGRATED PHRENIC NERVE ACTIVITY

30 sec

$P_{CO_2} = 31$ torr

CONTROL   HYPOXIA $P_aO_2 = 38$ torr   15   30   45   60

TIME AFTER HYPOXIA (minutes)

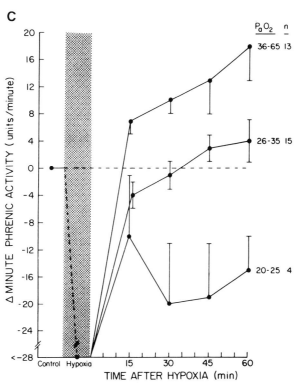

C

P_aO_2 n

36-65   13

26-35   15

20-25   4

Δ MINUTE PHRENIC ACTIVITY (units/minute)

Control   Hypoxia   15   30   45   60

TIME AFTER HYPOXIA (min)

severe hypoxia (P_aO_2 = 20–25 torr), moderate hypoxia (P_aO_2 = 26–35 torr), and mild hypoxia (P_aO_2 = 36–65 torr) are presented in Fig. 28.1C.

In order to locate the anatomical substrates for the long-lasting inhibition and the long-lasting facilitation of phrenic activity following hypoxia, we performed a series of experiments involving transection of the neuraxis. Figure 28.2A shows the response of one "brain intact" cat to mild (P_aO_2 = 40 torr) hypoxia, whereas Fig. 28.2B shows the response of the same cat to the same degree of hypoxia following high decerebration, a transection of the neuraxis just rostral to the mesencephalon. Figure 28.2C shows the response of the same cat to the same degree of hypoxia, this time following low decerebration, a midcollicular transection of the neuraxis that left the pons, but not the mesencephalon, intact. The phrenic response during hypoxia was qualitatively similar in the three trials. The change in arterial pressure was comparable in the three cases. However, the phrenic response following hypoxia differed dramatically before and after the transections. As expected, the response of the "brain intact" cat to mild hypoxia was a long-lasting facilitation. Following high decerebration, hypoxia resulted in a long-lasting inhibition of phrenic activity. After receiving a low decerebration, the same cat showed neither the long-lasting inhibition nor the long-lasting facilitation following hypoxia.

In all, nine cats underwent high decerebration. All of these cats responded with at least 60 min of inhibition of phrenic activity following even mild hypoxia. It should be stressed that, in the intact animals, this same range of P_aO_2 values led to facilitation. In other words, removal of higher brain structures both prevented the facilitation seen in the "brain intact" cats and allowed the expression of the inhibitory response. The low decerebration studies, performed in six cats, further defined the site of the inhibitory mechanism. The minute phrenic activity of these cats following hypoxia did not differ from the minute phrenic activity before hypoxia, although the same range of hypoxia had resulted in long-lasting inhibition in the high-decerebrate group. The averaged responses of high-decerebrate (P_aO_2 = 29–54 torr) and low decerebrate (P_aO_2 = 31–57 torr) are presented in Fig. 28.2D along with the averaged responses of "brain intact" cats to the same range of hypoxia (P_aO_2 = 29–52 torr).

Because the surgical trauma associated with low decerebration was similar to that associated with high decerebration, it cannot be argued that the inhibition exhibited by the high-decerebrate cats was trauma induced. Further, as we were unable to elicit the inhibitory response following hypoxia in low decerebrate cats, we suggest that the mesencephalon is necessary for the long-lasting inhibition of phrenic activity seen following acute hypoxia. Because we were able to elicit the long-lasting facilitation following hypoxia in "brain intact" but not in high-decerebrate cats, we believe that the facilitatory mechanism resides above the brainstem.

→

Fig. 28.2 Response of cats with intact brains, high decerebration, and low decerebration following hypoxia. **(A)** Effect on phrenic activity of 10 min of mild (40 torr) hypoxia in a cat with intact brain. **(B)** Response of the same cat to mild hypoxia following high decerebration. **(C)** Response of the same cat to hypoxia following low decerebration. **(D)** Averaged responses of cats with (●) intact brains (P_aO_2 = 29–52 torr), (■) high decerebration (P_aO_2 = 29–54 torr), and (▲) low decerebration (P_aO_2 = 31–57 torr) to 10 min of hypoxia. Means ± SEM.

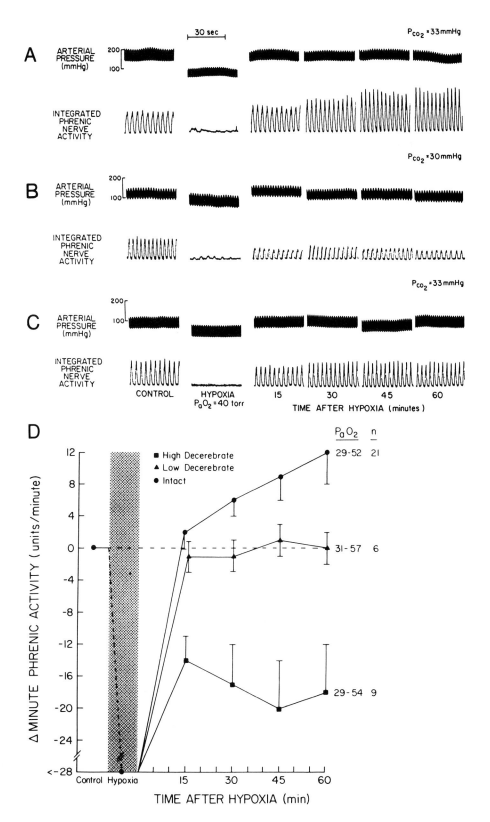

Preliminary observations in unanesthetized, decorticate cats indicate that this mechanism is still active and therefore does not require the presence of the cortex.

We believe that both the inhibitory and the facilitatory mechanisms are activated simultaneously, but that inhibition dominates at the most severe hypoxic levels whereas facilitation is the predominant response to mild hypoxia. The response to moderate hypoxia is a more even balance of the two mechanisms, resulting in little overall change from control. The fact that, following all three ranges of hypoxia, the minute phrenic activity increased between 30 and 60 min of recovery may indicate that after the first 30 min, the facilitatory mechanism begins to overcome any inhibition that is present. Interestingly, a similar finding was reported 40 years ago by Davenport et al. (2). In that early study, unanesthetized, chronically chemodenervated dogs responded to 20 min of hypoxia with an initial depression of respiration. However, within 10 min, respiratory rate increased sufficiently to bring ventilation close to control levels. During the 10 min immediately following hypoxia, respiration rose above control levels. The authors inferred that a central inhibition and a central stimulation added algebraically to produce the noted result.

Other reports have indicated that central stimulation of respiration during hypoxia is present but often masked by anesthesia (5,8). In particular, Tenney and co-workers (5,11) reported an increase in the rate of breathing during hypoxia which they were able to attribute to the diencephalon. Although it is encouraging that we have arrived at the same conclusion concerning the site of the long-lasting facilitation, there are important differences between our studies and these previous reports. First, the long-lasting inhibition we observed was present in high decerebrate cats that had received no anesthesia, and was therefore not due to anesthetic depression. Second, we concentrated on the 60 min following hypoxia rather than on the hypoxic period itself. We have, however, had occasion to observe the response of cats during hypoxia. In preliminary studies, unanesthetized, decorticate cats with diencephalon intact showed a decrease in both phrenic rate and peak phrenic activity during hypoxia.

A recent report (4) indicates that hypoxic stimulation of respiration which is lost following glomectomy may be partially restored over a period of time. The hypoxia-induced central facilitation that we have demonstrated provides a possible explanation for these observations.

At this time, we do not know the mechanism by which hypoxia causes a central facilitation of respiration. Evidence does exist for hypoxic excitation at the cellular level. Schiff and Somjen (10) have reported an increased excitability of hippocampal tissue slices for 40–55 min following exposure to hypoxia.

In conclusion, we have demonstrated two respiratory responses elicited following hypoxia. The first, long-lasting inhibition, resides in the mesencephalon; the second, long-lasting facilitation is found most likely in the diencephalon. Both mechanisms appear to be triggered simultaneously, the output of the central respiratory network reflecting the influence of each. The relative contribution of each mechanism may depend upon the degree of hypoxia, the time course of each mechanism, and the level of anesthesia. However, it is clear that both responses can be triggered in unanesthetized animals.

ACKNOWLEDGMENTS
These studies were supported by NIH Grant HL-33831 and AHA 881108. EAG was a recipient of a 1985 National SIDS Foundation Summer Fellowship. DEM is an Established Investigator of the American Heart Association and is now a Career Investigator of the American Lung Association.

REFERENCES

1. Cherniack, N. S., N. H. Edelman, and S. Lahiri. Hypoxia and hypercapnia as respiratory stimulants and depressants. *Respir. Physiol. 11:* 113–126, 1970.
2. Davenport, H. W., G. Brewer, A. H. Chambers, and S. Goldschmidt. The respiratory responses to anoxemia of unanaesthetized dogs with chronically denervated aortic and carotid chemoreceptors and their causes. *Am. J. Physiol. 148:* 406–416, 1947.
3. Lee, L-Y. and H. T. Milhorn. Central ventilatory response to O_2 and CO_2 at three levels of carotid chemoreceptor stimulation. *Respir. Physiol. 25:* 319–333, 1975.
4. Martin-Body, R. L., G. J. Robson, and J. D. Sinclair. Restoration of hypoxic respiratory responses in the awake rat after carotid body denervation by sinus nerve section. *J. Physiol. (Lond.) 380:* 61–73, 1986.
5. Miller, M. J., and S. M. Tenney. Hypoxia-induced tachypnea in carotid-deafferented cats. *Respir. Physiol. 23:* 31–39, 1975.
6. Millhorn, D. E., F. L. Eldridge, J. P. Kiley, and T. G. Waldrop. Prolonged inhibition of respiration following acute hypoxia in glomectomized cats. *Respir. Physiol. 57:* 331–340, 1984.
7. Millhorn, D. E., F. L. Eldridge, and T. G. Waldrop. Prolonged stimulation of respiration by a new central neural mechanism. *Respir. Physiol. 41:* 87–103, 1980.
8. Moyer, C. A., and H. K. Beecher. Central stimulation of respiration during hypoxia. *Am. J. Physiol. 136:* 13–21, 1942.
9. Rubio, R., R. M. Berne, E. L. Bockman, and R. R. Curnish. Relationship between adenosine concentration and oxygen supply in rat brain. *Am. J. Physiol. 228:* 1896–1902, 1975.
10. Schiff, S. J., and G. S. Somjen. Hyperexcitability following moderate hypoxia in hippocampal tissue slices. *Brain Res. 337:* 337–340, 1985.
11. Tenney, S. M., and L. C. Ou. Ventilatory response of decorticate and decerebrate cats to hypoxia and CO_2. *Respir. Physiol. 29:* 81–92, 1977.
12. Watt, J. G., P. R. Dumke, and J. H. Comroe, Jr. Effects of inhalation of 100 per cent and 14 per cent oxygen upon respiration of unanaesthetized dogs before and after chemoreceptor denervation. *Am. J. Physiol. 138:* 610–617, 1943.

Part VI
AIRWAY MECHANISMS

Introduction

A, M. TRZEBSKI AND H. M. COLERIDGE

The chapters in this section provide new perspectives on the peripheral neural control of airway mechanisms. In their report on sensory mechanisms, Coleridge and Coleridge (Chap.29) indicate the need for reevaluation of the role of rapidly adapting (irritant) receptors and revision of the concept that most are inactive at resting tidal volume (V_T). These investigators show that the receptors begin to discharge in inflation in response to small, physiological reductions in lung compliance and provide the respiratory centers with information regarding the progressive increase in the force required to expand the lung. In these circumstances, the receptors may have a facilitatory reflex function during quiet breathing. Evidence that C fiber input from the lungs has a tonic shortening effect on duration of expiration (T_E) is also presented.

Mitchell et al. (Chap.30), reporting data obtained from intracellular recordings of tracheal ganglion cell activity in vivo, provide insights beyond those obtained by use of in vitro recordings. Their correlation of physiological and morphological evidence indicates two distinct populations of ganglion cells, both discharging with a respiratory rhythm in the absence of any corresponding swings in membrane potential—the smaller ones with expiration, and the larger ones with inspiration. Numerous excitatory postsynaptic potentials were recorded in both types of cell, and the larger cells, but not the smaller ones, showed prominent postspike hyperpolarization lasting 90–100 ms. Correlation of activity with changes in smooth muscle tone suggests that the larger cells innervate airway smooth muscle, and that the cells, acting as low-frequency filters along the motor pathway, require multiple excitatory potentials to evoke an action potential. The smaller cells are thought to innervate tracheal glands.

In the last chapter in this section, Nadel explores a new aspect of peripheral neural control, namely the release of physiologically active peptides such as substance P from sensory terminals in the airways. He suggests that in health airways the presence of enkephalinase ensures that such peptides will be rapidly degraded, and describes the enhancement of the substance P-induced tracheal secretory response in ferrets after administration of an enkephalinase inhibitor. Nadel suggests that enkephalinase production is suppressed, for example, by viral infections, allowing full expression of the local inflammatory and other effects of neural peptide release. This emphasis on the key role of airway enkephalinase indicates important new directions in research related to airway disease.

29

Functional Role of Pulmonary Rapidly Adapting Receptors and Lung C Fibers

J. C. G. COLERIDGE AND H. M. COLERIDGE

This volume, in honor of Julius Comroe, has as its main theme the peripheral chemoreceptors of the carotid and aortic bodies and their role in respiratory regulation. This is an area in which Julius Comroe made important contributions, perhaps most notably his classic study in 1939 on the location and function of the aortic bodies. There are other sensory nerve endings, which although not chemoreceptors in the conventional sense since they do not signal changes in O_2 or CO_2, nevertheless are sensitive to a wide range of chemical agents and are capable of evoking pronounced respiratory effects. These chemosensitive vagal endings, located in the lower respiratory tract, play a part in the respiratory chemoreflexes, another topic that will always be associated with the name of Julius Comroe.

This brief review reassesses the functional significance of two such sensory pathways from the lower airways. One pathway comprises the vagal myelinated fibers of the rapidly adapting (irritant) receptors that supply the intra- and extrapulmonary airways. The other comprises the more numerous afferent C fibers present in the pulmonary and bronchial vagal branches. C fibers innervating the distal lung divisions, and with endings (corresponding to Paintal's J receptors) accessible to chemicals injected into the pulmonary circulation, are referred to as *pulmonary C fibers;* those innervating the conducting airways, and with endings accessible from the bronchial circulation, are referred to as *bronchial C fibers.*

Although rapidly adapting receptors (RARs) and C fibers are sensitive to a variety of mechanical stimuli, chemicals have been used frequently to investigate their properties. Activity in the fibers of both pathways is generally scanty and irregular, and hence difficult to identify, in recordings of afferent activity from normal lungs, and investigators have often used chemical irritants such as histamine (in studies of RARs) and phenyldiguanide and capsaicin (in studies of afferent C fibers) to reveal the presence of the fibers in vagal filaments, and to study their reflex properties. These chemicals were introduced largely as a matter of experimental convenience, but their extensive use since the mid-1960s and 70s has tended, not surprisingly, to draw attention away from other functions of these afferents, and to lead to an impression that both are essentially chemosensitive inputs whose primary function is to evoke protective (defense) reflexes. This brief review attempts in small part to redress the balance.

Thus although the reflex potentialities of a visceral afferent pathway can be explored by use of a chemical to excite the nerve endings, chemical stimulation may provide little indication of the functional significance of an afferent pathway. The functional importance of a given afferent input depends on the circumstances leading to its activation in the intact animal, and on the appropriateness of the evoked reflex response in those particular circumstances.

RAPIDLY ADAPTING RECEPTORS: BACKGROUND

Rapidly adapting or irritant receptors (RARs) were originally identified in cats, and, as the first of these two names implies, were described as rapidly adapting mechanoreceptors that were stimulated by rapid inflation or deflation of the lungs (13,30,31). That RARs had a reflex influence on respiratory events quite different from that of slowly adapting stretch receptors was suggested by the observation that both rapid inflation and rapid deflation, though opposite in sign, had excitatory effects on inspiratory motor output. On the basis of his early studies in cats, Widdicombe (30) suggested that RARs were most numerous in the extrapulmonary airways, particularly in the region of the carina, and became scarcer in the bronchial subdivisions. Those at the carina were exquisitely sensitive to the lightest touch, and stimulation of this region with a fine probe or bristle evoked vigorous coughing; hence receptors in this area were considered to be cough receptors. These extrapulmonary RARs were stimulated by insufflation of carbon particles, which also caused coughing, but they did not appear to be particularly sensitive to chemical irritants, such as sulfur dioxide, which rarely produced coughing when confined to the extrapulmonary airways.

The RARs described subsequently by Widdicombe and his colleagues in rabbits, and given the alternative (and increasingly popular) designation of "irritant receptor," were found in the intrapulmonary, rather than the extrapulmonary airways (16,28). These intrapulmonary receptors, like their extrapulmonary counterparts, were initially identified by their rapidly adapting response to inflation and deflation of the lungs. They were stimulated in a variety of pathological conditions of the lung, including microembolism, anaphylaxis, congestion, and pneumothorax; they were also stimulated by intravenous injection of histamine. A decrease in lung compliance was thought to play a part in stimulating the receptors in all the above conditions, although other factors appeared to be involved. Like the extrapulmonary RARs, the intrapulmonary RARs were held to be largely inactive, and hence without appreciable reflex influence, during normal quiet breathing, becoming active only when tidal volume increased considerably above the resting level, or in abnormal conditions such as those outlined above. Their primary reflex function was thought to be as a trigger for defense reflexes from the lungs, initiating both changes in breathing, and reflex bronchoconstriction (16).

Not surprisingly, the sensitivity of the intrapulmonary RARs to histamine rapidly became a focus of interest, especially to investigators concerned with the changes in breathing and airway caliber that accompany lung disease. The receptors were thought to be highly sensitive to chemical irritants, although this could not be confirmed for all species studied, and to be responsible for the effects evoked in humans when aerosols of a variety of autacoids were administered to the lower respiratory tract. The functional implications of the name "irritant receptor" led to the widespread inference that not only were these myelinated fibers principally responsible for the airway defense response (a constellation of reflex effects including cough, rapid shallow breathing, bronchoconstriction, and increased airway secretion) but also this was their principal function.

CHANGING VIEWS OF THE ROLE OF INTRAPULMONARY RAPIDLY ADAPTING (IRRITANT) RECEPTORS

A number of observations made since the 1970s have led to some reconsideration of the possible "irritant" role of RARs. In some species, RARs appear less sensitive to irritant chemicals than was originally thought (27). Certainly irritant receptors in rabbits and dogs are not stimulated by high concentrations of sulfur dioxide, and those in dogs show little response to bradykinin, a highly irritant substance. Even in the case of chemicals that activate RARs, the question remains open whether the endings are primarily sensitive to the chemical, or are stimulated secondarily by local mechanical changes. Many of the reflex responses attributed to RARs may in fact have been due to engagement of a nonmyelinated afferent input, since bronchial C fibers (see below) have a similar distribution in the airways, and are stimulated by chemicals that appear to have little effect on RARs.

Recent observations in our laboratory have served to reemphasize the mechanoreceptive properties of RARs, and have redirected our attention to Widdicombe's suggestion that decreased lung compliance could sensitize irritant receptors to phasic lung inflation (32). This led us to question the widely accepted view that RARs are necessarily inactive in the normal lung at resting tidal volume. While recording pulmonary afferent activity in open chest dogs with lungs ventilated at normal resting tidal volume, end-expiratory volume, and frequency, we found that the irregular activity of RARs often disappeared after we had hyperinflated the lungs in order to confirm the rapidly adapting nature of the receptors (22). The action potentials reappeared, and the receptors were clearly stimulated, when positive end-expiratory pressure (PEEP) was removed, and firing continued, often with regular bursts during inflation, when PEEP was restored. The reappearance of RAR activity under control ventilatory conditions coincided with a small increase in lung stiffness.

This method of removing PEEP for a few ventilatory cycles was used in subsequent studies in dogs, cats, and rabbits to produce a series of reductions in

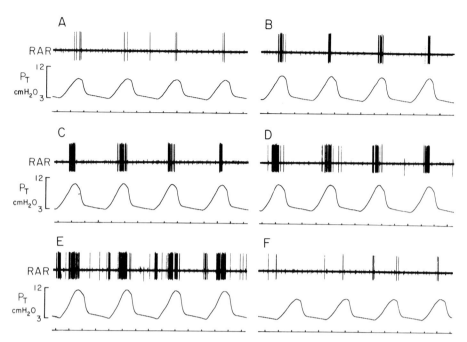

Fig. 29.1 Stimulation of a rapidly adapting receptor (RAR) by progressive reduction of dynamic lung compliance (C_{dyn}) in a rabbit with open chest and lungs ventilated at constant rate and tidal volume. **(A)** Control; C_{dyn} is maximal. **(B–E)** C_{dyn} is reduced in stages by removal of PEEP. In each panel, activity is recorded approximately 10 s after PEEP is restored. **(E)** C_{dyn} is 32% less than control. **(F)** C_{dyn} is restored to control by hyperinflation of the lung. P_T, tracheal pressure; time trace, 1 s. [Reproduced by permission from Yu et al., 1987 (33).].

dynamic lung compliance that were readily reversible. We began by hyperinflating the lungs to produce maximal compliance, and, after examining the receptor response to stepwise reduction in compliance to approximately 60% of the control value, we restored compliance to maximum by another hyperinflation. Small, successive changes in lung compliance increased RAR activity in a proportional manner, the response being reversible and reproducible (11,33). The conversion of the typically irregular, low-frequency pattern of discharge at maximal lung compliance to high-frequency bursts of activity at the peak of inflation (Fig. 29.1) is a striking feature of the response of intrapulmonary RARs to reduction of lung compliance. A similar response can be demonstrated during spontaneous breathing. The changes in receptor activity are not abolished by atropine and hence do not depend on changes in bronchial smooth muscle tone.

RARs are also known to be sensitive to the rate of inflation, their volume threshold decreasing and sensitivity increasing when inflation rate increases (19). It seems likely that these inflation rate effects, like those described above, are a function of the rate of change of transpulmonary pressure, and are not due to increased airflow per se. Nevertheless, when RAR activity is expressed as a function of transpulmonary pressure and its rate of change, a decrease in lung compliance often appears to be a more effective stimulus than an increase in tidal airflow (33). The reason for this difference may not be far to seek when the lungs are ventilated artificially by positive pressure, and the increase in transpulmonary pressure produced by an increase in tidal volume is partly spent in inflating the lungs against an inert chest wall. However, in preliminary studies we have observed similar effects on RARs in spontaneously breathing dogs (Pisarri, Jonzon, Coleridge, and Coleridge, unpublished). Lung compliance was reduced during spontaneous breathing by compression of the chest wall for periods of a minute or so with an inflatable cuirass; at the end of the experiment, compliance was restored to control by hyperinflation of the lungs. In one such experiment (Fig.29.2), we compared the increase in RAR discharge evoked by reduction of lung compliance with that evoked when CO_2 was added to the inspired gas to increase tidal airflow. In this

Fig. 29.2 Stimulation of a rapidly adapting receptor in a spontaneously breathing dog by progressive reduction of dynamic lung compliance (above, A–C) and by progressive increase in tidal volume (below, D–F). From top to bottom, traces represent RAR impulse frequency (IF), counted by ratemeter in 0.1-s bins; transpulmonary pressure (P_{TP}); and tidal volume (V_T). **(A)** Control; lung compliance is maximal. **(B, C)** Compliance is reduced by restriction of chest movement for 30 s (between A and B) and 60 s (between B and C); B and C are recorded approximately 30 s after restriction is removed. **(D)** Recorded after compliance is restored to control by hyperinflation of the lung. **(E, F)** The rate and depth of breathing are increased by addition of CO_2 to the inspired gas. Note that in relation to the transpulmonary pressure changes, a reduction in lung compliance was a more effective stimulus to the receptor than an increase in tidal volume and airflow.

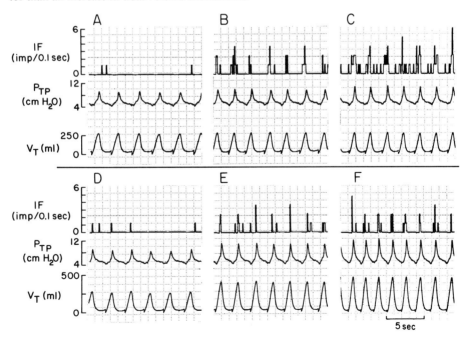

RAR in a spontaneously breathing dog, as in the majority of RARs in artificially ventilated cats and rabbits (33), a reduction in compliance was the more effective of the two stimuli.

Compliance is known to decrease spontaneously during quiet breathing (8). Hence a reflex facilitation of inspiratory drive will serve the homeostatic function of maintaining tidal ventilation as the lungs become stiffer. When compliance decreases to a critical level, reflex deep breaths or sighs become more frequent (23), and are thought to open up collapsed alveoli and increase the surfactant at the alveolar air–liquid interface (18). The sensitivity of RARs to a progressive decrease in lung compliance, together with their known excitatory effects on inspiratory motor output, suggests that they are responsible for these reflex effects. The notion that RARs have a homeostatic function during quiet breathing is a marked departure from the previous emphasis on their high mechanical threshold and their role in irritant reflexes.

AFFERENT C FIBERS: BACKGROUND

The development of ideas about the afferent C-fiber innervation of the lungs and airways has had a somewhat different history. It began with the observation that powerful reflex cardiovascular and respiratory effects, consisting of bradycardia, systemic hypotension, and apnea followed by rapid shallow breathing, and collectively called the "pulmonary chemoreflex," were evoked in anesthetized animals by the action of chemicals such as phenyldiguanide and capsaicin within the pulmonary vascular bed. The electrophysiological study of the vagal afferents responsible for the pulmonary chemoreflex was launched by Paintal in 1955 (20), and over the next 30 years bronchoconstriction, increased airway secretion, inhibition of spinal reflex mechanisms, and coronary vasodilation were added to the overall reflex picture (for literature review, see ref. 3). The pulmonary chemoreflex evoked by a bolus injection of chemical into the pulmonary artery is highly artificial, involving as it probably does the abrupt and simultaneous engagement of the total population of pulmonary C fibers (J receptors). Hence its functional significance, as such, is debatable. Nevertheless, it gives an indication of the widespread reflex mechanisms that can be triggered by pulmonary C fiber input. Without the use of exotic chemicals this important afferent pathway might have been overlooked.

In spite of the emphasis placed on chemical stimuli, it was known from early work that other stimuli were of potential importance. For example, pulmonary C fibers were known to be stimulated by acute distension of the lung, and for this reason were first characterized in the dog as "high-threshold inflation receptors" (4). On the basis of their possible juxtapulmonary capillary location and their response to acute, severe pulmonary edema, Paintal suggested that these C fiber endings act as interstitial stretch receptors in the alveolar walls (21). Nevertheless, although the powerful respiratory chemoreflex effects of pulmonary C fiber input were widely acknowledged, until recently their possible contribution to respiratory control mechanisms was generally overlooked in favor of the contributions of the more easily identified slowly and rapidly adapting receptors.

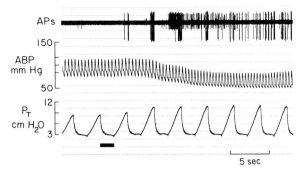

Fig. 29.3 Action potentials in a bronchial C fiber (smaller spikes) and in a myelinated fiber from a rapidly adapting receptor (larger spikes), recorded from the same vagal strand in a cat. Activity evoked by injection of histamine, 50 μg/kg, i.v. (at the signal). ABP, arterial blood pressure; P_T, tracheal pressure. Note that activity in the bronchial C fiber was irregular throughout, whereas the RAR fired initially in response to the increase in peak tracheal pressure.

Our ideas about the afferent C fiber innervation of the lower respiratory tract were extended by the identification of bronchial C fibers supplying the trachea and bronchi (2,5,25). Bronchial C fibers and RAR fibers are often found together in the vagus nerve, both innervate the conducting airways, and both are stimulated by histamine (Fig.29.3); hence, they could easily be thought to represent the nonmyelinated and myelinated counterparts of a single afferent system. This is not the case, however. Recent work indicates that bronchial C fibers are sensitive to endogenous chemicals in doses that have little or no effect on either RARs or pulmonary C fibers, so that their role in irritant conditions of the lower airways may surpass that of the original irritant receptors with myelinated fibers.

CHANGING VIEWS OF THE FUNCTIONAL ROLE OF AFFERENT C FIBERS

There has been much speculation about the significance of pulmonary C fibers in the regulation of breathing, but experimental evidence has often been scanty. The hypothesis that pulmonary C fibers are responsible for the dyspnea and tachypnea of pulmonary edema was proposed by Paintal, who found that activity in J receptors in cats increased in the acute pulmonary edema induced by chlorine and alloxan, and during brief obstruction of left ventricular outflow (21). In spite of recent challenges, the balance of evidence indicates that Paintal's overall hypothesis is likely to be correct, and that tachypnea is the typical respiratory outcome when bronchial and pulmonary C fibers are stimulated.

Brief reports suggested that stimulation of pulmonary C fibers did not cause tachypnea, but only apnea, and that the delayed tachypnea of the pulmonary chemoreflex was triggered by stimulation of nerve endings downstream to the pulmonary circulation (9). Thus injection of capsaicin into the isolated pulmonary circulation of one lung was found to cause apnea without subsequent tachypnea, and although reducing the injected dose reduced the duration of apnea, it never evoked tachypnea (1). Paintal had anticipated such a challenge by suggesting that apnea was due to the unnaturally abrupt and intense increase in afferent input evoked by the rapid injection of a powerful chemical (20). He believed that tachypnea was the usual response when pulmonary C fibers were stimulated under natural conditions, and would occur without preceding apnea in experimental situations if the chemical was injected slowly, or was given in small doses. Results of experiments in dogs in which the pulmonary and systemic circulations were perfused independently support Paintal's contention. Thus rapid injection of small doses of capsaicin into the isolated pulmonary circulation evoked apnea followed by rapid, shallow breathing, whereas slow infusions evoked rapid, shallow breathing without preceding apnea (10). These results provide clear evidence that pulmonary C fibers can evoke tachypnea. Tachypnea was also observed when bronchial C fibers in dogs were stimulated by slow infusion of bradykinin into the bronchial artery (5).

The tachypneic influence of C fibers is not confined to pathological situations. There is now evidence that the low-frequency background discharge in afferent C fibers from the lungs and airways has a tonic tachypneic influence during normal breathing. Changes in breathing pattern have been recorded in anesthetized rabbits and dogs while the vagus nerves were cooled (17,22). In neither species did the slow deep breathing characteristic of vagotomy develop fully until the nerves were cooled to a temperature below that required to block transmission in myelinated fibers, and in both species tonic activity in afferent vagal C fibers appeared to shorten expiratory time. The pulmonary origin of this tonic activity was confirmed in dogs by cooling the pulmonary vagal branches, the abdominal branches being cut (22). The phrenic neurogram provided an index of respiratory pattern (Fig. 29.4). Expiratory time did not increase maximally until the vagus nerves were cooled below 3°C, and the neural pattern of slow deep breathing obtained subsequently by interrupting the pulmonary vagal branches was unaffected by cutting the cervical vagus nerves. Hence the tonic tachypneic influence on breathing pattern originates in the lungs and not in other vagally innervated thoracic structures.

Recent studies have confirmed Paintal's hypothesis that vagal C fiber input increases in interstitial lung edema (24). Interstitial edema was induced in dogs by infusing Krebs–Henseleit solution intravenously in an amount equivalent to approximately 20% of body weight. Activity increased in slowly adapting pulmonary stretch receptors and RARs, as well as in pulmonary and bronchial C fibers, as long as pulmonary vascular pressures were high. At the end of the infusion, when pulmonary vascular pressures were reduced to control but interstitial edema remained, activity in myelinated fibers reverted to control or decreased below the control level, but activity in both pulmonary and bronchial C fibers remained elevated. The increase in activity in bronchial C fibers was associated with severe edema, and the presence of marked bronchial "cuffing."

The clinical observation that tachypnea and dyspnea are associated with pulmonary edema cannot always be confirmed in the laboratory. Thus Lloyd (14) and Wead et al. (29) were unable to repeat an early observation in anesthetized dogs that acute, severe unilateral pulmonary congestion and edema evoked a vagally mediated cardiovascular depression and apnea or tachypnea (7). The reasons for

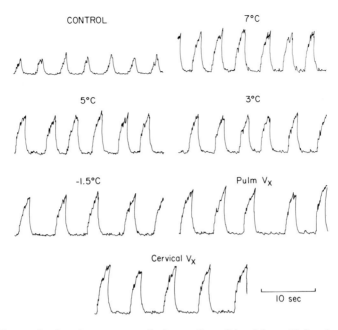

Fig. 29.4 Changes in phrenic neurogram during cooling of the right and left pulmonary vagal branches in a dog with open chest and lungs artificially ventilated at constant frequency and tidal volume (the thoracic vagus nerves were ligated above the diaphragm). Control: The temperature of the pulmonary vagal branches was 37°C; the branches were then cooled gradually to −1.5°C. Pulm. V_X: The pulmonary vagal branches were cut. Cervical V_X: The cervical vagus nerves were cut. Note the increase in amplitude of phrenic bursts at 7°C and below, and the increase in intervals between bursts when the temperature was reduced to below 3°C. Note also that cutting the pulmonary and cervical vagus nerves had no further effect on the timing of the phrenic neurogram. [Reproduced by permission from Pisarri et al., 1986 (22).]

this failure are still uncertain and may relate to the depth or type of anesthesia. Tachypnea is induced by acute unilateral pulmonary congestion in decerebrate cats; it is abolished after capsaicin, dissolved in alcohol, has been applied to the vagus nerve, a procedure that appears to abolish conduction in C fibers selectively (J. Hatridge, A. Haji, and J. E. Remmers, personal communication).

The afferent and reflex properties of bronchial C fibers have been examined in dogs by injection of bradykinin or prostacyclin into a bronchial artery. These autacoids, which are known to be formed and released in the airways, were found to stimulate bronchial C fibers but to have little or no effect on pulmonary C fibers, RARs, or pulmonary stretch receptors. The doses employed were small, so that the concentrations reaching bronchial C fiber endings were probably close to those that can occur naturally, and systemic side effects on arterial blood pressure were avoided. When bradykinin was infused slowly into a bronchial artery or delivered as an aerosol, bronchial C fibers were stimulated and rapid shallow breathing, bronchoconstriction, and increased airway secretion evoked. Effects could still be elicited when conduction in myelinated vagal fibers was blocked by cooling the vagus nerves to 7°C, but were abolished when conduction in nonmyelinated fibers was blocked by cooling to 0°C (5,6,12,25,26).

The functional significance of bronchial C fibers as an afferent pathway for the airway defense response has recently received an added dimension. These C fibers are believed to be involved in local inflammatory changes in the bronchial mucosa, analogous to those that cause the wheel-and-flare reaction in the skin. Local effects, which include an increase in tracheal vascular permeability and smooth muscle contraction, have been demonstrated in the lower airways of rats and guinea pigs. They are thought to be due to release of substance P, which is transported peripherally in the C fiber axons and released when the sensory terminals are depolarized (15). This afferent system is destroyed if very large doses of capsaicin (more than 2000 times larger than those that evoke pronounced reflex effects from the pulmonary or bronchial circulations) are administered by repeated subcutaneous injection to immature animals. So far these "axon-reflex" effects have not been demonstrated in the airways of larger animals, but their potential significance in the pathophysiology of lower airway function is an important direction for future research.

REFERENCES

1. Cassidy, S. S., W. B. Wead, M. P. Kaufman, J. H. Ashton, and Y. Monsereenusorn, Reflex responses caused by pulmonary C-fibers. *Physiologist 26:* 45, 1983.

2. Coleridge, H. M., and J.C.G. Coleridge. Impulse activity in afferent vagal C fibres with endings in the intrapulmonary airways of dogs. *Respir. Physiol. 29:* 124–142, 1977.

3. Coleridge, H. M., and J.C.G. Coleridge. Reflexes evoked from tracheobronchial tree and lungs. In: *Handbook of Physiology,* Sec. 3: *The Respiratory System,* Vol. 2: *Control of Breathing,* ed. N. S. Cherniack and J. G. Widdicombe. Bethesda: Am. Physiol. Soc., 1986, pp. 395–429.

4. Coleridge, H. M., J.C.G. Coleridge, and J. C. Luck. Pulmonary afferent fibres of small diameter stimulated by capsaicin and by hyperinflation of the lungs, *J. Physiol. (Lond.) 179:* 248–262, 1965.

5. Coleridge, H. M., J.C.G. Coleridge, and A. M. Roberts. Rapid shallow breathing evoked by selective stimulation of bronchial C fibres in dogs. *J. Physiol. (Lond.) 340:* 415–433, 1983.

6. Davis, B., A. M. Roberts, H. M. Coleridge, and J.C.G. Coleridge. Reflex tracheal gland secretion evoked by stimulation of bronchial C-fibers in dogs. *J. Appl. Physiol. 53:* 985–991, 1982.

7. Downing, S. E. Reflex effects of acute hypertension in the pulmonary vascular bed of the dog. *Yale J. Biol. Med. 30:* 43–56, 1957.

8. Ferris, B. G. Jr., and D. S. Pollard. Effect of deep and quiet breathing on pulmonary compliance in man. *J. Clin. Invest. 39:* 143–149, 1960.

9. Ginzel, K. H. The respiratory effect of vagal lung afferents ('J receptors') excited by phenyldiguanide (PDG). *Fed. Proc. 37:* 579, 1978.

10. Green, J. F., N. D. Schmidt, H. D. Schultz, A. M. Roberts, H. M. Coleridge, and J.C.G. Coleridge. Pulmonary C-fibers evoke both apnea and tachypnea of pulmonary chemoreflex. *J. Appl. Physiol. 57:* 562–567, 1984.

11. Jonzon, A., T. E. Pisarri, J.C.G. Coleridge, and H. M. Coleridge. Rapidly adapting receptor activity in dogs is inversely related to lung compliance. *J. Appl. Physiol. 61:* 1980–1987, 1986.

12. Kaufman, M. P., H. M. Coleridge, J.C.G. Coleridge, and D. G. Baker. Bradykinin stimulates afferent vagal C-fibers in intrapulmonary airways of dogs. *J. Appl. Physiol. 48:* 511–517, 1980.

13. Knowlton, G. C., and M. G. Larrabee. A unitary analysis of pulmonary volume receptors. *Am. J. Physiol. 147:* 100–114, 1946.

14. Lloyd, T. C. Cardiopulmonary baroreflexes: effects of pulmonary congestion and edema. *J. Appl. Physiol. 43:* 107–113, 1977.

15. Lundberg, J. M., and A. Saria, Capsaicin-induced desensitization of airway mucosa to cigarette smoke, mechanical and chemical irritants. *Nature 302:* 251–253, 1983.

16. Mills, J. E., H. Sellick, and J. G. Widdicombe. Activity of lung irritant receptors in pulmonary microembolism, anaphylaxis and drug-induced bronchoconstrictions. *J. Physiol. (Lond.) 203:* 337–357, 1969.

17. Miserocchi, G., T. Trippenbach, M. Mazzarelli, N. Jaspar, and M. Hazucha. The mechanism of rapid shallow breathing due to histamine and phenyldiguanide in cats and rabbits. *Respir. Physiol. 32:* 141–153, 1978.

18. Nicholas, T. E., J. H. Power, and H. A. Barr. The pulmonary consequences of a deep breath. *Respir. Physiol. 49:* 315–324, 1982.

19. Pack, A. I., and R. G. Delaney. Response of pulmonary rapidly adapting receptors during lung inflation. *J. Appl. Physiol. 55:* 955–963, 1983.

20. Paintal, A. S. Impulses in vagal afferent fibres from specific pulmonary deflation receptors. The response of these receptors to phenyl diguanide, potato starch, 5-hydroxytryptamine and nicotine, and their role in respiratory and cardiovascular reflexes. *Q. J. Exp. Physiol. 40:* 89–111, 1955.

21. Paintal, A. S. Mechanism of stimulation of type J pulmonary receptors. *J. Physiol. (Lond.) 203:* 511–532, 1969.

22. Pisarri, T. E., J. Yu, H. M. Coleridge, and J.C.G. Coleridge. Background activity in pulmonary vagal C-fibers and its effects on breathing. *Respir. Physiol. 64:* 29–43, 1986.

23. Reynolds, L. B., Jr. Characteristics of an inspiration-augmenting reflex in anesthetized cats. *J. Appl. Physiol. 17:* 683–688, 1962.

24. Roberts, A. M., J. Bhattacharya, H. D. Schultz, H. M. Coleridge, and J.C.G. Coleridge. Stimulation of pulmonary vagal afferent C-fibers by lung edema in dogs. *Circ. Res. 58:* 512–522, 1986.

25. Roberts, A. M., M. P. Kaufman, D. G. Baker, J. K. Brown, H. M. Coleridge, and J.C.G. Coleridge. Reflex tracheal contraction induced by stimulation of bronchial C-fibers in dogs. *J. Appl. Physiol. 51:* 485–493, 1981.

26. Roberts, A. M., H. D. Schultz, J. F. Green, D. J. Armstrong, M. P. Kaufman, H. M. Coleridge, and J.C.G. Coleridge. Reflex tracheal contraction evoked in dogs by bronchodilator prostaglandins E_2 and I_2. *J. Appl. Physiol. 58:* 1823–1831, 1985.

27. Sampson, S. R., and E. H. Vidruk. Properties of "irritant" receptors in canine lung. *Respir. Physiol. 25:* 9–22, 1975.

28. Sellick, H., and J. G. Widdicombe. The activity of lung irritant receptors during pneumothorax, hyperpnoea and pulmonary vascular congestion. *J. Physiol. (Lond.) 203:* 359–381, 1969.

29. Wead, W. B., S. S. Cassidy, and R. C. Reynolds. Pulmonary edema in dogs fails to cause reflex responses. *Am. J. Physiol. 252:* H89–H99, 1987.

30. Widdicombe, J. G. Receptors in the trachea and bronchi of the cat. *J. Physiol. (Lond.) 123:* 71–104, 1954.

31. Widdicombe, J. G. Respiratory reflexes excited by inflation of the lungs. *J. Physiol. (Lond.) 123:* 105–115, 1954.

32. Widdicombe, J. G. Modes of excitation of respiratory tract receptors. *Prog. Brain Res. 43:* 243–252, 1976.

33. Yu, J., J.C.G. Coleridge, and H. M. Coleridge. Influence of lung stiffness on rapidly adapting receptors in rabbits and cats. *Respir. Physiol.,* 68: 161-176, 1987.

30

Neurohumoral Regulation of Airway Smooth Muscle: Role of the Tracheal Ganglia

R. A. MITCHELL, D. A. HERBERT, AND C. A. RICHARDSON

The pattern of breathing in humans is adjusted to that requiring minimal work (26,28), indicating a link between the breathing pattern, compliance, and airway tone. In 1966, Widdicombe (26) recorded rhythmic respiratory-related activity in vagal efferent nerves innervating the trachea and bronchi. He suggested that these fibers might innervate the airway smooth muscle and provide a mechanism that integrates breathing and airway resistance to minimize the work of breathing. Furthermore, Widdicombe and Nadel (16,27) demonstrated that many respiratory reflexes that increase breathing also increase airway resistance, whereas reflex inhibition of breathing reduces airway smooth muscle tone. Subsequently, McAllen and Spyer (11) reported that inspiratory firing cells in the nucleus ambiguus innervate the airways. Anatomical verification of this conclusion came from the observations of Kalia (9), who reported that horseradish peroxidase injected into the trachea and bronchi retrogradely stained cells in the nucleus ambiguus.

The regulation of airway smooth muscle tone and mucous secretion are believed to result from the interaction of the parasympathetic and sympathetic nerves (2,7,17,30); the major input arising from the cholinergic (parasympathetic) nerves. Electrical stimulation of the vagus nerve evokes bronchoconstriction and mucous secretion, whereas atropine, which blocks the cholinergic pathway, abolishes these responses. In this report, we demonstrate that airway resistance, activity in tracheal ganglion cells identified as innervating tracheal smooth muscle, and tracheal smooth muscle tone all fluctuate with respiration; peak resistance, cell activity, and tone occur during inspiration, as judged from the activity of the phrenic nerve. During neural apnea (the absence of phrenic nerve activity), the firing of the ganglion cells decreased or was absent; the rhythmic fluctuations in tracheal smooth muscle tone and airway resistance disappeared; and the tone and resistance decreased to the same level as that achieved by administration of atropine or bilateral section of the vagi. However, in most instances the tracheal ganglion cells continued to fire, although at a reduced frequency, in the absence of phrenic activity and were quiescent during stimulation of the posterior nasopharynx which evoked bursts of activity in the phrenic nerve (sniff reflex).

We therefore conclude that the major excitatory input to the smooth muscle of the airways arises from cholinergic nerve fibers that fire during inspiration, and whose preganglionic cell bodies are in the nucleus ambiguus. Despite their close proximity in this nucleus to other motoneurons that innervate the phrenic and intercostal motor nerves, they do not share a common motor pool with them. However, during normal breathing, as well as during many evoked respiratory reflexes, the input to the ganglion cells may be modulated by the same central respiratory pattern generator that modulates phrenic nerve activity.

METHODS

All studies were done in cats, anesthetized with a mixture of α-chloralose (40 mg/kg) and urethan (200 mg/kg). We exposed the trachea through a midline incision from the mandible to the sternum. We identified the right phrenic nerve, freed it from the surrounding tissue, and cut and desheathed it for subsequent recording. We cannulated the trachea as low in the neck as possible, preserving the recurrent laryngeal nerve and the blood supply to the trachea. Using similar precautions, we removed a segment of the esophagus from the region of the trachea to be studied. We created a bilateral pneumothorax and ventilated the cat by a Harvard respiratory pump at a frequency of 60–70 breaths/min while maintaining an end-expiratory pressure of 2.5 cm of water. The volume of the inflations was set at a level sufficient to produce neural apnea when CO_2 was not added to the inspired gas. During control periods, CO_2 was added to the inspired gas to maintain the end-tidal CO_2 between 40 and 45 torr. Lung hyperinflation was produced by an increase in end-expiratory pressure. We incised the trachea ventrally along the midline from the larynx to the tracheal cannula and mounted the cat in a supine position in a spinal frame and head holder.

The methods employed in the measurement of tracheal smooth muscle tone, evoking respiratory reflexes, and the analysis of results are as described in detail in a previous publication (15).

To record intracellular potentials from tracheal ganglion cells, we rotated the tracheal cannula clockwise 90° and stabilized it by a clamp attached to the spinal frame. The incised trachea rostral to the tracheal cannula was rotated an additional 90°, and the cut edges were sewn to a Lucite platform which was rigidly attached to the spinal frame and illuminated by a fiberoptic lamp. Throughout the studies, the cat's body temperature was maintained at 38°C by a servo heating pad. Cotton pledgets saturated with 0.01% neutral red, a stain for tracheal ganglion cells that does not alter their function (23), were placed on the exposed adventitial surface of the trachea for 30 min. The connective tissue overlying the ganglia was removed and the ganglion cells were penetrated with beveled-glass electrodes containing 5% Lucifer Yellow or 5 M potassium acetate. Once the membrane potential stabilized, we recorded the spontaneous (control) activity of the cells. During the control period, we maintained the end-expiratory pressure at 2.5 cm H_2O and the end-tidal P_{CO_2} between 40 and 45 torr.

The methods employed to evoke the reflex responses to lung hyperinflation, hypocapnia, carotid body stimulation, and electrical stimulation of the vagi are as previously reported (15). We stimulated the posterior nasopharynx with a small plastic fiber to evoke the sniff reflex. We placed cuff electrodes on the cervical vagi to determine the conduction velocity of the preganglionic fibers and to evaluate the effect of vagal stimulation on the ganglion cells. Throughout the experiments, the end-tidal CO_2, tracheal pressure (transpulmonary pressure), ganglion cell membrane potential, and phrenic nerve activity were continuously recorded on a Grass polygraph and FM tape.

Statistical Analysis

The pooled data are reported as means $\pm$ SD averaged across cats. The statistical significance of the evoked reflex responses was tested by nonparametric statistical analysis (Wilcoxon signed-step test). Power spectral analysis of the synaptic input into the ganglion cells and the detection of the spectral peaks and their significance were done by the methods described by Richardson (19).

RESULTS

Tracheal Segment Tension

In all cats studied, the tracheal segment tension showed significant fluctuations, with the same rhythm as that observed in the phrenic nerve. During normal breathing at a frequency of 11 ± 0.9 breaths/min, the tension of the tracheal segment fluctuated 0.7 ± 0.1 g about a mean tension of 31.8 ± 1.6 g. Intravenous injection of atropine (0.5 mg/kg) or transection of the vagi eliminated the rhythmic oscillations in the tension and decreased the tension to 21.2 ± 1.8 g. Hypocapnia caused a decrease in the phrenic activity and a simultaneous decrease in the amplitude of the oscillations in tracheal tone as well as a reduction in the average tone. During neural apnea (absence of phrenic activity) produced by hypocapnia, the oscillations disappeared and tracheal tone decreased from 31.5 ± 2.0 g to 22.7 ± 1.3 g, a value not significantly different from that observed following the administration of atropine or bilateral section of the vagus nerves. Lung hyperinflation also decreased or abolished phrenic activity and caused a similar decrease in tracheal segment tone (Fig.30.1). However, during neural apnea induced by hypocapnia, lung hyperinflation caused no further decrease in tracheal tone. During the neural apnea produced by hyperinflation of the lung, the tracheal tension (23.1 ± 4.2) was not significantly different from that recorded during neural apnea induced by hypocapnia, the administration of atropine, or section of the vagi.

Carotid body stimulation evoked by intravenous administration of 200 μg of NaCN caused, in all cats tested, a significant increase in tracheal tension that paralleled the increase in phrenic activity (Fig. 30.1). (See refs. 15,20 for complete description of the above studies.)

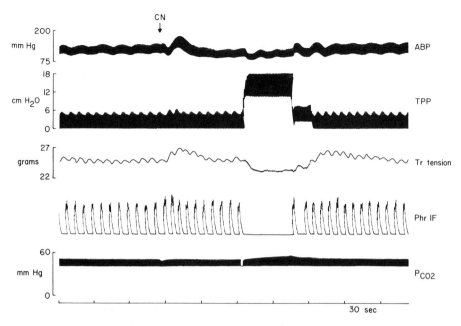

Fig. 30.1 Effects of stimulation of the carotid chemoreceptor by injection of 200 μg NaCN intravenously (arrow). Also demonstrated is the effect of lung hyperinflation on transpulmonary pressure, tracheal tension, and integrated phrenic activity. ABP, arterial blood pressure; TPP, transpulmonary pressure; Tr tension, tracheal segment tension; Phr IF, integrated phrenic firing; P_{CO_2}, tracheal CO_2 tension.

Firing Pattern of Tracheal Parasympathetic Ganglion Cells

We successfully recorded intracellularly the spontaneous activity of 122 tracheal parasympathetic ganglion cells in 66 cats. In our initial studies, in order to identify the ganglion cells and their axonal projections, we used microelectrodes containing Lucifer Yellow, which was injected intrasomally after the electrophysiological properties were recorded. In 28 cats we were able to record stable intracellular potentials for up to 30 min and then inject Lucifer Yellow. Two distinct types of ganglion cells were encountered, which could be distinguished by their anatomical and electrophysiological features. Compact clusters of small ganglion cells (diameter, 36 ± 6 μm, $n = 5$) were located primarily in the posterolateral tracheal adventitia near the intercartilaginous spaces, although occasionally clusters were located in apposition to the tracheal smooth muscle. These cells fired either with an expiratory rhythm or continuously with increased frequency during expiration (Fig. 30.2). During inspiration, small synaptic potentials could be observed that failed to elicit action potentials. These small cells were excited by lung hyperinflation, had an average membrane potential of 61 ± 8 mV, and had no significant (i.e., <3 mV) post-spike afterhyperpolarization. When injected with Lucifer Yellow, the cells' axonal projections could be traced into the intercartilaginous spaces toward the nerve plexus about the mucous glands, but the final termination of the axons could not be determined.

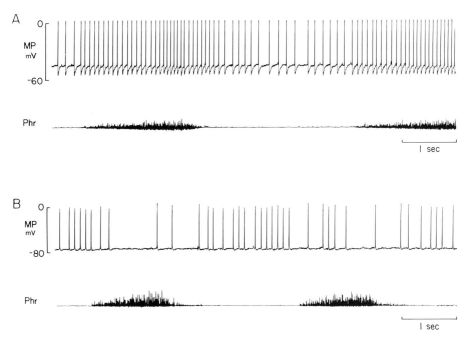

Fig. 30.2 Simultaneous intracellular recording of the spontaneous activity of the tracheal parasympathetic ganglion units and the phrenic nerve (Phr). **(A)** An inspiratory firing (large) parasympathetic cell (resting membrane potential, -62 mV). **(B)** An expiratory firing (small) cell (resting membrane potential, -58 mV). Note the continuous synaptic potentials throughout the respiratory cycle and the phasic action potentials in the absence of apparent inhibitory postsynaptic potentials (IPSPs). MP, membrane potential.

A second population of cells of larger diameter (63 ± 5 μm, $n = 27$) were located in the adventitia in close apposition to the trachealis muscle near its attachment to the tracheal cartilaginous rings. They fired either with an inspiratory rhythm or continuously with increased frequency during inspiration (Fig. 30.2). These cells had a membrane potential of 52 ± 12 mV, and a significant afterhyperpolarization of 10 ± 1.2 mV lasting 94 ± 18 ms. They fired at a peak frequency of 10–13 Hz, with numerous synaptic potentials in the interspike intervals which failed to reach a threshold sufficient to evoke an action potential during the postspike afterhyperpolarization. Also suppression of the action potentials and accentuation of the synaptic potentials by the injection of a hyperpolarizing current revealed that the regularly occurring synaptic potentials seen during inspiration persisted, but at a reduced amplitude, during expiration (Figs. 30.3 and 30.4). The action potentials were inhibited by lung hyperinflation, although in many instances synaptic potentials were seen during the inhibition of phrenic activity produced by lung hyperinflation. Neither long-lasting inhibitory postsynaptic potentials (IPSPs) nor excitatory postsynaptic potentials (EPSPs) were apparent during the spontaneous activity, nor did rhythmic inhibitory potentials acting at the level of the ganglia appear to play a role in the rhythmic firing of these cells. Axonal projections

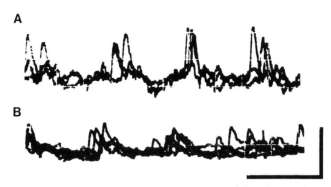

Fig. 30.3 Superimposed recordings of the membrane potential and synaptic potentials of five (one for each of five successive breaths) sweeps of the oscilloscope triggered by the synaptic potentials during inspiration (**A**) and during expiration (**B**). During the recording of these traces, a hyperpolarizing current was injected into the cell to accentuate the amplitude of the excitatory postsynaptic potentials (EPSPs) and inhibit action potentials. Calibrations: vertical bar = 10 mV; horizontal bar = 50 ms.

extended up to 6 mm from the cell bodies, had numerous varicosities over the last 5 mm, and were in close apposition to the trachealis muscle or projected into it.

The firing of the larger ganglion cells, for the most part, paralleled the activity of the phrenic nerve. Stimulation of the carotid chemoreceptors always caused an increase in both phrenic nerve and ganglion cell activity. Lung hyperinflation always caused a decrease in the activity of the phrenic nerves and ganglion cells. However, even when the phrenic nerve was silenced by hyperinflation, there was a range of responses in the ganglion cell activity: quiescence when the level of inflation was greatest, continuous synchronous synaptic potentials with a reduced amplitude at intermediate levels of inflation, and continuous synchronous synaptic potentials plus action potentials when the level of inflation was moderate. Hypocapnia, sufficient to eliminate phrenic activity, always reduced the firing of ganglion cells. However, in most cells studied, synaptic potentials as well as action potentials were recorded from ganglion cells during quiescence of phrenic activity (Fig.30.3B and 30.4). When end-tidal CO_2 was sufficiently reduced to quench both phrenic nerve and ganglion cell activity and then gradually raised to control values, there was a progressive increase in the amplitude of the synchronized synaptic potentials. This was followed by the onset of action potentials, which gradually increased in frequency but without a respiratory rhythm, prior to the onset of firing in the phrenic nerve. The response to the stimulation of the posterior nasopharynx, however, clearly dissociated the phrenic nerve activity from that of the ganglion cells. Such stimulation caused repetitive bursts of phrenic activity unaccompanied by firing in the ganglion cells.

Transmission Through Tracheal Parasympathetic Ganglion

Electrical stimulation of the vagus nerve evoked synaptic potentials in the ganglion cells. The conduction velocity of the vagal preganglionic fibers, calculated from the time interval between the shock artifact and the onset of a synaptic potential, was 2.1 ±0.2 m/s. Incremental increases in the strength of the electrical stimulation of the vagi caused a progressive increase in the amplitude of the evoked synaptic potential, with action potentials being elicited only after the summation of five or more synaptic potentials. During repetitive supermaximal stimulation of the vagi, action potentials were elicited following each stimulus up to a frequency of 10 Hz. At frequencies of 10 Hz or above, the cells failed to fire with each stimulus. We attribute the failure of these cells to follow electrical stimulation at frequencies above 10 Hz to the post-spike afterhyperpolarization. During normal breathing, spontaneous EPSPs of 5.5 ± 2.4 mV lasting 11.2 ± 2.6 ms occurred at regular intervals with a frequency of 24.9 ± 2.4 Hz. During expiration or during neural apnea, induced by hypocapnia or lung hyperinflation, many cells continued to exhibit synaptic potentials at the same intervals recorded during inspiration, but they were reduced in amplitude (Figs. 30.3 and 30.4).

DISCUSSION

These studies provide good evidence that the tone of airway smooth muscle in the cat is determined primarily by parasympathetic cholinergic nerves firing with an inspiratory rhythm, since atropinization has the same effect on tracheal tension as does transection of the vagi. We have also shown that airway smooth muscle tone fluctuates with a respiratory rhythm and parallels the activity of the phrenic nerves during normal breathing, as well as during inhibition of phrenic activity elicited by hypocapnia or lung hyperinflation, and during stimulation of breathing evoked by carotid body chemoreceptor stimulation. These findings confirm the observations of Widdicombe and Nadel (16,27), who reported that airway reflexes causing an increase or decrease in the level of breathing also caused parallel changes in airway resistance.

Although the function of airway smooth muscle tone is unknown, the following functions have been suggested (18). Rhythmic contractions of the airway

Fig. 30.4 Intracellular recording of an inspiratory firing ganglion cell (upper trace) during the injection of a hyperpolarizing current to enhance the amplitude of the synaptic potentials and inhibit action potentials. Note the waxing and waning of the amplitude of the synchronized synaptic potentials during inspiration and expiration, as indicated by the firing of the phrenic nerve (lower trace).

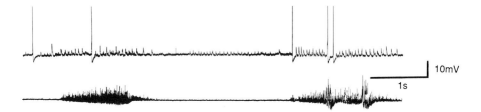

smooth muscle might oppose the forces occurring during inspiration and thereby provide a more stable airway and a balance of dead space against airway resistance to produce the most efficient breathing. Alternatively, the fluctuations in airway smooth muscle tone may be a vestige of a primitive system, reported to be present in lower animals, which employed the smooth muscle of the lung to assist in gas exchange.

We assume that the motor output to the tracheal smooth muscle arises from the nucleus ambiguus, since the bilateral destruction of the dorsal vagal nucleus, the only other source of vagal motor fibers, does not affect airway reflexes (10). This assumption is supported by the observations of Merrill (13), who reported that the inspiratory firing nerve fibers in the recurrent laryngeal nerve, the nerve innervating the trachea, had their origin in the nucleus ambiguus, as well as the work of McAllen and Spyer (11), who demonstrated that nerves projecting from this nucleus innervated the lung. Also, morphological evidence provided by Kalia (9) indicates that nerves arising from the nucleus ambiguus innervate the lung and trachea.

On the basis of the above reports, we suggested that the motor pathways to the diaphragm and airway smooth muscle are modulated by a common central respiratory pattern generator (15). However, several respiratory reflexes—for example, the aspiration reflex (25)—dissociate these pathways. We propose that these reflexes operate through a different central pattern generator, as has been suggested for the gasp reflex (19,24), and indicate that the pool of inspiratory neurons that innervate the phrenic and intercostal motoneurons is separate from that which innervates the airways.

The results obtained from the action potentials in ganglion cells, identified as innervating tracheal smooth muscle, support the above proposal. During normal breathing the firing of ganglion cells was modulated in phase with the phrenic nerve. Stimulation of the carotid body chemoreceptors caused a parallel increase in ganglion cell and phrenic nerve activity. Hypocapnia and lung hyperinflation caused a decrease in both ganglion cell and phrenic nerve activity. However, during step increases in lung hyperinflation it was possible to inhibit phrenic nerve activity while nonrhythmic firing of the ganglion cells persisted. Likewise, during hypocapnia sufficient to cause cessation of phrenic activity, synaptic potentials as well as action potentials persisted in the ganglion cells. Furthermore, following hypocapnic apnea, the gradual increase in end-tidal P_{CO_2} caused a progressive increase in the frequency of ganglion cell action potentials prior to the onset of rhythmic firing of the ganglion cells and phrenic nerve. Although the reflex responses of the ganglion cells and phrenic nerve to lung hyperinflation, carotid chemoreceptor stimulation, and hypocapnia resulted in an increase or decrease in both phrenic nerve and ganglion cell activity, the sniff reflex caused bursts of activity in the phrenic nerve unaccompanied by similar activity in the ganglion cells. These results are consistent with our view, as stated above, that the firing of the ganglion cells and the phrenic motoneurons are modulated by the same central pattern generator, but that separate upper motoneuron pools drive the phrenic nerve and the ganglion cells.

The firing pattern of the ganglion cells could result from the intrinsic properties of the ganglion cells (the post-spike afterhyperpolarization), the phasic activity of the synaptic input, or modulation of the membrane properties of the ganglion cells by other inputs, such as the sympathetic nerves.

Although the afterhyperpolarization that follows each action potential may be important in determining the peak firing frequency of the ganglion cells during inspiration, we believe the frequency and temporal summation of synchronized synaptic inputs, which are necessary to produce action potentials, are the primary determinants of their firing pattern.

The regular repetitive summed synaptic inputs into the ganglion cells, at a regular frequency of 25 Hz, are like the synchronized firing of synaptic input into other nerves exhibiting a respiratory rhythm. Rhythmic periodic action potentials or synaptic potentials have been reported in the phrenic nerves (4,6,21,31), in the sympathetic nerves (8), and in the cells of the dorsal and ventral respiratory groups (5,14). However, the frequency of periodic activity at these sites was not that observed in the ganglion cells. We suggest that meaningful synaptic transfer of information is dependent on the tight synchrony of the presynaptic fibers, resulting in temporal summation of the EPSPs sufficient to depolarize the postsynaptic ganglion cell to a level above its firing threshold, a level that could not be achieved by asynchronous, random firing of presynaptic fibers, even at the same or higher average firing rates.

In the one comparable in vivo study of the firing pattern of parasympathetic ganglion cells—in this case, in the ciliary ganglia—the investigators reported firing rates of 10–15 Hz, synaptic potentials at frequencies in excess of firing frequencies, and post-spike afterhyperpolarization lasting about 100 ms (22). This is in marked contrast to the afterhyperpolarization observed in the enteric ganglia, which has an onset of 45–80 ms and a duration up to 20 s (29). Although there have been no comparable anatomical or electrophysiological studies in the cat, our observations are similar to those from in vitro studies in the ferret trachea. Baker et al. (1) describe two anatomically distinct populations of cells in the ferret; one consists of large cells along the longitudinal nerve trunks, analogous to the inspiratory firing cells in the cat, and a second consists of smaller cells in a deeper plexus associated with the trachealis muscle and laterally with the submucosal glands. These latter cells were similar in location to the expiratory firing cells in the cat. Cameron and Coburn (3), in in vitro studies in the ferret, identified two cell types, not anatomically identified as being different, in the paratracheal ganglia. In one type there was a significant post-spike afterhyperpolarization; in the second type orthodromic stimulation produced only a slow EPSP or rarely a fast IPSP. We found no comparable cells similar to the second group in the cat.

The continuing synaptic input we observed in the inspiratory firing ganglion cells during inhibition induced by lung hyperinflation was similar to the continuous synaptic input reported by Melnichenko and Skok (12) in the ciliary ganglion during a depression of firing, in the absence of IPSPs, produced by illumination of the eye. Our results are consistent with Skok's observations as well as his conclusion that multiple, synchronous inputs are required to elicit an action potential in parasympathetic ganglia (22), and that the modulation of the activity of the parasympathetic ganglia is achieved by regulation, in the central nervous system, of the number of active excitatory preganglionic fibers innervating the ganglion cells, not by IPSPs acting at the level of the ganglion cells.

The origin of the synchronized firing or synaptic potentials in respiratory related nerves is unknown. We have proposed that this synchrony arises from the respiratory pattern generator and results from mechanisms intrinsic to the generation of the respiratory rhythm (14). This hypothesis has been challenged on the basis that synchronized firing of the phrenic nerve is not always observed, and that synchronization may be abolished without affecting the gross aspects of the respiratory pattern. Our studies neither support nor refute the possibility that the synchronous firing of respiratory neurons results from the intrinsic properties of the central respiratory pattern generators.

Alternatively, the synchronized firing of the preganglionic nerve fibers, which appears to be essential for activation of action potentials in the postganglionic nerves, may result from modulation by a central respiratory pattern generator of an intermediate group of neurons associated with, but not part of, the neural network essential for the generation of rhythmic respiration. This latter hypothesis is consistent with our observations that the synchronized synaptic inputs recorded in inspiratory firing tracheal ganglion cells with a frequency of about 25 Hz may occur, although at a reduced amplitude, throughout the respiratory cycle, during expiration as well as during neural apnea induced by lung inflation or hypocapnia.

In summary, the rhythmic firing of the parasympathetic ganglion cells innervating tracheal smooth muscle, paralleling the firing of the phrenic nerves, appears to result from rhythmic modulation in the central nervous system of the number of active synchronously firing preganglionic nerves.

REFERENCES

1. Baker, D.G., D.M. McDonald, C.B. Basbaum, and R.A. Mitchell. The architecture of nerves and ganglia of the ferret trachea as revealed by acetylcholinesterase histochemistry. *J. Comp. Neurol. 246:* 513–526, 1986.
2. Cabezas, G.A., P.D. Graff, and J.A. Nadel. Sympathetic versus parasympathetic nervous regulation of airways in dogs. *J. Appl. Physiol. 31:* 651–655, 1971.
3. Cameron, A.R., and R.F. Coburn. Electrical and anatomical characteristics of the ferret paratracheal ganglion. *Am. J. Physiol. 246:* c450–c458, 1984.
4. Cohen, M.I. Synchronization of discharge, spontaneous and evoked, between inspiratory neurons. *Acta Neurobiol. Exp. (Warsz.) 33:* 189–218, 1973.
5. Cohen, M.I., and J.L. Feldman. Discharge properties of dorsal medullary inspiratory neurons: relation to pulmonary and phrenic efferent discharge. *J. Neurophysiol. 51:* 753–776, 1984.
6. Dittler, R., and S. Garten. Die zeitliche Folge der Aktionstrome in Phrenicus und Zwerchfell bei der naturlichen Innervation. *Z. Biol. 58:* 420–450, 1912.
7. Gallagher, J.T., P.W. Kent, M. Passatore, R.J. Phipps, and P.S. Richardson. The composition of tracheal mucous and the nervous control of its secretion in cats. *Proc. R. Soc. Lond. [Biol.] 192:* 49–76, 1976.
8. Gootman P.M., and M.I. Cohen. Sympathetic rhythms in spinal cats. *J. Auton. Nerv. Syst. 3:* 397–387, 1981.
9. Kalia, M. Brain stem localization of vagal preganglionic neurons. *J. Auton. Nerv. Syst. 3:* 451–481, 1981.
10. Kerr, F.W.L. Preserved vagal visceromotor function following destruction of the dorsal motor nucleus. *J. Physiol. (Lond.) 202:* 755–769, 1969.
11. McAllen, R.M., and K.M. Spyer. Two types of vagal preganglionic motoneurons projecting to the heart and lungs. *J. Physiol. (Lond.) 282:* 353–364, 1978.

12. Melnichenko, L.V., and V.I. Skok. Natural electrical activity in mammalian parasympathetic ganglion cells. *Brain Res. 23:* 277–279, 1970.

13. Merrill, E.G. The lateral respiratory neurons of the medulla: their association with the nucleus ambiguus, nucleus retroambigualis, the spinal accessory nucleus and the spinal cord. *Brain Res. 24:* 11–28, 1970.

14. Mitchell, R.A., and D.A. Herbert. Synchronized high frequency synaptic potentials in medullary respiratory neurons. *Brain Res. 75:* 350–355, 1974.

15. Mitchell, R.A., D.A. Herbert, and D.G. Baker. Inspiratory rhythm in airway smooth muscle tone. *J. Appl. Physiol. 58:* 911–921, 1985.

16. Nadel, J.A. and J.G. Widdicombe. Effect of changes in blood gas tensions and carotid sinus pressure on tracheal volume and total lung resistance to airflow. *J. Physiol. (Lond.) 163:* 13–33, 1962.

17. Olsen, C.R., H.J.H. Colebatch, P.E. Mebel, J.A. Nadel, and N.C. Staub. Motor control of pulmonary airways studied by nerve stimulation. *J. Appl. Physiol. 20:* 202–208, 1965.

18. Otis, A.B. A perspective of respiratory mechanics. *J. Appl. Physiol. 54:* 1183–1187, 1983.

19. Richardson, C.A. Unique spectral peak in the phrenic nerve activity characterizes gasps in decerebrate cats. *J. Appl. Physiol. 60:* 782–790, 1986.

20. Richardson, C.A., D.A. Herbert, and R.A. Mitchell. Modulation of pulmonary stretch receptors and airway resistance by parasympathetic efferents. *J. Appl. Physiol. 57:* 1842–1849, 1983.

21. Richardson, C.A., and R.A. Mitchell. Power spectral analysis of inspiratory nerve activity in the decerebrate cat. *Brain Res. 233:* 317–336, 1982.

22. Skok, V.I. Spontaneous and reflex activities: general characteristics. In: *Autonomic and Enteric Ganglia,* ed. A.G. Karczamar, K. Koketsu, and S. Nishi. New York: Plenum, 1986, pp. 425–438.

23. Skoogh, B.-E., M.A. Grillo, and J.A. Nadel. Neutral red stains ganglia in the vagal motor pathway to ferret trachea without affecting ganglionic transmission. *J. Neurosci. Methods 8:* 33–39, 1983.

24. St. John, W.M., and K.V. Knuth. A characterization of the respiratory pattern of gasping. *J. Appl. Physiol. 50:* 984–993, 1981.

25. Tomori, Z., and J.G. Widdicombe. Muscular, bronchomotor and cardiovascular reflexes elicited by mechanical stimulation of the respiratory tract. *J. Physiol. (Lond.) 200:* 25–49, 1969.

26. Widdicombe, J.G. Action potentials in parasympathetic and sympathetic efferent fibers to the trachea and lungs of dogs and cats. *J. Physiol. (Lond.) 186:* 56–88, 1966.

27. Widdicombe, J.G., and J.A. Nadel. Reflex effects of lung inflation on tracheal volume. *J. Appl. Physiol. 18:* 681–686, 1963.

28. Widdicombe, J.G. and J.A. Nadel. Airway volume, airway resistance and work and force of breathing: theory. *J. Appl. Physiol. 18:* 863–868, 1963.

29. Wood, J.D., and C.J. Mayer. Intracellular study of electrical activity of Auerbach's plexus in guinea pig small intestine. *Pflügers Arch. 374:* 265–275, 1978.

30. Woolcock, A.J., P.T. Macklem, J.C. Hogg, and N.J. Wilson. Influence of autonomic nervous system on airway resistance and elastic recoil. *J. Appl. Physiol. 26:* 814–818, 1969.

31. Wyss, O.A.S. Synchronization of inspiratory motor activity as compared between phrenic and vagus nerves. *Yale J. Biol. Med. 28:* 471–480, 1956.

31

Modulation of Neuropeptide Effects by Enkephalinase

J. A. NADEL

Neural regulation of lungs and airways has classically been ascribed to the parasympathetic (muscarinic) and sympathetic (adrenergic) nervous systems. However, it has long been recognized that noncholinergic, nonadrenergic neural effects occur in such tissues as airway smooth muscle, and recently a new class of molecules, the neuropeptides, has been described. These peptides are believed to play important roles as transmitters or modulators in the nervous system.

Although many key discoveries in neuropeptide research have been made in other tissues including brain and intestine (40), skin (15), eye (29), dental pulp (31), and other tissues (32), the present discussion will focus on airways. However, the present observations are likely to be relevant to the modulation of all tissues where neuropeptide release and neuropeptide actions exist.

There is substantial evidence that neuropeptide-containing nerves play a role in airway responses: Substance P (SP) immunoreactivity occurs in sensory nerves of the lower respiratory tract in various species including man; the SP is located in the lining epithelium, within the smooth muscle layer, and near blood vessels (21). Radioimmunoassay shows that SP can be detected in airways in ferrets (5), and also humans (20). SP has potent effects on airway tissue; for example, it contracts smooth muscle (23), increases capillary permeability (24,26), and stimulates gland secretion (2,10,12). Because neuropeptide-containing neurons exist in airways, and because the neuropeptides have potent airway effects, various investigators have attempted to determine which airway effects are due to the neural release of SP or other tachykinins. Two pharmacological tools have been used for this purpose: Capsaicin, the homovanillylamide derivative of red pepper, has a neurotoxic effect on afferent C fibers, depletes the lungs of SP (20), and inhibits the increased vascular permeability that usually occurs following the application of various irritants in the airways (25) and in the nose (22). SP antagonists are the second tool used to examine tachykinin effects (33). Generally, these antagonists are not specific but antagonize effects of all tachykinins (3).

The combination of the presence of tachykinin-producing nerves in airways, the potent effects of these tachykinins on various target cells in the airways, and the inhibition of the effects of various locally applied irritants in airways by capsaicin and by SP antagonists provides powerful evidence that tachykinins are neurotransmitters or mediators of multiple airway functions. We reasoned that degradative mechanisms should be present and could play an important role in modulating effects of tachykinins, just as in the cholinergic and adrenergic systems. Although the metabolism of tachykinins has not been studied in airways, studies in the gut provide evidence for SP degradation. Thus, SP is rapidly degraded in the ileum, suggesting that endogenous proteinases or peptidases degrade SP (13). The responsible enzymes were not identified, but several enzymes are known to degrade tachykinins; these include kininase II (angiotensin converting enzyme; ref. 7), acetylcholinesterase (9), serine proteases (14), and enkephalinase (38). The purpose of the studies presented here was to determine whether endogenous peptidases or proteinase regulate the responses to tachykinins. I limit the discussion to the airways, including studies of secretion and smooth muscle contraction. Our strategy was based on the idea that if endogenous peptidases degrade tachykinins, then inhibitors of proteolytic enzymes might increase the responses.

METHODS

The methods are described in detail in the original publications and will be described only briefly.

1. *Mucus secretion* (see refs. 4,5 for methods). We mounted segments of ferret trachea in Ussing-type chambers, added 0.167 mCi $Na_2{}^{35}SO_4$ to the mucosal side, and sampled on the luminal side at 15-min intervals. Then, we dialyzed and counted the $^{35}SO_4$-labeled macromolecules as a reflection of secretion.

2. *Smooth muscle contraction* (see ref. 41 for methods). We removed transverse rings (8 mm long) from ferret tracheas, mounted them in glass chambers, attached them to strain gauges to measure isometric tension, and placed the rings between two rectangular platinum electrodes for electrical field stimulation (EFS).

RESULTS

Mucus Secretion

Substance P (SP) increased the flux of bound SO_4 in a concentration-dependent fashion (5). The C-terminal fragment SP_{6-11} caused a potent release of bound SO_4, but the N-terminal fragment SP_{1-9} did not. When we added enzyme inhibitors alone to the submucosal side of the chamber, none of them stimulated secretion significantly. However, when we added thiorphan or phosphoramidon (inhibitors

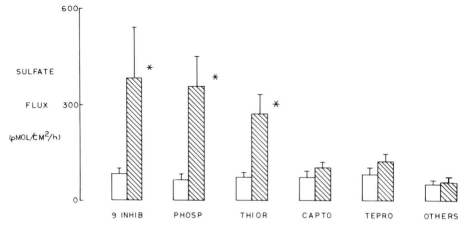

Fig. 31.1 Effects of proteinase inhibitors on the substance P (SP)-induced change in sulfate flux (mean ± SE) from tissues from ferret tracheas. Open bars: response to SP 10^{-6} M in control tissues from each group. Hatched bars: responses to SP 10^{-6} M in tissues pretreated with nine proteinase inhibitors (9 INHIB; 10 μg/ml), phosphoramidon (10^{-5} M; PHOSP), thiorphan (10^{-4} M; THIOR), captopril (10^{-4} M; CAPTO), teprotide (10^{-4} M; TEPRO), or other inhibitors (OTHERS) including leupeptin, aprotonin, bacitracin, bovine serum albumin (each inhibitor, 10 μg/ml), or bestatin (10^{-5} M). *$p<.05$. [Reproduced by permission from Borson et al., 1987 (5).]

Fig. 31.2 Effects of substance P (SP) and of leucine-thiorphan (leu-thiorphan) on active tension in isolated segments of ferret tracheal smooth muscle. Results are reported as mean ± SE of 12 ferrets (SP ≤ 10^{-6} M) or 6 ferrets (SP ≥ 5×10^{-6} M). Significant differences from corresponding control values are indicated by *$p < .05$; **$p < .01$; ***$p < .001$. Substance P alone (□) increased tension, but only at concentrations of 5×10^{-6} M and higher. Leucine-thiorophan (♦) caused a shift in the dose–response curve to lower concentrations of SP. [Reproduced by permission from Sekizawa et al., in press (1987).]

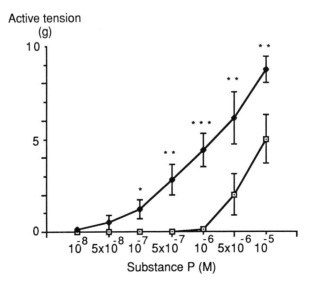

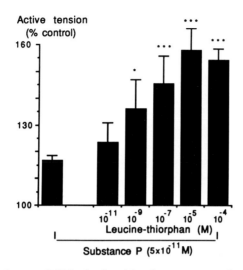

Fig. 31.3 Effects of substance P (SP) plus leu-thiorphan on contractions produced by electrical field stimulation (EFS; 5 Hz). Data are expressed as the percentage of control responses to EFS without added drugs and are reported as means $\pm$ SE ($n = 10$ at $\leq 10^{-5}$ M; $n = 4$ at 10^{-4} M). Significant differences from SP alone or SP plus leu-thiorphan are indicated by $*p < .05$; $***p < .001$. Substance P alone augmented contractile responses to EFS, and this augmentation was potentiated by leu-thiorphan. [Reproduced by permission from Sekizawa et al., in press (1987).]

of enkephalinase), SP-induced secretion was potentiated (Fig. 31.1). These effects of thiorphan were dose dependent. In contrast to inhibitors of enkephalinase, inhibitors of other enzymes did not potentiate SP-induced secretion (Fig. 31.1). Thus, captopril and teprotide (inhibitors of kininase II), leupeptin, aprotinin, bacitracin, BSA, and bestatin did not potentiate SP-induced secretions.

Smooth Muscle Contraction

SP alone caused an increased muscle tension, but only at concentrations of 5×10^{-6} M or greater (Fig. 31.2). Addition of leucine-thiorphan (leu-thiorphan, 10^{-5} M) had no significant effect on resting tension, but it shifted the dose–response relationship to SP to lower concentrations by approximately 1 log unit (Fig. 31.2). The N-terminal fragment, SP_{1-9} (10^{-5} M) had no significant effect on resting tension. The SP antagonist [D-Pro^2-D-Trp^{7,9}]-SP (10^{-6} M) reduced the contraction produced by SP (10^{-6} M) in the presence of leu-thiorphan (10^{-5} M) to 36% of control.

Concentrations of SP that had no effect on resting tension (e.g., as low as 5×10^{-11} M) augmented the responses to EFS (Fig. 31.3). Addition of increasing concentrations of leu-thiorphan in the presence of SP produced dose-related increases in the responses to EFS (Fig. 31.3). To determine whether endogenously released tachykinins normally modulate the bronchomotor response to EFS, we examined the response to EFS in the presence of leu-thiorphan. Leu-thiorphan potentiated

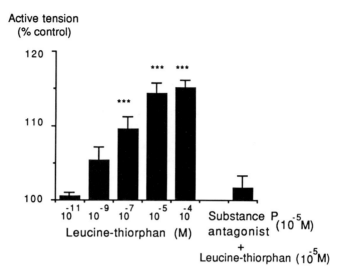

Fig. 31.4 Effects of leucine-thiorphan (leu-thiorphan) and the substance P antagonist, [D-Pro²-D-Trp⁷,⁹]-SP, on contractions produced by electrical field stimulation (EFS; 5 Hz). Data are expressed as the percentage of control responses to EFS without added drugs and are reported as mean $\pm$ SE ($n = 5$). Significant differences from control values are indicated by ***$p < .01$. Leu-thiorphan-augmented contractions produced by EFS, and this augmentation was inhibited by the SP antagonist (10^{-5} M). [Reproduced by permission from Sekizawa et al., in press (1987).]

the response to EFS in a concentration-dependent fashion (Fig. 31.4). The tachykinin antagonist [D-Pro²-D-Trp⁷,⁹]-SP (10^{-5} M) inhibited the increase in response to EFS induced by leu-thiorphan. In contrast to leu-thiorphan, captopril (10^{-5} M), bestatin (10^{-5} M), and leupeptin (10^{-5} M) did not affect SP-induced augmentation of responses to EFS.

DISCUSSION

The present studies provide evidence that enkephalinase (neutral metalloendopeptidase; EC 3.4.24.11) in airways degrades SP to inactive metabolites and thus provides an important mechanism for modulating the effects of this neuropeptide on secretion and on smooth muscle contraction. This conclusion is based on the finding that phosphoramidon, thiorphan, and leucine-thiorphan—inhibitors of enkephalinase (27,34)—potentiated the secretory and smooth muscle responses to exogenous SP. In contrast to enkephalinase, other peptidases possibly present in airways do not appear to be important in regulating SP-induced secretion or smooth muscle contraction. Thus, although kininase II is present in the lung and degrades SP (7), neither captopril nor teprotide potentiated SP-induced responses, suggesting that kininase II does not regulate the SP effects in airways. Furthermore, although serine proteinases from neutrophils, mast cells, and bacteria may act in airways, leupeptin and aprotinin (serine proteinase inhibitors) did not potentiate SP effects, we conclude that serine proteinases do not modulate SP effects under normal conditions. Finally, we conclude that aminopeptidases do not regulate SP effects in airways because the aminopeptidase inhibitor, bestatin (8), was without effect.

Enkephalinase cleaves SP between the 9 and 10 positions (38), generating the fragment, SP_{1-9}, which we have shown to be ineffective in stimulating secretion (5) or smooth muscle contraction (36) in airways. When such a cleavage of SP occurs in the airways, the amount of "active" SP reaching the target cell receptors will be less than the SP concentration in the medium. Preventing degradation of SP would therefore increase the concentration of SP at the tissue receptors, thereby increasing the response to SP.

Enkephalinase has been discovered in the kidney (17), but no physiological role for the enzyme in the kidney has been identified. The identical enzyme has been identified in brain (28), where it has been suggested to modulate the actions of opioids (35). Recently, enkephalinase has been shown to exist in other peripheral organs and cells including lungs (19). The exact distribution in specific lung cells is not yet known. However, enkephalinase concentrations are reported to be higher in airways than in alveoli (16). In airways, we have demonstrated enkephalinase activities in the vagus nerves, tracheal epithelium and smooth muscle, tracheal submucosal glands, and the area of submucosal glands (6).

The enzyme is found in particulate fractions of tissues (18,27,38) and is membrane-bound. Proximity of the enzyme to sites of release (e.g., sensory and motor nerves) and to sites of action (e.g., glands and smooth muscle) could promote rapid degradation of SP near effector cells in the airways, and thus be important in modulating peptide-induced responses.

In addition to SP, enkephalinase can hydrolyze a variety of neuropeptides, including the tachykinins (1,11,30,39), bradykinin, and other peptides, and is likely to modulate their effects in airways.

SUMMARY

Recently, a new class of small peptides, the tachykinins, have been described and shown to exist in sensory nerves. These peptides cause neutrophil chemotaxis, mast cell release, increased capillary permeability, airway smooth muscle contraction, and submucosal gland secretion. The present studies evidence that a membrane-bound endopeptidase, enkephalinase, by cleaving tachykinins at sites near their receptors in such tissues as airway submucosal glands, smooth muscle, and vagal motor nerves, modulates the effects of tachykinins. Perhaps it is appropriate to reconsider the nomenclature of this enzyme!

ACKNOWLEDGMENTS
This work has been supported by the NIH Program Project Grant HL+24136 and the Cystic Fibrosis Foundation Component I Development Program Award.

REFERENCES

1. Almenoff, J., and M. Orlowski. Membrane-bound kidney neutral metalloendopeptidase: interaction with synthetic substrates, natural peptides, and inhibitors. *Biochemistry* 22: 590–599, 1983.
2. Baker, A. P., L. M. Hillegass, D. A. Holden, and W. J. Smith. Effect of kallidin, substance P and other basic polypeptides on the production of respiratory macromolecules. *Am. Rev. Respir. Dis. 115:* 811–817, 1977.
3. Bjorkroth, U., S. Rosell, T.-C. Xu and K. Folkers. Pharmacological characterization of four related substance P antagonists. *Acta Physiol. Scand. 116:* 167–173, 1982.
4. Borson, D. B., M. Charlin, B. D. Gold, and J. A. Nadel. Neural regulation of $^{35}SO_4$-macromolecule secretion from tracheal glands of ferrets. *J. Appl. Physiol. 57:* 457–466, 1984.
5. Borson, D. B., R. Corrales, S. Varsano, M. Gold, N. Viro, G. Caughey, J. Ramachandran, and J. A. Nadel. Enkephalinase inhibitors potentiate substance P-induced secretion of $^{35}SO_4$-macromolecules from ferret trachea. *Exp. Lung Res. 12:* 21–36, 1987.
6. Borson, D. B., B. Malfroy, M. Gold, J. Ramachandran, and J. A. Nadel. Tachykinins inhibit enkephalinase activity from tracheas and lungs of ferrets. *Physiologist 29:* 174, 1986.
7. Cascieri, M. A., H. G. Bull, R. A. Mumford, A. A. Patchett, N. A. Thornberry, and T. Liang. Carboxy-terminal tripeptidyl hydrolysis of substance P by purified rabbit lung angiotensin-converting enzyme and the potentiation of substance P activity in vivo by captopril and MK-422. *Mol. Pharmacol. 25:* 287–293, 1984.
8. Chaillet, P., H. Marcais-Collado, J. Costentin, C.-C. Yi, S. De La Baume, and J. C. Schwartz. Inhibition of enkephalin metabolism by, and antinociceptive activity of, bestatin, an aminopeptidase inhibitor. *Eur. J. Pharmacol. 86:* 329–336, 1983.
9. Chubb, I. W., A. J. Hodgson, and G. H. White. Acetylcholinesterase hydrolyzes substance P. *Neuroscience 5:* 2065–2072, 1980.
10. Coles, S. J., K. R. Bhaskar, D. D. O'Sullivan, K. H. Neill, and L. M. Reid. Airway mucus: composition and regulation of its secretion by neuropeptides in vitro. In: *Mucus and Mucosa, Ciba Found. Symp.* Vol. 109, ed. J. Nugent and M. O'Connor. London: Pitman, 1984, pp. 40–60.
11. Gafford, J. T., R. A. Skidgel, E. G. Erdos, and L. B. Hersh. Human kidney "enkephalinase," a neutral metalloendopeptidase that cleaves active peptides. *Biochemistry 22:* 3265–3271, 1983.
12. Gashi, A. A., D. B. Borson, W. E. Finkbeiner, J. A. Nadel, and C. B. Basbaum. Neuropeptides degranulate serous cells of ferret tracheal glands. *Am. J. Physiol. 20:* C223–C229, 1986.
13. Growcott, J. W., and A. V. Tarpey. Effects of substance P-(1–9) nonapeptide amide on inactivation of substance P in vitro. *Eur. J. Pharmacol. 84:* 107–109, 1982.
14. Hanson, G. R., and W. Lovenberg, Elevation of substance P-like immunoreactivity in rat central nervous system by protease inhibitors. *J. Neurochem. 35:* 1370–1374, 1980.
15. Jancso, G., E. Kiraly, and A. Jancso-Gabor. Pharmacologically induced selective degeneration of chemosensitive primary sensory neurons. *Nature 270:* 741–743, 1977.
16. Johnson, A. R., J. Ashton, W. W. Schulz, and E. G. Erdos. Neutral metalloendopeptidase in human lung tissue and cultured cells. *Am. Rev. Respir. Dis. 132:* 564–568, 1985.
17. Kerr, M. A., and A. J. Kenny. The purification and specificity of a neutral endopeptidase from rabbit kidney brush border. *Biochem. J. 137:* 477–488, 1974.
18. Lee, C. M., B.E.B. Sandberg, M. R. Henley, and L. L. Iversen. Purification and characterization of a membrane-bound substance P degrading enzyme from human brain. *Eur. J. Biochem. 114:* 315–327, 1981.

19. Llorens, C., and J.-C. Schwartz. Enkephalinase activity in rat peripheral organs. *Eur. J. Pharmacol. 69:* 113–116, 1981.

20. Lundberg, J. M., E. Brodin, and A. Saria. Effects and distribution of vagal capsaicin-sensitive substance P neurons with special reference to the trachea and lungs. *Acta Physiol. Scand. 119:* 243–252, 1983.

21. Lundberg, J. M., T. Hokfelt, C.-R. Martling, A. Saria, and S. Cuello. Substance P-immunoreactive sensory nerves in the lower respiratory tract of various animals including man. *Cell Tissue Res. 235:* 251–261, 1984.

22. Lundberg, J. M., L. Lundblad, A. Saria, and A. Anggard. Inhibition of cigarette smoke-induced oedema in the nasal mucosa by capsaicin pretreatment and a substance P antagonist. *Naunyn Schmiedebergs Arch. Pharmacol. 326:* 181–185, 1984.

23. Lundberg, J. M., C. R. Martling, and A. Saria. Substance P and capsaicin-induced contraction of human bronchi. *Acta Physiol. Scand. 119:* 49–53, 1983.

24. Lundberg, J. M., and A. Saria. Capsaicin-sensitive vagal neurons involved in control of vascular permeability in rat trachea. *Acta Physiol. Scand. 115:* 521–523, 1982.

25. Lundberg, J. M., and A. Saria. Capsaicin-induced desensitization of airway mucosa to cigarette smoke, mechanical and chemical irritants. *Nature 302:* 251–253, 1983.

26. Lundberg, J. M., A. Saria, E. Brodin, S. Rosell, and K. Folkers. A substance P antagonist inhibits vagally induced increase in vascular permeability and bronchial smooth muscle contraction in the guinea pig. *Proc. Natl. Acad. Sci. U.S.A. 80:* 1120–1124, 1983.

27. Malfroy, B., and J.-C. Schwartz. Comparison of dipeptidyl carboxypeptidase and endopeptidase activities in the three enkephalin-hydrolysing metallopeptidases: "angiotensin-converting enzyme," thermolysin and "enkephalinase." *Biochem. Biophys. Res. Commun. 130:* 372–378, 1985.

28. Malfroy, B., J. P. Swerts, A. Guyon, B. P. Roques, and J.-C. Schwartz. High-affinity enkephalin-degrading peptidase in mouse brain and its enhanced activity following morphine. *Nature 276:* 523–526, 1978.

29. Mandahl, A., and A. Bell. Ocular responses to antidromic trigeminal stimulation, intracameral prostaglandin E_1 and E_2 capsaicin and substance P. *Acta Physiol. Scand. 112:* 331–338, 1981.

30. Matsas, R., A. J. Kenny, and A. J. Turner. The metabolism of neuropeptides: the hydrolysis of peptides, including enkephalins, tachykinins and their analogues, by endopeptidase-24.11. *Biochem. J. 223:* 433–440, 1984.

31. Olgart, L., B. Gazelius, E. Brodin, and G. Nilsson. Release of substance P-like immunoreactivity from the dental pulp. *Acta Physiol. Scand. 101:* 510–512, 1977.

32. Pernow, B. Substance P. *Pharmacol. Rev. 35:* 85–141, 1983.

33. Pernow, B. Role of tachykinins in neurogenic inflammation. *J. Immunol. 135:* 812S–815S, 1985.

34. Roques, B. P., C. M. Fournie-Zaluski, E. Soroca, J. M. Lecomte, B. Malfroy, C. Llorens, and J.-C. Schwartz. The enkephalinase inhibitor thiorphan shows antinociceptive activity in mice. *Nature 288:* 286–288, 1980.

35. Schwartz, J.-C., J. Costentin, and J.-M Lecomte. Pharmacology of enkephalinase inhibitors. *TIPS Rev. 6:* 472–476, 1985.

36. Sekizawa, K., J. Tamaoki, J. A. Nadel, and D. B. Borson. Enkephalinase inhibitor (leucine-thiorphan) potentiates mammalian tachykinin-induced contraction in ferret trachea. *Fed. Proc. 46:* 650, 1987.

37. Sekizawa, K., J. Tamaoki, J. A. Nadel, and D. B. Borson. Enkephalinase inhibitor potentiates substance P- and electrically induced contraction in ferret trachea. *J. Appl. Physiol. 63:* 1401–1405, 1987.

38. Skidgel, R. A., A. Engelbrecht, A. R. Johnson, and E. G. Erdos. Hydrolysis of substance P and neurotensin by converting enzyme and neutral endoproteinase. *Peptides 5:* 769–776, 1984.

39. Stephenson, S. L., and A. J. Kenny. Metabolism of neuropeptides. *Biochem. J. 241:* 237–247, 1987.

40. von Euler, U. S., and J. H. Gaddum. An unidentified depressor substance in certain tissue extracts. *J. Physiol. (Lond.) 72:* 74–87, 1931.

41. Walters, E. H., P. M. O'Byrne, L. M. Fabbri, P. D. Graf, M. J. Holtzman, and J. A. Nadel. Control of neurotransmission by prostaglandins in canine trachealis smooth muscle. *J. Appl. Physiol. 57:* 129–134, 1984.

Part VII
CENTRAL MECHANISMS AND EFFECTORS

Introduction

A. I. Pack

As outlined in the chapter by Anderson and Swanson, Comroe suggested that to solve problems related to respiratory control required good neurophysiologists and good control-system engineers. This section contains contributions from both. Anderson and Swanson extend Comroe's ideas and indicate that there is another potential signal that the system can use for feed-forward control. This signal is based on the comparison between changes in arterial P_{CO_2} that result from changes in ventilation. This allows computation of metabolic CO_2 production. Thus, there are now a number of possible signals that can produce feed-forward control, either singly or in combination.

The neural control system is currently being extensively examined by neurophysiologists, and major insights into the organization of the system are being obtained. Such investigators are studying each stage of the neural process—afferent relays (Spyer), the central pattern generator (Ballantyne et al.), and the phrenic motor nucleus (Berger et al.).

The central projections of chemoreceptor afferents in the nucleus tractus solitarius have been mapped with the major projection being to the commissural subnucleus. In the nucleus tractus solitarius, convergence occurs between different afferent systems and there is modification of the activity of afferent relay cells by inputs from other areas (Spyer). Thus, as in the dorsal horn of spinal cord, the nucleus tractus solitarius is not simply a relay station but rather there is both integration and control of the strength of afferent inputs.

These afferents are likely to project in a highly specific way to cells in the central pattern generator. The cellular basis for the known effect of different afferent stimuli on respiratory rhythmogenesis is now being investigated. The specific effect of chemoreceptor activation is described by Ballantyne et al. The importance of the recently recognized postinspiratory phase of the respiratory cycle is again indicated.

This exquisite neural organization also occurs at the level of the phrenic motor nucleus. Here the organization is not to subserve the function of rhythm generation but rather to control the pattern of activation of the diaphragm. Using elegant neuroanatomical and neurophysiological techniques, Berger et al. have revealed important neural mechanisms. Synchrony of activation of different motor units seems to be maximized by the anatomical arrangement of clusters of motoneurons into which axon collaterals project. During resting ventilation, slowly contracting diaphragmatic muscle fibers are used almost exclusively. Faster units are reserved for more forceful contractions. Recruitment order was found to be in accord with Henneman's "size principle." Such results have implications not only for respiration but also for motor control in general. Indeed, the diaphragm with its continued rhythmic contraction in anesthetized animals, offers a convenient tool to study the neurophysiology of a motor system.

Unfortunately, less is known about the neurobiology of development of this neural system. Evidence presented by Gootman et al. suggests that the development is somewhat staggered. In particular, the upper airway motoneuron pool seems to develop slower than that for activation of the respiratory pump muscles. The obvious inherent importance and insights that can be gained from such studies suggests that they will become more extensive in the future.

These chapters indicate that modern neurobiology, with its panoply of neurophysiological, neuroanatomical, and neuropharmacological techniques holds the promise, as Comroe surmised, of understanding the neural basis of that most essential of rhythmic behaviors—respiration.

32

The Central Integration of Sino-aortic Reflexes

K. M. SPYER

The nature of the central processes that are involved in mediating both arterial baroreceptor and chemoreceptor reflex inputs are as yet unresolved. However, it is clear that the nucleus tractus solitari (NTS) is the site of termination of the sinus (SN) and aortic (AN) nerves (9,17). It has also been shown that suprabulbar areas—for example, regions of the hypothalamus and the amygdala—that are implicated in cardiovascular control innervate the NTS (18). In this context, it is known that stimulation within the "defense" region of the hypothalamus (HDA) and central nucleus of the amygdala (CN) in the cat elicits a pattern of behavioral, somatic, and autonomic response that includes tachycardia and a maintained pressor response (8,19). These cardiovascular changes include a suppression of the baroreceptor reflex. Furthermore, the NTS receives a marked innervation from vagal afferent fibers with endings in the airways and lungs (2,9). As there are numerous indications in the literature that the performance of both cardiovascular and respiratory reflexes, and particularly sino-aortic reflexes, are modified by respiratory activity (1), it has often been implied that the NTS has a role in "respiratory-gating" of these reflexes. These observations imply that the NTS may be the site of integration of inputs that are of importance in cardiovascular and respiratory homeostasis.

With this background in mind, a series of neurophysiological investigations were undertaken in my laboratory over a number of years. These were designed to determine (a) the regional distribution of sino-aortic afferent inputs to the NTS, (b) the morphological and physiological characteristics of those NTS neurons that mediate these reflexes, (c) the action of inputs related to respiratory activity on their synaptic responses to AN and SN stimulation, and finally (d) whether stimulation within the perifornical region of the hypothalamus, which evokes the "defense" reaction, modifies transmission of the baroreceptor reflex at a site within the NTS.

METHODS

The studies to be reported were all conducted in anesthetized, paralyzed, and artificially ventilated cats (full experimental details are given in refs. 3–6,11,13,14,16). They involved studies on the central projections of individual carotid sinus (4) and aortic (5) baroreceptor afferents using an antidromic mapping technique with the activity of the afferent being recorded extracellularly by microelectrodes positioned in the petrosal and nodose ganglia, respectively. In the second series, we sought to identify with intracellular recording techniques those nonrespiratory neurons of the NTS whose activity is modified by SN and AN stimulation (3). Furthermore, we selectively stimulated the baroreceptors of the carotid sinus by advancing a balloon-tipped catheter through the external carotid artery into the carotid sinus. Chemoreceptor afferents were selectively activated by injection of CO_2-saturated physiological saline retrogradely through the lingual artery into the arterial supply of the carotid body.

Recordings were made from NTS neurons by using electrodes filled with either 4 M KCl, 0.2 M K acetate, or 4% horseradish peroxidase (HRP) in Tris buffer. We analyzed the influence of (a) central respiratory activity, monitored by recording phrenic nerve discharge, and (b) lung inflation on the postsynaptic potentials (PSPs) evoked by SN and AN stimulation. These two influences could be examined separately in these experiments as the animals were ventilated at a rate dissociated from central respiratory discharge and all animals were given a bilateral pneumothorax. In a proportion of neurons characterized on the basis of responses to SN, AN, and baroreceptor inputs, the effects of HDA stimulation have been assessed. Sites in the hypothalamus were selected by stimulation (70 Hz, 1-ms pulses at 150 μA) which evoked the cardiovascular components of the defense reactions including a suppression of the reflex responses to SN stimulation. Once identified we examined the effects of stimulation (2–15 pulses at 500 Hz, 1 ms, 150 μA) on the activity of NTS neurons. Furthermore, this stimulus was used as a conditioning stimulus to test stimuli delivered to the SN (and AN) to determine its influence on the PSPs evoked from these nerves. A selection of these neurons were labeled intracellularly with HRP. The histological and histochemical procedures used to reveal these cells were as described in ref. 12.

RESULTS

A series of extracellular recording studies dating back to the early 1970s led to the current investigations. In these, we established that baroreceptor activation led to excitatory responses in a significant number of NTS neurons, particularly in those located rostral to the obex and in lateral, ventrolateral, and dorsal aspects of the nucleus (10). Subsequently, we showed that respiratory neurons of the NTS, both Rα and Rβ inspiratory neurons, were activated only by the arterial chemoreceptors if the stimulus was timed to occur during inspiration (11). The equivalent stimulus delivered in expiration failed to excite them, but it tended to increase the expiratory

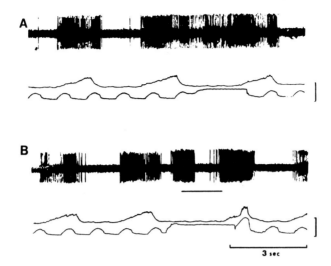

Fig. 32.1 (**A**) The control response of this neuron to lung inflation without chemoreceptor stimulation. (**B**) Effects of chemoreceptor stimulation on an Rβ unit during maintained expiratory firing induced by lung inflation. [Modified by permission from Lipski et al., 1977 (11).]

pause. Indeed, as illustrated in Fig. 32.1, when the Rβ inspiratory neuron was made to discharge tonically by a maintained lung inflation, chemoreceptor stimulation inhibited the cell. Similar effects were evoked in both Rα and Rβ inspiratory neurons when these were made to fire tonically by the microiontophoresis of excitant amino acids. This led us to believe that the major excitatory influences of the arterial chemoreceptors must be mediated by a group of nonrespiratory neurons of the NTS, and thus we were impelled to make a detailed analysis of the pattern of projection of individual baroreceptor and chemoreceptor afferents.

Central Projections of Baroreceptors and Chemoreceptors

Baroreceptors
In the cat we showed that aortic baroreceptor afferents with myelinated axons (conduction velocity, 12.5–22.0 m/s) innervate the ipsilateral NTS at levels rostral to the obex (5). This evidence was based on observations made using an antidromic mapping technique and an analysis of the depth-threshold contours derived from serial stimulating electrode tracks through the medulla. With regard to carotid sinus baroreceptors, the pattern of projection of both those with myelinated or unmyelinated axons were mapped by use of equivalent techniques (4). All gave ipsilateral projections, and for *all* baroreceptor afferents it appears that the densest innervation is of the dorsolateral and dorsomedial regions of the NTS at levels rostral to the obex, with a marked innervation of lateral and to a lesser extent, ventrolateral areas.

Chemoreceptor Afferents

To date, we have mapped the central projections of 13 carotid body chemoreceptor afferents, all of which were discharging under eupneic conditions. To our surprise, all were activated with latencies indicating that they relayed to the CNS with unmyelinated axons (4). Their patterns of termination derived by antidromic activation were markedly different from those of the arterial baroreceptors (see Fig. 32.2). They innervated the medial subnucleus, and particularly its dorsomedial aspect, at levels rostral to the obex (see Fig. 32.2A). The major projection was, however, to the commissural nucleus (Fig. 32.2A,B). Some input to the lateral subnucleus was also observed, but no evidence of a projection to the ventrolateral region of the nucleus was found.

Postsynaptic Responses

Baroreceptor Inputs

In an ongoing intracellular recording study, we have identified NTS neurons in which electrical stimulation of the SN and AN evoke PSPs (3,13,14,20), and a proportion of these have been shown to receive input from the baroreceptors of the carotid sinus.

The PSPs evoked on SN stimulation fell into three distinct categories: an excitatory PSP (EPSP), an excitatory PSP–inhibitory PSP (EPSP–IPSP) sequence, and an IPSP. The latency, rise time, and amplitudes of the PSPs indicated that excitatory responses included both mono and disynaptic inputs whereas the inhibitory responses had characteristics of a dispersed disynaptic action. In a large number of those neurons showing EPSPs or EPSP–IPSP sequences in response to SN stimulation, a convergent excitatory input from the AN, among other inputs, was revealed. A number of these neurons were also excited on inflation of a balloon-tipped catheter within the ipsilateral carotid sinus (13,20). In the case of those neurons receiving an IPSP on SN stimulation, several were inhibited by baroreceptor stimulation. On the basis of a limited number of neurons that have been labeled intracellularly with HRP (15), it appears that the majority of these neurons were localized within the dorsolateral, lateral, and ventrolateral regions of the NTS 0.5–2.0 mm rostral to the obex.

We investigated whether the PSPs evoked on SN stimulation were in any way modified by lung inflation or the timing of the stimulus in the central respiratory cycle (14). No changes in the latency, rise time, or amplitude of these postsynaptic responses were observed. Together with our earlier description of an absence of presynaptic depolarizations in response to these respiratory events in baroreceptor afferents (16, Fig. 32.3), this makes it unlikely that the respiratory "gating" of the baroreceptor reflex is occurring at this level of the NTS.

Chemoreceptor Inputs

Several of the neurons tested for a baroreceptor input were unaffected although they received SN (and AN) inputs; thus it is possible that this population of neurons studied included some neurons with chemoreceptor inputs. Consequently, in an as yet unpublished study, we made recordings from NTS neurons and observed their responses to SN stimulation and activation of the chemoreceptors of the

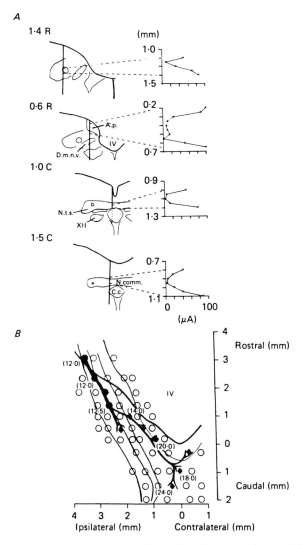

Fig. 32.2 Nonmyelinated chemoreceptor afferent (conduction velocity, 1.2 m/s). **(A)** Penetrations and depth-threshold profiles; **(B)** Schematic map of full projections. Scales indicate distances (in mm): rostral (R), caudal (C), and lateral to the obex (o). Sites of stimulating electrode penetrations are indicated, classed according to the type of depth-threshold profile obtained; that is, point (●), field (◆), or no response (○). Numbers in parentheses indicate the antidromic latency. A possible course of the main axon is shown by the bold line connecting point types, and regions of branching or termination by the fine lines. Abbreviations: area postrema (A. p.), dorsal motor nucleus of vagus (D.m.n.v.), nucleus commissuralis (N. Comm.), nucleus tractus solitarii (N.t.s.), central canal (C. c.), hypoglossal nucleus (XII), and fourth ventricle (IV). [Reproduced by permission from Donoghue et al., 1984 (3).]

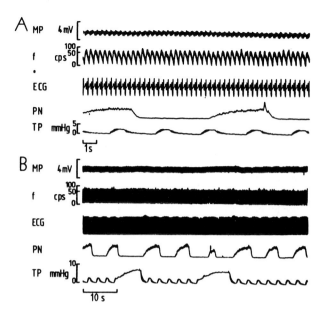

Fig. 32.3 Membrane potential of two aortic baroreceptor fibers recorded within the NTS in the cat. The membrane potential (MP) of the afferent fibers shown in **A** and **B** did not show any fluctuation in synchrony with the central respiratory activity, as indicated by the phrenic nerve activity (PN), or with artificial lung inflation or during static inflation test. ECG, electrocardiogram; f, discharge frequency of the baroreceptor; TP, tracheal pressure. [Reproduced by permission from Richter et al., 1986 (16).]

carotid body (P. Izzo, D. W. Richter, and K. M. Spyer, unpublished observations). Such neurons were also labeled by intracellular injection of HRP. These neurons were located at or caudal to the obex, with their cell bodies just dorsal and lateral to the NTS. They had dendrites extending laterally and also medially into the commissural nucleus where we showed chemoreceptor afferents to project (Fig. 32.2 and see above). Experiments are in progress to determine their physiological and morphological characteristics in more detail.

"Defense" Area Input to NTS

Stimulating with brief trains of pulses in the perifornical region of the hypothalamus evoked a long-lasting IPSP (82–195 ms) in a number of NTS neurons (13). This was a Cl^--dependent IPSP since it could be reversed to a wave of depolarization by the injection of Cl^- or DC hyperpolarizing currents. These IPSPs were observed in NTS neurons which received EPSPs on SN stimulation (and also in those receiving an EPSP–IPSP sequence). This action of the hypothalamic defense area was able to maintain SN effects at subthreshold levels through the evoked hyperpolarization and reduced membrane input resistance. This mechanism would appear to account, at least in part, for the suppression of the baroreflex during the defense reaction. Conversely, several NTS neuron receiving IPSPs on SN stimulation received EPSPs on HDA stimulation. Clearly, interactions between these pools of neurons with distinctive patterns of response localized within the NTS are going to play an important role in the integration of baroreceptor inputs.

DISCUSSION

The data reviewed in this report show that the intermediate region of the NTS receives a patterned innervation from the arterial baroreceptors and chemoreceptors. The description of afferent projection derived from the antidromic mapping studies (9) has been substantiated in terms of the distribution of NTS interneurons seen to be affected by these reflex inputs. Chemoreceptor-sensitive neurons have been located at the level of, and caudal to, the obex, whereas baroreceptor-sensitive neurons appear concentrated at levels rostral to the obex.

With respect to neurons receiving a baroreceptor input, evidence has been obtained that many receive convergent inputs from a range of other afferents; for example, vagal afferents and afferents in the superior laryngeal nerve, and, as demonstrated here, many are also affected by descending inputs activated by stimulation in the hypothalamus. Clearly they have the potential to subserve an integrative role in cardiovascular control. This does not, however, extend to an interaction with inputs related to respiration. Given that lung inflation appears to exert profound influences on sino-aortic reflexes in several species (1), and since slowly adapting pulmonary afferents relay to the NTS (6), this is perhaps surprising. However, in the case of the baroreceptor–vagal reflex in the anesthetized cat, Gilbey et al. (7) were unable to observe any influence of lung inflation although cardiac vagal motoneurons were inhibited in phase with inspiratory activity. The effects of rapid and large inflations have not been tested, but it is notable that NTS neurons excited by SN and baroreceptor inputs were never seen to be inhibited on vagal nerve stimulation at intensities 2.0–5.0 times the threshold for inhibiting inspiratory discharge. This would seem to suggest that any influence of lung inflation on that particular component of the baroreceptor–vagal reflex must be mediated at an as yet undisclosed synapse(s) between the NTS and vagal cardio-inhibitory neurons.

The role of the NTS neurons receiving an excitatory chemoreceptor input remains to be examined. The restricted distribution of these neurons may well reflect the limited sample so far investigated. It would, however, seem essential to determine the connections of these neurons, if any, with the classical pools of premotor respiratory neurons of the medulla as it is likely that they will be found to play an important role in the chemoreceptor control of respiration.

CONCLUSIONS

These studies have revealed that the NTS is an essential site in the integration of sino-aortic reflexes. The behavioral modifications of these reflexes appear to be accomplished, at least in part, at this level. A combination of physiological and morphological methods seems essential to resolve the integrative functions of the NTS.

ACKNOWLEDGMENTS

I wish to acknowledge the contributions of many of my collaborators in furthering these studies. The financial support of the British Heart Foundation and Medical Research Council is gratefully acknowledged.

REFERENCES

1. Daly, M. de Burgh. Interactions between respiration and circulation. In: *Handbook of Physiology,* Sec. 3: *The Respiratory System,* Vol. 2: *Control of Breathing,* ed. N. S. Cherniack and J. G. Widdicombe. Bethesda, MD: Am. Physiol. Soc., 1985 pp. 529–594.

2. Davies, R. O. and L. Kubin. Projection of pulmonary rapidly adapting receptors to the medulla of the cat: an antidromic mapping study. *J. Physiol. (Lond.) 373:* 63–86, 1986.

3. Donoghue, S., R. B. Felder, M. P. Gilbey, D. Jordan, and K. M. Spyer. Post-synaptic activity evoked in the nucleus tractus solitarius by carotid sinus and aortic nerve afferents in the cat. *J. Physiol. (Lond.) 360:* 261–273, 1985.

4. Donoghue, S., R. B. Felder, D. Jordan, and K. M. Spyer. The central projections of carotid baroreceptors and chemoreceptors in the cat: a neurophysiologcal study. *J. Physiol. (Lond.) 347:* 397–410, 1984.

5. Donoghue, S., M. Garcia, D. Jordan, and K. M. Spyer. Identification and brain-stem projections of aortic baroreceptor afferent neurones in nodose ganglia of cats and rabbits. *J. Physiol. (Lond.) 322:* 337–352, 1982.

6. Donoghue, S., M. Garcia, D. Jordan, and K. M. Spyer. The brain-stem projections of pulmonary stretch afferent neurones in cats and rabbits. *J. Physiol. (Lond.) 322:* 353–363, 1982.

7. Gilbey, M. P., D. Jordan, D. W. Richter, and K. M. Spyer. Synaptic mechanisms involved in the inspiratory modulation of vagal cardio-inhibitory neurones in the cat. *J. Physiol. (Lond.) 356:* 65–78, 1984.

8. Hilton, S. The central nervous contribution to vasomotor tone. In: *Central and Peripheral Mechanisms of Cardiovascular Regulation,* ed. A. Magro, W. Osswald, D. Reis, and P. Vanhoutte. New York: Plenum, 1986, pp. 465–486.

9. Jordan, D., and K. M. Spyer. Brainstem integration of cardiovascular and pulmonary afferent activity. *Prog. Brain Res. 67:* 295–314, 1986.

10. Lipski, J., R. M. McAllen, and K. M. Spyer. The sinus nerve and baroreceptor input to the medulla of the cat. *J. Physiol. (Lond.) 251:* 61–78, 1975.

11. Lipski, J., R. M. McAllen, and K. M. Spyer. The carotid chemoreceptor input to the respiratory neurones of the nucleus of the tractus solitarius. *J. Physiol. (Lond.) 269:* 797–810, 1977.

12. Mesulum, M.-M. Tracing neural connections with horseradish peroxidase. *Methods in the Neurosciences.* New York: John Wiley, 1982.

13. Mifflin, S. W., K. M. Spyer, and D. J. Withington-Wray. Hypothalmic inhibition of baroreceptor inputs in the nucleus of the tractus solitarius of the cat. *J. Physiol. (Lond.) 373:* 58P, 1986.

14. Mifflin, S. W., K. M. Spyer, and D. J. Withington-Wray. Lack of respiratory modulation of baroreceptor inputs in the nucleus of the tractus solitarius of the cat. *J. Physiol. (Lond.) 376:* 33P, 1986.

15. Mifflin, S. W., K. M. Spyer, and D. J. Withington-Wray. Intracellular labelling of neurones receiving carotid sinus nerve inputs in the cat. *J. Physiol. (Lond.) 387:* 60P, 1987.

16. Richter, D. W., D. Jordan, D. Ballantyne, M. Meesmann, and K. M. Spyer. Presynaptic depolarization in myelinated vagal afferent fibres terminating in the nucleus of the tractus solitarius in the cat. *Pflügers Arch. 406:* 12–19, 1986.

17. Spyer, K. M. Neural organisation and control of the baroreceptor reflex. *Rev. Physiol. Biochem. Pharmacol. 88:* 23–124, 1981.

18. Spyer, K. M. Central nervous integration of cardiovascular control. *J. Exp. Biol. 100:* 109–128, 1982.

19. Spyer, K. M. Central control of the cardiovascular system. In: *Recent Advances in Physiology,* Vol. 10, ed. P. F. Baker. Edinburgh: Churchill Livingstone, 1984, pp. 163–200.

20. Spyer, K. M., S. W. Mifflin, and D. J. Withington-Wray. Diencephalic control of the baroreceptor reflex at the level of the nucleus of the tractus solitarius. In: *Organisation of the Autonomic Nervous System: Central and Peripheral Mechanisms,* ed. F. R. Calaresu, J. Ciriello, and C. Polosa. New York: Alan R. Liss, 1987, pp. 307–314.

33

How Arterial Chemoreceptor Activity Influences the Respiratory Rhythm

D. BALLANTYNE, E. E. LAWSON, P. M. LALLEY,
AND D. W. RICHTER

Changes in the intensity or timing of the respiratory pattern produced by activation of peripheral chemosensory afferents may be presumed to reflect both the way the afferents are connected to respiratory neurons within the brainstem and the way these neurons are themselves connected. There is, at present, only limited evidence that any (conventionally defined) medullary respiratory neurons form part of the pool of second-order chemosensory neurons (see refs. 8,13). However, there is abundant evidence for a nongated chemosensory activation of interneurons in the general region of termination of sinus nerve afferents (reviewed by Spyer, Chap. 32, this volume), which includes a region of high concentration of medullary respiratory neurons. These interneurons may constitute the immediate source of the chemosensory signal for the medullary respiratory network. If this is the case, their response and transmission characteristics are evidently sufficiently fast, on the respiratory time scale, to preserve phase information supplied by their input (3,4) since the response of the respiratory network to a brief chemosensory stimulus depends on when in the cycle the stimulus is given (5,6,9–12,15–18). This naturally places much of the emphasis of chemosensory processing on the internal connectivity of the network and the way this connectivity controls the synaptic rhythm of its various components.

An important feature that has emerged from analysis of the synaptic activity of various selected categories of medullary respiratory neurons is the provision which the network makes for the insertion of delays into the rhythm (20–22). These delays take the form of inhibitory inputs to respiratory neurons during the "active" phase of their rhythm—for example, in (some) inspiratory neurons during the early stage of inspiration (1), and in (some) expiratory neurons during the early stage of expiration (postinspiratory inhibition) (2). The manner in which these inhibitory inputs respond to chemoreceptor stimulation is unknown. In the following account, we describe one aspect of the control of caudal medullary expiratory neurons which depends on the interaction between chemoreceptor-mediated excitation and network-controlled postinspiratory inhibition.

METHODS

The experiments were performed on 17 cats anesthetized with sodium pentobarbitone (initial dose, 35–40 mg/kg, i.p.), paralyzed with gallamine triethiodide, and artifically ventilated with oxygen-enriched air. End-tidal CO_2 was maintained at 3–5%. A bilateral pneumothorax was established to minimize respiratory movements of the brainstem, and an end-expiratory pressure of 1–3 cmH_2O was maintained. Blood pressure was continuously monitored via a femoral artery cannula.

The general surgical preparation, arrangements for nerve stimulation and recording, and exposure of the medulla have been described in detail elsewhere (2). The animals were bilaterally vagotomized and the respiratory rhythm was monitored by recording the phrenic nerve activity. Bulbospinal expiratory neurons were identified by their antidromic response to intraspinal stimulation at segments C2–3. To stimulate carotid body chemoreceptors, a catheter was placed in the lingual artery and small volumes (0.03–0.3 ml) of solution—1 M $NaHCO_3$ or Ringer's—equilibrated with 95% O_2–5% CO_2 or 100% CO_2 were injected by hand; the time course of injection was monitored from the time course of the pressure change within the catheter. The sinus nerves on one or both sides were usually prepared for stimulation or recording. Sympathetic activity (not shown here) was recorded in the renal nerve to control for the absence of short latency (0.2–0.3 s), baroreceptor-mediated inhibition following lingual artery injection, and confirmation that the injection activated the chemoreceptors. Stimulation parameters for electrical stimulation of the sinus nerve were selected on the basis of the phrenic and sympathetic nerve responses; since such stimulation must almost invariably activate baroreceptor as well as chemoreceptor afferents, these data are included here only when they were wholly consistent with the responses produced by chemical stimulation.

Stable intracellular recordings (micropipettes filled with 3 M KCl or 2 M K-acetate) were obtained from 19 expiratory neurons (12 bulbospinal) located in the caudal region of the ventral group of medullary respiratory neurons (2).

RESULTS

Modification of Inspiratory IPSP Activity in Response to Chemoreceptor Stimulation

Figure 33.1 shows recordings from an expiratory neuron, together with phrenic nerve activity, and illustrates two aspects of the synaptic control exerted by chemoreceptor inputs over expiratory activity. Under control conditions, the membrane potential rhythm of this neuron lay well within the range of variation nor-

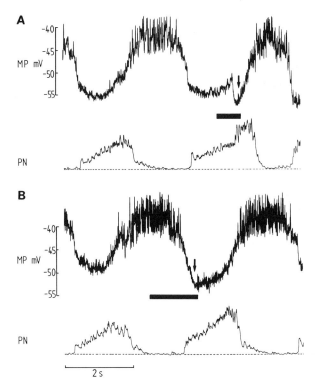

Fig. 33.1 Integrated phrenic nerve (PN) activity and membrane potential (MP) pattern, recorded from an expiratory neuron in response to lingual artery injections (0.2 ml) (horizontal bars) during inspiratory discharge **(A)**, and at the expiratory-to-inspiratory transition **(B)**. There was an intensification of IPSP activity (arrows) after chemoreceptor stimulation.

mally encountered in intracellular sampling from this population; there was a well-developed hyperpolarization, due to inhibitory postsynaptic potential (IPSP) activity (2,19), during the phrenic inspiratory discharge and depolarization during the intervening expiratory interval. It is, however, worth noting that in this neuron the rapid phase of membrane hyperpolarization at the transition to inspiration was preceded by a slower hyperpolarization and, at the average membrane potential prevailing in this record (see below), expiratory discharge ceased up to 200 ms before the onset of inspiration (see also ref. 7).

In the test illustrated in Fig. 33.1A, the injection was delivered toward the end of the phrenic inspiratory ramp discharge. The first detectable response to the injection was an abrupt increase in the amplitude of discharge in the phrenic nerve and a corresponding rapid and large (ca. 7 mV) hyperpolarizing wave (arrow) in the neuron, these two effects occurring about 0.6 s after the onset of injection. This intensified wave of IPSPs (readily reversed by intracellular chloride injection) was followed by a more rapid pattern of depolarization and a brief and more intense phase of expiratory discharge than was seen in the prestimulus control; the corresponding expiratory interval was shortened and there was a rapid decline in the intensity of the phrenic discharge.

Figure 33.1B shows the same neuron but at an earlier stage in the recording when there was a slightly lower average membrane potential (see calibration) so that the average frequency of discharge during the expiratory burst was higher; the underlying pattern of membrane potential changes was the same. In this test, the injection was delivered during the second half of the expiratory interval and extended into the early stage of inspiration. Neither in this, nor in other similar tests on this neuron, were we able to detect an obvious change in the shape of the membrane potential trajectory during expiration coincident with the injection, but the rapid pattern of hyperpolarization normally accompanying the onset of phrenic discharge (see control cycles in A and B) was replaced by a more gradual and larger amplitude hyperpolarization (arrow). The accompanying decline in the intensity of inspiratory inhibition was manifested by a small increase in the rate of rise and a larger peak amplitude of the phrenic discharge. The subsequent pattern of expiratory depolarization followed a path essentially similar to that prior to stimulation, with no change in discharge threshold.

Lengthening of the Postinspiratory Delay in Response to Chemoreceptor Stimulation

Figure 33.2 shows recordings from two late expiratory neurons that illustrate the sensitivity of the membrane potential trajectory during the expiratory phase to a brief stimulus delivered during the immediately preceding inspiration. In Fig. 33.2A, the injection was delivered in the second half of inspiration, resulting in a "sharpening" of the late inspiratory discharge in the phrenic nerve. This effect was insufficient to change the pattern of arrival of inspiratory IPSPs compared with the prestimulus control. There was, however, a quite distinct change in the subsequent pattern of events, the inspiratory-to-expiratory transition in the membrane potential record being followed by a short (ca. 300-ms) postinspiratory plateau component to the expiratory potential trajectory and a correspondingly delayed approach to discharge threshold (arrow) (see also ref. 17). The length of the expiratory interval was increased by about 25% compared with the preceding control interval.

Because of the quite variable time course of increased sinus nerve activity following injections into the lingual artery (not shown here), it was important to determine whether the lengthened time course of expiration was due to a persistent high level of chemoafferent activity or to events within the central neuronal network triggered by the timing of the stimulus. Although we cannot exclude the former, it was possible to produce a similar effect on the shape and time course of the expiratory trajectory by brief electrical stimulation of the sinus nerve. In Fig. 33.2B, stimulation (30 Hz; 0.4 s) was delivered shortly after the onset of inspiratory discharge in the phrenic nerve. This resulted in a rapid growth in the amplitude of discharge, the total duration of which was reduced by about 25% compared with the preceding inspiration (see also ref. 10). This rapid intensification of inspiratory discharge was accompanied by a large increase in the amplitude of inspiratory hyperpolarization and, at the transition to expiration, by a subsequent postinspiratory plateau (arrow) in the expiratory trajectory. As with the lingual artery injection in Fig. 33.2A, the onset of the expiratory burst was delayed and the concurrent expiratory interval increased in length. The conclusions drawn from these observations are that activation of chemoreceptor afferents (only presumed in the case

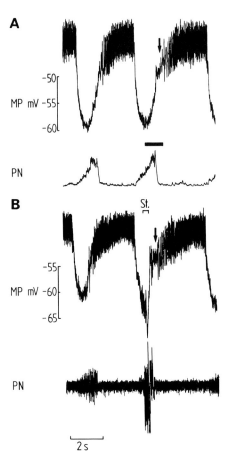

Fig. 33.2 Membrane potential (MP) patterns recorded from two expiratory bulbospinal neurons in response to **(A)** lingual artery injection (0.15 ml), and **(B)** carotid sinus nerve stimulation (St., 2 V; 0.05 ms; 30 Hz; 0.4 s) There was a delayed onset to expiratory discharge after chemoreceptor stimulation. PN, phrenic nerve activity (integrated in A; original in B). The arrows point to the postinspiratory delays inserted into the expiratory membrane potential trajectories.

of electrical stimulation) shortly before the inspiratory-to-expiratory transition inserts a postinspiratory delay into the rhythm and that the occurrence of this delay is not dependent on *concurrent* activity in chemoreceptor afferents.

Synaptic Excitation of Expiratory Bulbospinal Neurons in Response to Chemoreceptor Stimulation

The intensification or introduction of a postinspiratory delay into the rhythm appeared to be largely dependent on events occurring in late inspiration and was thus associated mostly with a late inspiratory stimulus. Stimuli delivered at other times could intensify or advance the onset of the expiratory burst (see also ref. 14). This feature is illustrated in Fig. 33.3A, where the injection was delivered toward the end of the expiratory interval, and, in a different neuron, in Fig. 33.3B, where the injection was made early in inspiration. The most immediate effect in both cases was a moderate increase in the amplitude of the phrenic discharge. The most significant feature, however, was the replacement of the prevailing postinspiratory pattern of depolarization by a rapid onset and large wave of depolarization upon which was superimposed an intense discharge in the neurons. This effect was not dependent on the shape or amplitude of the immediately preceding inspiratory wave of membrane hyperpolarization, but the effect was more intense in A than in B, possibly because of the intensification of inspiratory inhibition in the former. We assume that this effect was due to prolonged chemoafferent activity since equivalently timed electrical stimulation (Fig. 33.4D, below) did not cause a similar effect.

Figure 33.4 shows the response of a bulbospinal neuron to electrical stimulation of the sinus nerve at various times in the respiratory cycle. This particular neuron was initially tested for its responses to brief chemical stimulation of carotid body chemoreceptors; these responses were qualitatively similar to those illustrated in Fig. 33.2A, in that there was an intensification of the postinspiratory delay following a late inspiratory stimulus. The main objective of this experiment was to determine whether the excitatory input, inferred from the response shown in Fig.

Fig. 33.3 Advanced onset to expiratory discharge following chemoreceptor stimulation. Membrane potential (MP) pattern in two expiratory bulbospinal neurons and corresponding activity recorded from the phrenic nerve (PN) in response to lingual artery injection (0.1 ml) toward the end of the expiratory interval (horizontal bar) **(A)**, and during the early stage of inspiration **(B)**.

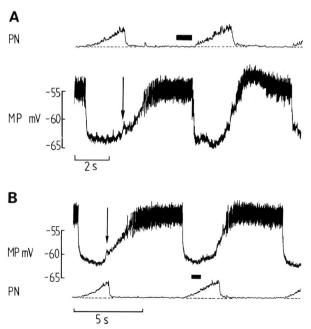

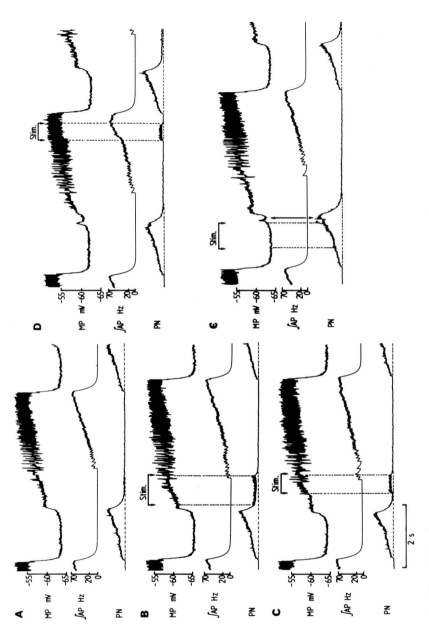

Fig. 33.4 Excitatory effect of electrical stimulation of the contralateral carotid sinus nerve on the membrane potential (MP) pattern and discharge frequency (AP) of an expiratory bulbospinal neuron. PN, integrated phrenic nerve activity. (**A**) Control cycle (no stimulation). (**B–E**) Stimulation (Stim., 30 Hz) delivered at various points in the respiratory cycle (cf. Figs. 33.4D and 33.1A). The arrow in E signifies intensified IPSP activity.

33.3 (see also refs. 14,18), has "access" to the neuron during the course of the postinspiratory delay.

Figure 33.4A shows the normal cycle of the membrane potential pattern, which provided a good control on which to test for postinspiratory "gating" of the sinus nerve input because there was a well-developed postinspiratory plateau and a delayed expiratory burst. We assume (without proof in this case, see ref. 2) that this delay involved postinspiratory IPSP activity. In Fig. 33.4B and C, the sinus nerve was stimulated at the same intensity and frequency but for different lengths of time during the course of the postinspiratory delay. In both tests, the effect of the stimulus was to increase the rate at which threshold for expiratory discharge was approached so that the onset of the expiratory burst was advanced. This effect was fairly gradual in B but quite abrupt in C. This observation indicates that the sinus nerve excitatory input (presumed chemosensory) has "access" to the neuron during the phase of postinspiratory inhibition. Note that in B, immediately after cessation of stimulation there was a slight hyperpolarizing shift in membrane potential, suggesting that the excitatory input was largely confined to the duration of stimulation. The effect of this hyperpolarization was to generate a distinct plateaulike component to expiratory discharge so that the ramp component (stage II; see refs. 20–22) was delayed relative to the control in A. In both tests, the lengths of the expiratory interval and the concurrent expiratory burst were increased compared with control.

Figure 33.4D shows that a stimulus sequence delivered toward the end of the expiratory interval evoked a large wave of depolarization and a much increased rate of rise of discharge frequency which did not, however, exceed the maximum frequency attained under control conditions (in this particular test it was slightly less). Figure 33.4E shows that a stimulus train confined to the ramp phase of phrenic discharge increased the amplitude of this discharge. About 40 ms following stimulation, there was a renewed wave of IPSP activity, generating a large hyperpolarizing transient and an accompanying burst of activity in the phrenic nerve (see also record D in Fig. 33.4). The subsequent pattern of development of the expiratory potential trajectory resembled that seen under control conditions (Fig. 33.4A).

DISCUSSION

In this study we have shown that appropriately timed activation of carotid body chemoreceptors causes an intensification of inspiratory IPSP activity in expiratory neurons, resulting in several different effects on the form of the expiratory phase membrane potential trajectory. The questions of interest, then, concern the mechanisms underlying these effects and their functional significance.

It has long been recognized that the form of the respiratory response to incoming chemoafferent activity varies during the course of the respiratory cycle, and the nature of this variation suggests that the "sensitivity" of both the inspiratory and expiratory components of the network increases progressively during each half-cycle of the oscillation (see ref. 18). The present results reveal an additional aspect to this variation in showing that the intensity of postinspiratory activity within the network may vary following stimulation.

The insertion of a postinspiratory delay into the rhythm forms part of the response to several afferent inputs which have, as part of their effect, an intensification of late inspiratory discharge in phrenic motoneurons or medullary inspiratory neurons. The most striking similarity with the present results is seen in the response produced by laryngeal inputs (2,20). In both cases, the effect of a stimulus arriving toward the end of inspiration is to initiate a postinspiratory delay in expiratory neurons and to excite medullary postinspiratory neurons. To this extent then, the activation of the delay illustrated in Fig. 33.2 would appear to reflect the operation of network properties that may be utilized by a variety of inputs, rather than being a specific expression of the response to chemoreceptor input.

The intense pattern of postinspiratory synaptic excitation shown in Fig. 33.3 presumably reflects failure of the stimulus to activate the postinspiratory delay. Part of the explanation for the difference between Figs. 33.2 and 33.3 may reside in the timing of the stimulus and the form of the response in the phrenic nerve: In Fig. 33.2, the critical feature preceding the postinspiratory delay was the development of a sharp peak in late inspiratory discharge. Of course, this does not necessarily imply that the occurrence of postinspiratory inhibition is generally dependent on the detailed form of the immediately preceding inspiration (cf. ref. 2). In both examples shown in Fig. 33.3, there was clearly a moderately well-developed postinspiratory delay prior to stimulation, but the level of inhibition setting this delay was evidently insufficient to gate out the intense synaptic excitation resulting from chemoreceptor stimulation. The result shown in Fig. 33.4B and C would also suggest that where the chemoreceptor input is superimposed on a given prevailing level of postinspiratory IPSP input, the two inputs simply summate.

The question then arises as to the significance of incorporating into the network a mechanism capable of postinspiratory gating of the chemoreceptor input— one which, moreover, is dependent on a fairly narrow time "window" in late inspiration for its activation. There is no direct evidence as to why this feature is part of the design of the network, but because of the apparently quite general use to which it is put, the answer probably lies in the consequences that it has for the timing of the expiratory burst. A rapid, steplike onset to expiratory discharge is probably not a useful feature, except possibly in transient states. So far as the response to chemoreceptor input is concerned, it seems likely that the effect of postinspiratory inhibition is mainly one of preserving a ramplike (rather than steplike) character to expiratory discharge over a wide range of average frequencies.

Stimulation of (presumed) chemoafferents in the sinus nerve has at least two effects on ongoing, expiratory-related, synaptic events: It produces an excitatory effect on expiratory neurons which appears to summate with the level of postinspiratory inhibition and which may be sufficient to reach discharge threshold; and it results in a lengthening of the postinspiratory plateau so that, although the neuron may very well discharge at this time, the ramplike component to this discharge (stage II) is delayed in onset. This effect may be mediated by the excitation of medullary postinspiratory neurons (the presumed source of the delay) which is elicited by both sinus nerve stimulation (19) and chemoreceptor stimulation (unpublished data). The critical feature governing expiratory duration following a chemoreceptor stimulus may be the level of discharge developed by the stage II pattern rather than the length of the postinspiratory delay. For example, in some circumstances where chemoreceptor stimulation *shortens* the expiratory interval, this shortening may also be accompanied by a brief but intense phase of postinspiratory inhibition; the release from this inhibition, however, is followed by a very much more rapid pattern of expiratory depolarization so that discharge frequency may come close to that reached at the end of an expiration of normal length. In this circumstance, the functionally significant effect may be one of ensuring high-frequency expiratory neuronal discharge in the much shorter time available for discharge. In this connection, it is of interest that the powerful wave of inhibition illustrated in Fig. 33.1A may be considered to represent inspiratory IPSP activity (on the basis of its relationship to phrenic nerve activity), but that from its timing and consequence for the subsequent pattern of expiratory discharge, it may be considered to represent postinspiratory IPSP activity. The significant feature in either case is that the release from inhibition constitutes a significant mechanism controlling the pattern of expiratory depolarization which immediately follows.

We conclude that chemoreceptor stimulation results in intensified inspiratory activity and inspiratory inhibition of expiratory neurons, and intensified expiratory synaptic excitation of expiratory neurons. The membrane potential trajectory during the expiratory phase and the timing of the expiratory discharge are dependent on whether chemoreceptor stimulation also intensifies postinspiratory IPSP activity; this intensification, in turn, depends on events occurring in the respiratory network in the late stage of inspiration. Under steady-state conditions, the combination of intensified postinspiratory IPSPs and chemoreceptor-mediated excitation probably constitutes a means of controlling the rate of increase of expiratory discharge. Any rapid shifts in the time of arrival of chemoafferent activity during the course of the respiratory cycle may result in more intense expiratory excitation (for shifts in the stimulus maximum away from late inspiration) or more intense postinspiratory inhibition (for shifts toward late inspiration).

ACKNOWLEDGMENTS
This work was supported by the DFG.

REFERENCES

1. Ballantyne, D., and D. W. Richter. Post-synaptic inhibition of bulbar inspiratory neurones in the cat. *J. Physiol. (Lond.) 348:* 67–87, 1984.
2. Ballantyne, D., and D. W. Richter. The non-uniform character of expiratory synaptic activity in expiratory bulbospinal neurones of the cat. *J. Physiol. (Lond.) 370:* 433–456, 1986.
3. Band, D. M., I. R. Carmeron, and S.J.G. Semple. The effect on respiration of abrupt changes in carotid artery pH and P_{CO_2} in the cat. *J. Physiol. (Lond.) 211:* 479–494, 1970.
4. Biscoe, T. J., and M. J. Purves. Observations on the rhythmic variation in the cat carotid body chemoreceptor activity which has the same period as respiration. *J. Physiol. (Lond.) 190:* 389–412, 1967.
5. Black, A.M.S., N. W. Goodman, B. S. Nail, P. S. Rao, and R. W. Torrance. The significance of the timing of chemoreceptor impulses for their effect upon respiration. *Acta Neurobiol. Exp. (Warsz.) 33:* 139–147, 1973.

6. Black, A.M.S., and R. W. Torrance. Chemoreceptor effects in the respiratory cycle. *J. Physiol. (Lond.) 189:* 59–61P, 1967.

7. Cohen, M. L., J. L. Feldman, and D. Sommer. Caudal medullary expiratory neurone and internal intercostal nerve discharges in the cat: effects of lung inflation. *J. Physiol. (Lond.) 368:* 147–178, 1985.

8. Davies, R. O., and M. W. Edwards. Medullary relay neurons in the carotid body chemoreceptor pathway of cats. *Respir. Physiol. 24:* 69–79, 1975.

9. Eldridge, F. L. The importance of timing on the respiratory effects of intermittent carotid sinus nerve stimulation. *J. Physiol. (Lond.) 222:* 297–318, 1972.

10. Eldridge, F. L. The importance of timing on the respiratory effects of intermittent carotid body chemoreceptor stimulation. *J. Physiol. (Lond.) 222:* 319–333, 1972.

11. Eldridge, F. L. Expiratory effects of brief carotid sinus nerve and carotid body stimulations. *Respir. Physiol. 26:* 395–410, 1976.

12. Howard, P., B. Bromberger-Barnea, R. S. Fitzgerald, and H. N. Bane. Ventilatory responses to peripheral nerve stimulation at different times in the respiratory cycle. *Respir. Physiol. 7:* 389–398, 1969.

13. Kirkwood, P. A., N. Nisimaru, and T. A. Sears. Monosynaptic excitation of bulbospinal respiratory neurones by chemoreceptor afferents in the carotid sinus nerve. *J. Physiol. (Lond.) 293:* 35–36P, 1979.

14. Koepchen, H.-P., D. Klussendorf, and U. Phillip. Mechanisms of central transmission of respiratory reflexes. *Acta Neurobiol. Exp. (Warsz.) 33:* 287–299, 1973.

15. Lipski, J. Central organization of chemoreceptor input. In: *Central Interaction Between Respiratory and Cardiovascular Control Systems,* ed. H.-P. Koepchen, S. M. Hilton, and A. Trzebski. Berlin: Springer-Verlag, 1977, pp. 93–96.

16. Lipski, J., R. M. McAllen, and K. M. Spyer. The carotid chemoreceptor input to the respiratory neurones of the nucleus of the tractus solitarius. *J. Physiol. (Lond.) 269:* 797–810, 1977.

17. Lipski, J., A. Trzebski, J. Chodobska, and P. Kruk. Effects of carotid chemoreceptor excitation on medullary expiratory neurons in cats. *Respir. Physiol. 57:* 279–291, 1984.

18. Marek, W., and N. R. Prabhakar. Electrical stimulation of arterial and central chemosensory afferents at different times in the respiratory cycle of the cat: II. Responses of respiratory muscles and their motor nerves. *Pflügers Arch. 403:* 422–428, 1985.

19. Mitchell, R. A., and D. A. Herbert. The effect of carbon dioxide on the membrane potential of medullary respiratory neurons. *Brain Res. 75:* 345–349, 1974.

20. Remmers, J. E., D. W. Richter, D. Ballantyne, C. R. Bainton, and J. P. Klein. Reflex prolongation of stage I of expiration. *Pflügers Arch. 407:* 190–198, 1986.

21. Richter, D. W. Generation and maintenance of the respiratory rhythm. *J. Exp. Biol. 100:* 93–107, 1982.

22. D. Richter, and D. Ballantyne, A three-phase theory about the basic respiratory pattern generator. In: *Central Neuron Environment and the Control Systems of Breathing and Circulation,* ed. M. E. Schlafke, H-P. Koepchen, W. R. See. Berlin: Springer-Verlag, 1983, pp. 164–174.

34

Phrenic Motoneurons: Descending Inputs, Electrical Properties, and Recruitment

A. J. BERGER, T. E. DICK, J. S. JODKOWSKI, AND F. VIANA

A major research goal of studies investigating spinal respiratory motor control is to explain the basis for spinal respiratory motoneuronal behavior. The phrenic motor system is an ideal model for study of respiratory motor control as it receives both inspiratory-phase excitatory and expiratory-phase inhibitory inputs, and its target muscle, the diaphragm, is the principal muscle of breathing (1,4,16,18). Inputs to phrenic motoneurons arise predominantly from bulbospinal neurons in two subpopulations of medullary respiratory neurons. One source of input is associated with the dorsal respiratory group (DRG) of neurons in the dorsomedial medulla and the other, with the ventral respiratory group (VRG) of neurons located in the ventrolateral medulla (8,22).

Since the mid-1970s, this laboratory has been pursuing several avenues of research that are centered around the phrenic motor system. We investigated descending inputs to the phrenic motor column using recently developed anatomical and electrophysiological techniques. We also analyzed morphological and electrophysiological properties of the phrenic motoneurons themselves. Although these studies represent a variety of experimental approaches, the goal of our research has remained the same: to understand the spinal neural mechanisms controlling the function of the main respiratory muscle.

METHODS

These studies were performed in anesthetized, paralyzed, artifically ventilated adult cats. Whole phrenic nerve activity was recorded and was used as an index of central respiratory drive.

The results from three different studies are described. In all experiments the animals were placed in a stereotaxic head-holder and spinal frame. The dorsal surface of the cervical spinal cord was exposed via a dorsal laminectomy extending generally from C3 or C4 to C7.

One study investigated the projection of axons from inspiratory (I) neurons in the VRG to the spinal cord (5). For this purpose, extracellular activity was recorded from these I-neurons after exposure of the dorsal surface of the medulla. A second extracellular electrode was inserted into the contralateral white matter of the spinal cord at C3–C4 to map the location of single descending VRG I-axons by employment of antidromic microstimulation and the recording of extracellular axonal potentials using spike-triggered averaging (STA).

In a second series of experiments, intraaxonal injection of the enzyme horseradish peroxidase (HRP) was used for the labeling and later the reconstruction of the trajectories and terminations within the phrenic motor column of single I-axons and expiratory (E)-axons (6). High-impedance microelectrodes filled with HRP were inserted in the spinal white matter at the C5 or C6 level. Axons were impaled and identified as I or E by monitoring their spontaneous activity. HRP was injected in these axons only if they could not be evoked by stimulation of the ipsilateral C5–C6 phrenic nerve roots. Many of these axons could be evoked at short latency by electrical stimulation in the midline of the medulla at the level of the obex. A standard histochemical protocol for detecting HRP was followed (3). Stained stem axons, their collaterals, terminal arbors, and synaptic terminals were located at the light microscopic level and reconstructed with the aid of a camera lucida attached to the microscope.

In a third set of experiments, phrenic motoneurons were impaled with glass microelectrodes filled with 4 M potassium acetate (14). Several electrical properties of these motoneurons, including input resistance (R_n) and rheobase (I_{rh}) were determined during hypocapnic apnea (end-tidal CO_2 < 3%). After these determinations, end-tidal CO_2 was increased to initiate rhythmic respiratory neural activity and to allow study of the effect of increased synaptic activity on membrane potential trajectories and the firing of action potentials.

RESULTS

Descending Pathways

Using extracellular STA and antidromic microstimulation in the cervical spinal cord, we determined that bulbospinal VRG I-neurons have descending axons located primarily in the ventral and to a lesser degree in the lateral columns. Figure 34.1 shows the location of these axons and also shows that descending axonal trajectories are linear and maintain their relative positions in the white matter as the axons descend in the spinal cord. Further, we found that neighboring bulbospinal somata have descending axons in close proximity to one another in the white matter. Other recent results (7a) concerning descending axons arising from DRG I-neurons have shown that these axons are located somewhat more laterally and dorsally in the white matter of the cervical spinal cord than are axons arising from VRG I-neurons. The functional significance, if any, of this spatial segregation awaits determination.

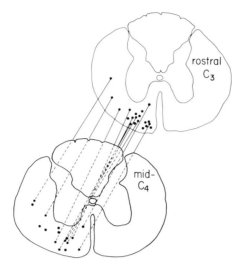

Fig. 34.1 Locations of inspiratory bulbospinal axons in rostral C3 and mid-C4 were determined by minimizing microstimulation current intensities and maximizing STA axonal potentials. Note that the 10 axons were located at both C3 and C4 (connected symbols), where solid and dashed lines connect the corresponding points for the same axons. [Reproduced by permission from Dick and Berger, 1985 (5).]

Recently we injected HRP into single respiratory axons (12 stem axons: 5 I and 7 E) in the ventral and ventrolateral columns in the C5–C6 spinal cord. We confirmed the linear trajectories of the stem axons that were observed neurophysiologically (see Fig. 34.1). In six of 12 axons we observed that collaterals (1–4 per axon) emerged from the stem axons at approximately right angles and proceeded directly to the ventral horn. All of these collaterals were found at the level of the phrenic motor column (C5–C6). Both I-axons ($n = 4$) and E-axons ($n = 2$) had collaterals. Also, for those stem axons having collaterals, the number of collaterals present varied inversely with the distance of the axon from the ventral horn. In other words, the closer to the ventral horn that an axon resided, the greater was the number of collaterals. The average intercollateral distance was 1.0 mm. Previously it was demonstrated that in cat, the somata of phrenic motoneurons cluster along the longitudinal axis of the spinal cord with an average intercluster distance of 0.95 mm (2).

All collaterals were observed to bifurcate very close to the ventral edge of the ventral horn. Nine I-collaterals and one E-collateral were stained sufficiently to trace their terminal arborizations within the ventral horn of the C5–C6 segments. Two different types of varicosities were seen on the finer terminals, and we assumed these to indicate the presence of both *en passant* and *terminaux* types of synaptic boutons. Inspiratory axon collaterals had an average of 27 boutons per collateral and most boutons were located within the rostrocaudally oriented phrenic motor column, suggesting that monosynaptic—presumably excitatory— contacts are present between these I-axons and phrenic motoneurons. Additionally, boutons were seen outside of the phrenic motor column, but always within the ventral horn. For the one E-collateral exhibiting a terminal arborization, only two synaptic boutons were observed, and both were located within the phrenic motor column.

Electrical Properties and Recruitment

In another series of experiments, we investigated the role of electrical properties of phrenic motoneurons in determining motoneuronal behavior. During hypocapnic apnea and in the absence of respiratory rhythm, we observed a significant negative linear correlation ($r = -.85$; $p < .0001$; $n = 38$ cells) between phrenic motoneuronal I_{rh} and R_n. This correlation resulted from the grouping of motoneurons into two subpopulations: (a) type L with low R_n and high I_{rh}, and (b) type H with high R_n and low I_{rh}. An R_n of 1.3 megohm (MΩ) served to separate the two types of phrenic motoneurons (type L, <1.3 MΩ, and type H, >1.3 MΩ).

For 14 phrenic motoneurons, we were able to elevate end-tidal CO_2 and induce rhythmic I-phase phrenic nerve activity while maintaining stable intracellular recording from these cells. As end-tidal CO_2 rose, we observed rhythmic membrane potential depolarizations to be in phase with phrenic nerve activity. Maximal synaptic depolarization (the difference between the peak depolarization during I and the end-expiratory membrane potential) was measured for each of these cells. Figure 34.2 is a three-dimensional plot derived from these data. It shows that at similar levels of end-tidal CO_2 (mean end-tidal CO_2 of 6.6% for type H and 7% for type

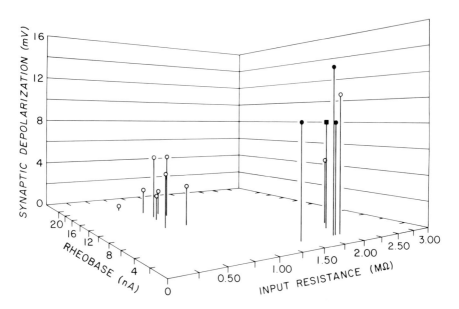

Fig. 34.2 Magnitude of I-phase CO_2-induced synaptic depolarization versus I_{rh} and R_n for 14 phrenic motoneurons. Each symbol represents a different cell: (O) cells that did not fire action potentials; (●, ■) cells that fired during I. For further information, see text. [Reproduced by permission from Jodkowski et al., *J. Neurophysiol.* 1987 (14).]

L) and end-expiratory membrane potentials (mean values: -71 mV and -70 mV, respectively), type H phrenic motoneurons had greater synaptic depolarization as compared to that of type L motoneurons. Furthermore, only type H phrenic motoneurons exhibited I-phase spike discharge. These experiments demonstrate that during modest hypercapnia in anesthetized cats, only type H phrenic motoneurons and their corresponding motor units are active. Thus on the basis of differences in electrical properties alone, the phrenic motor pool can be separated into two types of phrenic motoneurons. These two types have different behaviors in response to descending respiratory related drives.

DISCUSSION

Spinal respiratory motoneurons are activated rhythmically during breathing. A primary objective of our studies was to investigate the basis for rhythmic activation and recruitment of spinal motoneurons, and to establish anatomical and functional relationships between synaptic inputs and their target cells. Descending respiratory bulbospinal pathways and the phrenic motor system were chosen for this investigation.

Phrenic motoneurons undergo active excitation and inhibition during the respiratory cycle. Inspiratory-phase excitation is partly derived from monosynaptic excitatory inputs from bulbospinal I-neurons (4,16). Inhibition can be observed in many phrenic motoneurons during the E-phase (1) and monosynaptic inhibitory inputs from bulbospinal E-neurons have been demonstrated (18).

Descending Pathways

We determined the exact location of single I-axons by maximizing the orthodromic extracellular averaged potential and minimizing the antidromic stimulation current. I-axons were found in the ventral and lateral columns. Previous neuroanatomical and neurophysiological investigations have revealed a similar distribution of bulbospinal respiratory axons in the cervical spinal cord (9,17,20,21).

The neurophysiological evidence has shown that in the transverse plane, single I-axons from VRG neurons remain in approximately the same relative locations in the white matter as they descend in the cervical cord. This was confirmed for single I-axons that were labeled intracellularly with HRP, and also E-axons when they were labeled.

Based upon our anatomical results, axonal collaterals were observed to emerge perpendicularly from stem axons and then to traverse directly to the ventral horn where they arborized extensively within the phrenic motor column. We observed that the average intercollateral distance was approximately the same as the average distance between clusters of phrenic motoneurons (2). The close agreement of these two anatomical measurements may have functional significance. In particular, it may reflect a close anatomical–functional linkage between this input system and the presumptive target cells, the phrenic motoneurons. Our results may indicate that for these respiratory axons there is a one collateral:one motoneuronal cluster relationship. We have no evidence at present, however, to support this hypothesis.

Synaptic terminals of I-axons were found within the phrenic motor column, and to a lesser extent outside of the motor column in regions of the ventral horn that are known to contain phrenic motoneuronal dendrites (3). These results are consistent with known monosynaptic excitatory connections between I bulbospinal neurons and phrenic motoneurons (4,16,19), although synaptic interactions between the labeled axonal terminals to other ventral horn cells cannot be excluded.

The results reported here regarding the respiratory axons in the cervical spinal cord are remarkably similar to those reported for other descending motor systems, such as the corticomotoneuronal system (11,15). Both systems have stem axons with linear trajectories in the white matter, and have collaterals that emerge perpendicularly from stem axons, which then bifurcate very close to the border between the white and gray matter, then show extensive arborization and termination in the target regions, and, in some cases, lie parallel to the rostrocaudal axis of the spinal cord.

Electrical Properties and Recruitment

A study of the electrical properties of phrenic motoneurons during hypocapnic apnea revealed that the range of values of electrical properties (including R_n, I_{rh}, and the duration and amplitude of afterhyperpolarization) generally were similar to those seen in lumbosacral motoneurons (10,12). Of importance with regard to the issue of recruitment was the finding that an inverse relationship between I_{rh} and R_n arose as a result of the presence of two groups of phrenic motoneurons, the type L and the type H phrenic motoneurons. Zengel et al. (23), in their study of medial gastrocnemius motoneurons, concluded that the ratio of I_{rh} to R_n could be used to predict the type of motor unit without the measurement of motor unit contractile properties. In our own studies, because we used a paralyzed artificially ventilated preparation, we were unable to classify the phrenic motoneurons into types based upon motor unit contractile properties. However, the extrapolation of the results of Zengel et al. (23) to the phrenic motor pool leads to the conclusion that type H phrenic motoneurons (those with an $R_n > 1.3$ MΩ and $I_{rh}/R_n < 7$) innervate slowly contracting diaphragmatic muscle fibers, and type L phrenic motoneurons (those with an $R_n < 1.3$ MΩ and $I_{rh}/R_n > 7$) innervate fast-contracting diaphragmatic muscle fibers.

None of the type L phrenic motoneurons in our study could be recruited to fire during "normal" breathing. Only the type H motoneurons fired, and these motoneurons had significantly greater I-phase synaptic depolarization. Although the type L phrenic motoneurons, which probably innervate fast-contracting muscle fibers, were not active, they are active during increased demand for diaphragmatic muscle contraction as, for example, during the aspiration reflex (mechanical stimulation of the epipharynx). The set of phrenic motoneurons active in "normal" breathing, therefore, is not equivalent to the entire phrenic motor pool, but is a specific subset of that pool.

Previously we demonstrated the applicability of Henneman's (13) size principle to the subset of phrenic motoneurons active during "normal" breathing (7). To do this, we recorded activity from single motor units and precisely measured motor unit axonal conduction velocity using two-point, delayed spike-triggered averaging. For almost 95% of the simultaneously recorded diaphragmatic motor unit pairs, we observed that the axonal conduction velocity of the earlier recruited motor unit of the pair was less than that of the later recruited motor unit. Thus phrenic motoneuron axonal conduction velocity is an accurate predictor of motor unit recruitment order.

CONCLUSIONS

1. Descending bulbospinal respiratory axons have linear trajectories that parallel the longitudinal axis of the cervical spinal cord. Stem axons, as they descend, stay in approximately the same relative positions in the white matter.
2. Respiratory axonal collaterals emerge perpendicularly from the stem axons and traverse directly to the ventral horn. Many I-axons have multiple axonal collaterals, which terminate in synaptic boutons located primarily, but not exclusively, in the phrenic motor column.
3. In "normal" respiration in anesthetized cats, the active population of phrenic motoneurons are those with an $I_{rh}:R_n$ ratio <7. This population probably is made up almost exclusively of slowly contracting motor units.
4. Henneman's size principle predicts the recruitment order of phrenic motoneurons active in "normal" respiration.

ACKNOWLEDGMENTS
The authors thank William Satterthwaite for technical assistance, Hanna Atkins for editing and illustrations, and Patrick Roberts for photography. This research was supported by a U.S.P.H.S. Javits Neuroscience Investigator Award NS-14857 to A.J.B.; a fellowship from the Spanish Comité Conjunto Hispano-Norteamericano para la Cooperación Cultural y Educativa to F.V.; and a Parker B. Francis Fellowship from the Puritan-Bennett Foundation to T.E.D.

REFERENCES

1. Berger, A. J. Phrenic motoneurons in the cat: subpopulations and nature of respiratory drive potentials. *J. Neurophysiol. 42:* 76–90, 1979.
2. Berger, A. J., W. E. Cameron, D. B. Averill, R. C. Kramis, and M. D. Binder. Spatial distributions of phrenic and gastrocnemius motoneurons in the cat spinal cord. *Exp. Neurol. 86:* 559–575, 1984.
3. Cameron, W. E., D. B. Averill, and A. J. Berger. Morphology of cat phrenic motoneurons as revealed by intracellular injection of horseradish peroxidase. *J. Comp. Neurol. 219:* 70–80, 1983.
4. Davies, J.G.McF., P. A. Kirkwood, and T. A. Sears. The distribution of monosynaptic connexions from inspiratory bulbospinal neurones to inspiratory motoneurones in the cat. *J. Physiol. (Lond.) 368:* 63–87, 1985.
5. Dick, T. E., and A. J. Berger. Axonal projections of single bulbospinal inspiratory neurons revealed by spike-triggered averaging and antidromic activation. *J. Neurophysiol. 53:* 1590–1603, 1985.

6. Dick, T. E., J. S. Jodkowski, F. Viana, and A. J. Berger. Projections and terminations of single respiratory axons in the cervical spinal cord of the cat. *Brain Res.* 449:201–212, 1988

7. Dick, T. E., F.-J. Kong, and A. J. Berger. Correlation of recruitment order with axonal conduction velocity for supraspinally driven diaphragmatic motor units. *J. Neurophysiol. 57:* 245–259, 1987.

7a. Dick, T. E., F. Viana, and A. J. Berger. Electrophysiological determination of the axonal projections of single dorsal respiratory group neurons to the cervical spinal cord of cat. Brain Res. (in press).

8. Feldman, J. L. Neurophysiology of breathing in mammals. In: *Handbook of Physiology,* Sec. 1: *The Nervous System,* Vol. 4: *Intrinsic Regulatory Systems of the Brain,* ed. F. E. Bloom. Bethesda: Am. Physiol. Soc., 1986, pp. 463–524.

9. Feldman, J. L., A. D. Loewy, and D. F. Speck. Projections from the ventral respiratory group to phrenic and intercostal motoneurons in cat: an autoradiographic study. *J. Neurosci. 5:* 1993–2000, 1985.

10. Fleshman, J. W., J. B. Munson, G. W. Sypert, and W. A. Friedman. Rheobase, input resistance, and motor-unit type in medial gastrocnemius motoneurons in the cat. *J. Neurophysiol. 46:* 1326–1338, 1981.

11. Futami, T., Y. Shinoda, and J. Yokota. Spinal axon collaterals of corticospinal neurons identified by intracellular injection of horseradish peroxidase. *Brain Res. 164:* 279–284, 1979.

12. Gustafsson, B., and M. J. Pinter. An investigation of threshold properties among cat spinal α-motoneurones. *J. Physiol. (Lond.) 357:* 453–483, 1984.

13. Henneman, E. Relation between size of neurons and their susceptibility to discharge. *Science 126:* 1345–1347, 1957.

14. Jodkowski, J. S., F. Viana, T. E. Dick, and A. J. Berger. Electrical properties of phrenic motoneurons in the cat: correlation with inspiratory drive. *J. Neurophysiol., 58:* 105–124, 1987.

15. Lawrence, D. G., R. Porter, and S. J. Redman. Corticomotoneuronal synapses in the monkey: light microscopic localization upon motoneurons of intrinsic muscles of the hand. *J. Comp. Neurol. 232:* 499–510, 1985.

16. Lipski, J., L. Kubin, and J. Jodkowski. Synaptic action of Rβ neurons on phrenic motoneurons studied with spike-triggered averaging. *Brain Res. 288:* 105–118, 1983.

17. Merrill, E. G. Finding a respiratory function for the medullary respiratory neurons. In: *Essays on the Nervous System,* ed. R. Bellairs and E. Gray. Oxford: Clarendon, 1974, pp. 451–486.

18. Merrill, E. G., and L. Fedorko. Monosynaptic inhibition of phrenic motoneurons: a long descending projection from Bötzinger neurons. *J. Neurosci. 4:* 2350–2353, 1984.

19. Monteau, R., M. Khatib, and G. Hilaire. Central determination of recruitment order: intracellular study of phrenic motoneurons. *Neurosci. Lett. 56:* 341–346, 1985.

20. Nakayama, S., and R. von Baumgarten. Lokalisierung absteigender Atmungsbahnen im Rückenmark der Katze mittels antidromer Reizung. *Pflügers Arch. 281:* 231–244, 1964.

21. Newsom Davis, J., and F. Plum. Separation of descending spinal pathways to respiratory motoneurons. *Exp. Neurol. 34:* 78–94, 1972.

22. Speck, D. F., and J. L. Feldman. The effects of microstimulation and microlesions in the ventral and dorsal respiratory groups in medulla of cat. *J. Neurosci. 2:* 744–757, 1982.

23. Zengel, J. E., S. A. Reid, G. W. Sypert, and J. B. Munson. Membrane electrical properties and prediction of motor-unit type of medial gastrocnemius motoneurons in the cat. *J. Neurophysiol. 53:* 1323–1344, 1985.

35

Responses of Phrenic, Recurrent Laryngeal, and Hypoglossal Motoneurons to Hypoxia in Neonatal Swine

P. M. GOOTMAN, A. L. SICA, A. M. STEELE,
AND H. L. COHEN

Evidence of a long-term interest in the effects of asphyxia or hypoxia on respiration in both the adult and neonate can be concluded from Boyle's experiments using the "exhausted receiver" on ducks, cats, vipers, and kitlings (newborn kittens) in 1670 (4). His studies showed that both species and age-related differences existed concerning survival in lack of air. We now know that one of the most characteristic phenomena of neonatal respiration is the presence of the biphasic response to hypoxia. This biphasic pattern is seen in neonatal humans (17,18,24,29), kittens (3), pigs (15,20), rabbits (16), and monkeys (19,32). The suggestion has even been made that a biphasic response is present in adult humans (13). However, the pattern is different, with the steady-state response remaining above control levels for tidal volume and frequency (17). On the other hand, newborn lambs apparently have this adult pattern of response (2,9). The mechanisms involved in the biphasic response have been postulated to involve failure of the peripheral chemoreceptors (9) or failure within the respiratory rhythm generator (RRG). Recently, Blanco et al. (3), recording directly from chemoreceptor fibers during hypoxia in kittens, found that activity was maintained for the duration of hypoxia; that is, failure was not occurring at the level of the chemoreceptor. These results are essentially similar to those reported about 20 years ago in lambs (2).

In eupnea, motoneurons innervating the various muscles of inspiration receive excitatory inputs from the respiratory rhythm generator (RRG), and thereby have phasic discharges. However, such modulation by common neural networks does not exclude the possibility that other central and/or peripheral inputs are needed to shape functionally appropriate activities for innervated musculatures. Frequently, such inputs preferentially facilitate the activity of specific motoneurons.

For example, it is known from studies of adult animals that hypoglossal and recurrent laryngeal motoneurons are more markedly affected by removal of lung volume afferents than are phrenic motoneurons (12,14,26,27,31). Hypoglossal motoneurons show greater sensitivity to hypoxia than either phrenic or recurrent laryngeal motoneurons (5,31). In newborn animals, however, there is little information regarding these modulatory influences on upper-airway motoneurons (6). Thus, in the present investigation, we have examined the changes of hypoglossal, recurrent laryngeal, and phrenic nerve discharges in newborn pigs during hypoxia, before and after bilateral vagotomy.

METHODS

Experiments were carried out in 25 piglets ranging in age from birth to 40 days, anesthetized with alphaxalone (Saffan; 2–6 mg/kg/h), paralyzed with decamethonium Br, tracheotomized, and artificially ventilated on 100% O_2 (P_{O_2} > 200 torr) except during specific experimental protocols; hydration was maintained on 5% dextrose in 0.9% NaCl. Blood gases and pH were monitored throughout the course of the experiment and maintained within normal limits except during protocols. Body temperatures were maintained at 39°C by a heating blanket. End-tidal CO_2 was continuously monitored throughout the experiment, along with arterial blood pressure, ECG, and intratracheal pressure. Phrenic (PHR), recurrent laryngeal (RL), and hypoglossal (HYP) nerves were recorded in various combinations, monophasically with bipolar, platinum electrodes (bandpass, 10 Hz to 10 kHz). For polygraphic display, nerve signals were full-wave-rectified and integrated (time constant, 100 ms). The integrated PHR was used to obtain marking pulses for the onsets of the central inspiratory (I) and expiratory (E) phases. Vagi were prepared for sectioning during the experiment. Nerve activities along with end-tidal CO_2, intratracheal pressure, aortic pressure, and ECG were stored on magnetic tape for off-line data analyses.

Hypoxia was induced by ventilating the animals with various combinations of O_2 in N_2. The actual degree of hypoxia was determined by blood gas analysis on a Radiometer microsystem. The duration of the different degrees of hypoxia varied between 1 and 10 min. Depending upon age, 21% O_2 resulted in P_{O_2} values of 55–80 torr; 15% O_2, P_{O_2} values of 35–50 torr; and 10% O_2, P_{O_2} values of 25–32 torr.

Two types of analyses of the nerve signals were performed: averaging and power spectra on IBM computers. Respiratory I-triggered histograms (10-ms time bins) were constructed from PHR, RL, and HYP nerve signals during hyperoxia and hypoxia. Nerve signals were successively full-wave-rectified and integrated. Pulses marking the onset of PHR activity were used as synchronizing events for I-triggered histograms of nerve activities. Each histogram represented the average activity in 30 or more central I phases. For power spectral analysis, the PHR discharge was low-pass-filtered (1 kHz) and acquired at 4096 Hz. Autopower spectral estimates were obtained for each PHR burst by a fast Fourier transform routine (1024 points) triggered by pulses marking the onset of I. Final autopower spectra were constructed by ensemble averaging of all spectral estimates. Averages of 50–

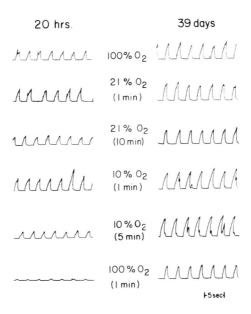

Fig. 35.1 Integrated phrenic activity (t.c., 100 ms) from a 20-h-old piglet (left traces) and a 39-day-old piglet (right traces) during hyperoxia and two degrees of hypoxia. Steady-state pH and arterial blood gases for these two animals were as follows:

	F_IO_2, 20-h-old piglet				F_IO_2, 39-day-old piglet			
	100%	21%	10%	100%	100%	21%	10%	100%
pH	7.40	7.395	7.42	7.35	7.406	7.409	7.410	7.409
P_aCO_2	44.8	43.0	39.7	44.1	42.8	38.0	36.5	34.6
P_aO_2	224.5	58.2	25.2	158.1	212.6	82.2	32.8	261.1

200 epochs were plotted as peak power versus frequency interval. (For further details of the methods, see refs. 11,15,28,30.)

RESULTS

Biphasic responses to two levels of hypoxia (21% and 10% O_2) were observed in our youngest piglets. After 2 weeks of age, the biphasic response to hypoxia was usually absent. Examples of the patterns of responses seen in our youngest and older piglets are shown in Fig. 35.1. Note that the biphasic response was obtained to two different degrees of hypoxia in the 20-h-old piglet (left panel). Hyperoxia, on the other hand, had a more profound inhibitory effect on the RRG, as indicated by marked depression of PHR discharge in the younger piglets. Power spectral analysis showed that the depression of integrated activity was a function of the decrease in total activity since there was a decline in energy in the high-frequency range (ca. 90–150 Hz, depending upon age; see ref. 15). An example of the changes in power

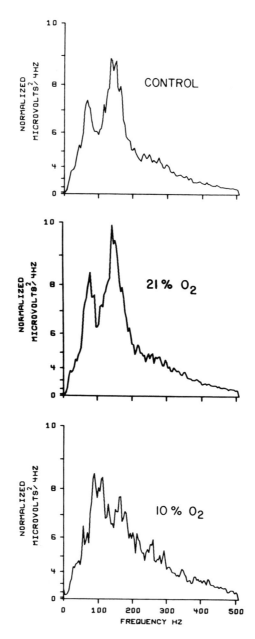

Fig. 35.2 Effects of changes in inspired O_2 on phrenic power spectra from a 34-day-old piglet. [Adapted by permission from Cohen et al., 1986 (11).]

observed during hypoxia is shown in Fig. 35.2. In this example, from a >2-week-old pig, power first increased at 21% inspired O_2 and then declined to about control levels.

In another series of experiments, the discharges of PHR, RL, and HYP nerves were compared during hyperoxia and hypoxia with vagi intact and following bilateral vagotomy. In no case was spontaneous HYP I activity observed with intact vagi. Therefore, comparison of activity patterns between the nerves is restricted to PHR and RL nerves with vagi intact, and to HYP and PHR following bilateral vagotomy. Utilizing averaging techniques, we found that under hyperoxic conditions the discharge pattern of the RL was usually I plateau, which is similar to that of adult cat (12,27), whereas the PHR was I augmenting. In some instances, RL also had a prominent early-expiratory (e-E) discharge. Figure 35.3 shows an example of the effects of hyperoxia and hypoxia on RL and PHR activities. This figure shows that the PHR had a biphasic response to hypoxia (Fig. 35.3, left) while RL inspiratory activity was not as markedly affected (right). The RL discharge became more of an augmenting pattern during hypoxia (Fig. 35.3, right) and remained augmenting while the PHR amplitude returned to control level (100% O_2). In addition, hypoxia elicited e-E activity (Fig. 35.3, INT RL N. during hypoxia).

Following bilateral vagotomy, spontaneous HYP activity rarely appeared (2/10 animals). In contrast, HYP I activity in the remaining 8 piglets was observed only during hypoxic drive. The response of HYP motoneurons to hypoxia was stereotypical. Figure 35.4 (top) shows a typical pattern of recruitment of I activity in HYP discharge. Such activity arose from a background of low-level, tonic activity and reached its maximum amplitude within 2 min. The amplitudes of both PHR and HYP nerve discharges decreased in the final 2–3 min of hypoxia; the decrease in PHR amplitude fell below that of control activity (biphasic response), while the HYP I discharge became tonic. Two different patterns of HYP activity were observed in response to the hypoxic stimulus (Fig. 35.4, solid curves): (a) a decrementing discharge pattern (left); (b) an augmenting discharge pattern (right). Of 8 animals, 5 showed the decrementing discharge patterns and 3 showed the augmenting discharge pattern.

DISCUSSION

Schwieler (25) has suggested that the biphasic response in kittens is due either to hyperpolarization of the chemoreceptor afferent nerve terminals in NTS or to alteration in response of the RRG to afferent stimulation. Because we have shown that the RRG can respond biphasically to two levels of hypoxia, failure of the chemoreceptors to respond (i.e., fatigue) is probably not the explanation. Further, 100% O_2 following hypoxia is a much greater inhibitory input in younger than in older piglets. This is unlike the reported responses in lambs (7) in which a greater depression in ventilation was observed in the older lambs. These investigators suggested that the smaller decline to 100% O_2 in the younger lambs was due to the degree of sensitivity of the O_2 chemoreceptors. Bureau et al. (8) have also reported that the hypoxic response was almost eliminated in lambs after carotid body denervation.

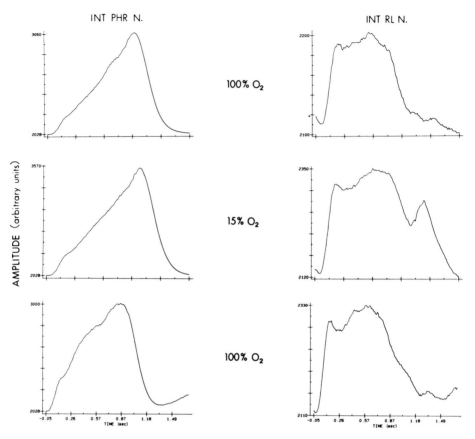

Fig. 35.3 Respiratory I-triggered histograms of integrated phrenic (INT PHR N.; left) and recurrent laryngeal nerve (INT RL N.; right) discharges. Comparison of amplitudes and discharge patterns in control (hyperoxia, 100% O$_2$), hypoxia (15% O$_2$), and recovery (hyperoxia, 100% O$_2$). Histograms of INT PHR N. show a typical augmenting pattern; however, activity in hypoxia has a greater amplitude than that of the control. Histogram of INT RL N. activity in the control condition has a slight augmenting pattern which becomes more pronounced in hypoxia. The increase of INT RL N. amplitude is not as marked as that of INT PHR N. Note the recruitment of a prominent burst of early-expiratory activity in INT RL N. discharge during hypoxia. All histograms are of average integrated activity in 30–40 central I-phases.

On the other hand, the greater depression seen in our younger piglets might be a reflection of the need of the RRG for continued chemoreceptor input to maintain a given level of excitability. Nishino and Honda (22) reported that changes in CO$_2$ and O$_2$ can indeed alter the level of excitability of the RRG in adult mammals. Thus the two different patterns in these two different species might be a reflection of the degree of maturation of the brainstem reticular formation at birth.

    We have also examined the changes of activity of nerves supplying upper-airway muscles during control respiratory cycles and during hypoxia. Unlike the discharge of the RL nerve, the HYP discharge lacked I modulation in central I phases

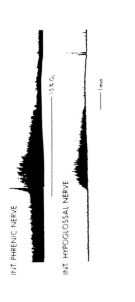

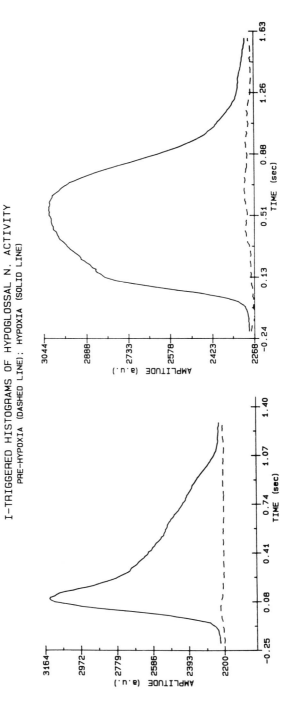

Fig. 35.4 (Upper panel) Comparison of integrated (t.c., = 100 ms) phrenic and hypoglossal nerve discharges in control (hyperoxia), hypoxia (15% O_2), and recovery (hyperoxia). Note that the phrenic discharge shows a biphasic response to hypoxia; the hypoglossal inspiratory discharge is recruited by hypoxia and returns to baseline activity toward the end of the hypoxic episode. **(Lower panel)** Respiratory I-triggered histograms of recruited hypoglossal inspiratory activity. Left: I-decrementing pattern; right: I-augmenting pattern. Histograms are of average integrated activity in 40–50 central I phases.

with pulmonary afferent inputs. This finding suggested a more profound depressant (inhibitory or disfacilitatory) influence of pulmonary afferent inputs on HYP motoneurons than on RL I motoneurons. This lack of I-modulation of HYP discharge has also been observed in experiments with anesthetized newborn kittens (6–70 days old) (6). On the other hand, spontaneous HYP I activity appears after bilateral vagotomy (6). In contrast, HYP I activity did not appear after bilateral vagotomy in our animals. This difference in the strength of I modulation of HYP discharge may be due to greater maturation of HYP motoneurons in kittens than in pigs. Another indication of immaturity in these motoneurons from piglets was that recruited HYP I activity often had an I-decrementing discharge pattern. This finding was surprising since, in adult cats, HYP decrementing pattern became augmenting when pulmonary afferent inputs were removed by withholding of inflation (26). The response observed in adult cats was due to disinhibition or facilitation of HYP I discharge (26). Thus, the observation of more decrementing patterns provides evidence for immaturity of the hypoglossal motoneuron pool in many of our animals. Such immaturity might be due to (a) membrane characteristics, (b) pattern of synaptic arrangements between motoneurons, or (c) incomplete synaptic connections with other brainstem regions.

There are differences in strength of I modulation of efferent nerves supplying upper-airway muscles. The appearance of spontaneous RL nerve activity supplies evidence of the functional integrity of these motoneurons; that is, they would produce appropriate contractions of the innervated muscles. Thus, the plateaulike pattern of RL I activity is similar to the pattern of glottic dilation (1) which provides for laryngeal patency. On the other hand, the absence of spontaneous HYP I activity (and consequently of its innervated muscles, the genioglossi) suggests that oropharyngeal patency may be compromised in these animals since such activity is necessary to oppose the collapsing forces due to diaphragmatic contraction. This absence of HYP I activity may be qualitatively similar to observations made in sleeping, preterm infants; that is, genioglossus muscles do not discharge in every central I phase (10). This may be due to the well-known depression of genioglossus I activity in certain central neural states (21,23). A similar phenomenon may be responsible for the lack of HYP I activity in unperturbed I phases.

CONCLUSIONS

Thus, neonatal swine are an excellent subprimate model of newborn infants, given the presence of a biphasic response to hypoxia and the absence of appropriate discharge patterns in the hypoglossal nerve. The maturation of such responses to the adult pattern within approximately one month permits detailed examination of postnatal maturation of respiratory responses to hypoxia.

ACKNOWLEDGMENTS
     The authors would like to thank Glaxo, Inc. for the generous gift of Saffan. The studies were supported by USPHS NIH Grant HL-20864 (PMG). ALS is a Parker B. Francis Research Fellow. The authors would like to thank the skilled assistance of computer programers L. P. Eberle and M. R. Gandhi and the skilled technical assistance of P. G. Griswold and Dr. P. P. Rao.

REFERENCES

1. Bartlett, D., Jr., J. E. Remmers, and H. Gautier. Laryngeal regulation of respiratory airflow. *Respir. Physiol. 18:* 194–204, 1973.
2. Biscoe, T. J., and M. J. Purves. Carotid body chemoreceptor activity in the new-born lamb. *J. Physiol. (Lond.) 190:* 443–454, 1967.
3. Blanco, C. E., M. A. Hanson, P. Johnson, and H. Rigatto. Breathing pattern of kittens during hypoxia. *J. Appl. Physiol. 56:* 12–17, 1984.
4. Boyle, R. New pneumatrical experiments about respiration. *Philos. Trans. 5:* 473–479, 1670.
5. Brouillette, R. T., and B. T. Thach. Control of genioglossus muscle inspiratory activity. *J. Appl. Physiol. 49:* 801–808, 1980.
6. Bruce, E. N. Hypoglossal and phrenic nerve responses to chemical stimuli in kittens. In: *Neurobiology of the Control of Breathing,* ed. C. von Euler and H. Lagercrantz. New York: Raven Press, 1986, pp. 75–80.
7. Bureau, M. A., and R. Begin. Postnatal maturation of the respiratory response to O_2 in awake newborn lambs. *J. Appl. Physiol. 52:* 428–433, 1982.
8. Bureau, M. A., J. LaMarche, P. Foulon, and D. Dalle. The ventilatory response to hypoxia in the newborn lamb after carotid body denervation. *Respir. Physiol. 60:* 109–119, 1985.
9. Bureau, M. A., R. Zinman, P. Foulon, and R. Begin. Diphasic ventilatory response to hypoxia in newborn lambs. *J. Appl. Physiol. 56:* 84–90, 1984.
10. Carlo, W. A., M. J. Miller, and R. J. Martin. Differential responses of respiratory muscles to airway occlusion in infants. *J. Appl. Physiol. 59:* 847–852, 1985.
11. Cohen, H. L., A. M. Steele, L. P. Eberle, and P. M. Gootman. Development of central respiratory function in swine. In: *Swine in Biomedical Research,* Vol. 2, ed. M. E. Tumbleson. New York: Plenum, 1986, pp. 1289–1295.
12. Cohen, M. I. Phrenic and recurrent laryngeal discharge patterns and the Hering–Breuer reflex. *Am. J. Physiol. 228:* 1489–1496, 1975.
13. Easton, P. A., L. J. Slykerman, and N. R. Anthonisen. Ventilatory response to sustained hypoxia in normal adults. *J. Appl. Physiol. 61:* 906–911, 1986.
14. Fukuda, Y., and Y. Honda. Role of vagal afferents on discharge patterns and CO_2-responsiveness of efferent superior laryngeal, hypoglossal, and phrenic respiratory activities in anesthetized rats. *Jpn. J. Physiol. 32:* 689–698, 1982.
15. Gootman, P. M., A. M. Steele, H. L. Cohen, and L. P. Eberle. Postnatal maturation of the respiratory rhythm generator. In: *The Physiological Development of the Fetus and Newborn,* ed. C. T. Jones and P. W. Nathaniels. London: Academic Press, 1985, pp. 223–228.
16. Grunstein, M. M., T. A. Hazinski, and M. A. Schlueter. Respiratory control during hypoxia in newborn rabbits: implied action of endorphins. *J. Appl. Physiol. 51:* 122–130, 1981.
17. Haddad, G. G., and R. B. Mellins. Hypoxia and respiratory control in early life. *Annu. Rev. Physiol. 46:* 629–643, 1984.
18. Jansen, A. H., and V. Chernick. Development of respiratory control. *Physiol. Rev. 63:* 437–483, 1983.
19. LaFramboise, W. A., and D. E. Woodrum. Elevated diaphragm electromyogram during neonatal hypoxic ventilatory depression. *J. Appl. Physiol. 59:* 1040–1045, 1985.
20. Lawson, E. E., and W. A. Long. Central origin of biphasic breathing pattern during hypoxia in newborns. *J. Appl. Physiol. 55:* 483–488, 1983.
21. Megirian, D., C.F.L. Hinrichsen, and J. H. Sherrey. Respiratory roles of genioglossus, sternothyroid, and sternohyoid muscles during sleep. *Exp. Neurol. 90:* 118–128, 1985.

22. Nishino, T., and Y. Honda. Effects of P_aCO_2 and P_aO_2 on threshold for the inspiratory-augmenting reflex in cats. *J. Appl. Physiol. 53:* 1152–1157, 1982.

23. Remmers, J. E., W. J. de Groot, E. K. Sauerland, and A. M. Anch. Pathogenesis of upper airway occlusion in sleep. *J. Appl. Physiol. 44:* 931–938, 1978.

24 Rigatto, H., J. P. Brady, and R. de la Torre Verduzco. Chemoreceptor reflexes in preterm infants: I. The effect of gestational and postnatal age on the ventilatory response to inhalation of 100% and 15% oxygen. *Pediatrics 55:* 604–613, 1975.

25. Schwieler, G. H. Respiratory regulation during postnatal development in cats and rabbits and some of its morphological substrate. *Acta Physiol. Scand. 72* (Suppl. 304): 3–123, 1968.

26. Sica, A. L., M. I. Cohen, D. F. Donnelly, and H. Zhang. Hypoglossal motoneuron responses to pulmonary and superior laryngeal afferent inputs. *Respir. Physiol. 56:* 339–357, 1984.

27. Sica, A. L., M. I. Cohen, D. F. Connelly, and H. Zhang. Responses of recurrent laryngeal motoneurons to changes of pulmonary afferent inputs. *Respir. Physiol. 62:* 153–168, 1985.

28. Sica, A. L., D. F. Donnelly, A. M. Steele, and M. R. Gandhi. Discharge properties of dorsal medullary inspiratory neurons in newborn pigs. *Brain Res.,* 408:222–226, 1987.

29. Steele, A. M. Developmental changes in neural control of respiration. In: *Developmental Neurobiology of the Autonomic Nervous System,* ed. P. M. Gootman. Clifton, NJ: Humana Press, 1986, pp. 327–401.

30. Steele, A. M., P. M. Gootman, H. L. Cohen, L. P. Eberle, and M. R. Gandhi. Maturational changes in phrenic nerve discharge. *Pediatr. Res. 20:* 442A, 1986.

31. Weiner, D., J. Mitra, J. Salome, and N. S. Cherniack. Effect of chemical stimuli on nerves supplying upper airway muscles. *J. Appl. Physiol. 52:* 530–536, 1982.

32. Woodrum, D. E., T. A. Standaert, D. E. Mayock, and R. D. Guthrie. Hypoxic ventilatory response in the newborn monkey. *Pediatr. Res. 15:* 367–370, 1981.

36

A Structure of the Respiratory Controller: Implications of Comroe's "Clogging" Theory

S. J. ANDERSON AND G. D. SWANSON

Numerous respiratory physiologists, beginning with Geppert and Zuntz in 1888, have been searching for the elusive "exercise" signal, which is correlated with metabolic CO_2 production that appropriately drives the respiratory controller. Julius Comroe suggested that one reason this problem remained unsolved is that "respiratory physiologists are not necessarily good neurophysiologists or good control-system engineers, and maybe they should be to solve the problem" (1). Comroe went on to suggest that arterial P_{CO_2} may be regulated at 40 mmHg during exercise by the controller "because its job is to control P_{CO_2} and keep it at a set level." He likened the controller structure to an "efficient air conditioner system" that regulates room temperature at 70°F as long as the system is not "clogged." He reasoned that when CO_2 is added to the inspired air, it "clogs" the mechanism for CO_2 elimination, and arterial CO_2 must therefore rise. Thus, he concluded that an explicit "exercise" signal might not be necessary.

The purpose of this chapter is to explore the plausibility of such a respiratory controller structure. We shall first outline a feedforward/feedback control system in which an explicit "exercise" signal is part of the feedforward structure. We shall then explore the concept that a feedforward signal is actually embedded implicitly in the lung gas exchange system in terms of the randomlike variation in ventilation and the corresponding arterial CO_2 response. With the brain dictating these variations in ventilation and sensing the arterial CO_2 response via the chemoreceptors, it can determine indirectly the CO_2 production via the concept of gas exchange efficiency. With this information, the brain can then respond with an appropriate ventilatory drive to both a metabolic CO_2 load via exercise and an airway CO_2 load via inspired CO_2—all without an explicit "exercise" signal.

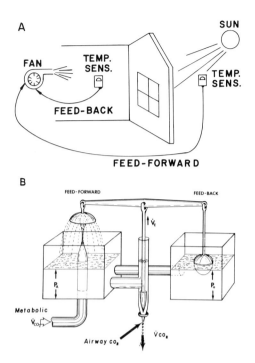

Fig. 36.1 **(A)** Feedforward/feedback structure for an air-conditioning system. **(B)** Fluid regulator to illustrate the feedforward/feedback structure of the respiratory controller (11).

CONTROL-SYSTEM STRUCTURE

Returning to Comroe's air conditioner analogy, consider the feedforward/feedback control system shown in Fig. 36.1A (11). We usually think of an air conditioner regulating room air temperature via *feedback* from a thermostat inside a room. That is, if the temperature in the room should begin to rise, the thermostat activates a cooling fan to bring the room air temperature back toward 70°F. However, a *feed-forward* signal could also facilitate temperature regulation. In this case, an outside temperature sensor feeds information forward to activate the cooling fan as the outside air temperature begins to rise.

The action of the respiratory controller can be visualized in terms of this feed-forward/feedback structure via the fluid regulator shown in Fig. 36.1B (11). The inflow of fluid is analogous to metabolic CO_2 production. An increase in the fluid flow causes an increase in the pressure exerted on the concave surface attached to the left-hand lever arm. The outflow valve, analogous to ventilation, opens, and if the system is calibrated correctly, the increase in the outflow will just equal the increase in the inflow. Thus the fluid level will remain constant, resulting in perfect regulation of arterial CO_2 during exercise. In contrast, when the inspired CO_2 is added via the airway, the fluid is forced up the outflow spout. This flow causes the fluid level to increase in both reservoirs. The increase in fluid level is sensed by the float attached to the right-hand lever, causing the lever arm to rise. This opens the outflow valve. The level of the fluid must rise until the valve opening is sufficient so that the outflow now compensates for the added inflow. Thus, a degraded regulation results, with arterial CO_2 rising during an airway CO_2 load.

This feedforward/feedback control system encodes the way we traditionally think about the respiratory controller. The feedback pathway involves the chemoreceptors that sense arterial CO_2 tension. The feedforward pathway encodes the "exercise" signal—a signal correlated to metabolic CO_2 production. A variety of mechanisms have been proposed for this signal, including CO_2 (pH) oscillations, a central neural stimulus from the motor cortex, afferent inputs from exercising muscles, lung CO_2 flux receptors, blood gas disequilibrium theories, etc.

These mechanisms could all be part of the feedforward stimulus; in the physiological literature we can find studies suggesting the involvement of each mechanism. However, we can also find evidence to suggest that each mechanism is not involved, because regulation can be demonstrated without that particular mechanism intact. We would have to conclude with Comroe, that after 100 years of intensive investigation, we still do not know the source of an exclusive "exercise" signal (1).

COMROE'S CLOGGING THEORY

Comroe's clogging theory has certain implications for an *implicit* "exercise" signal not previously considered. The concept is that lung gas exchange efficiency is directly related to CO_2 production. If gas exchange efficiency is monitored by the brain, then it can determine CO_2 production implicitly without an explicit "exercise" signal.

Let us define gas exchange efficiency as a change in arterial CO_2 tension divided by a given change in ventilation. Then gas exchange is highly efficient when a small change in ventilation leads to a large change in CO_2 tension. Gas exchange is most efficient at rest, with breathing of room air. As an airway CO_2 load is added via inspired CO_2, the difference between the arterial CO_2 level and the inspired CO_2 level narrows. This tends to "clamp" the arterial CO_2 so that a change in ventilation produces minimal change in arterial CO_2 tension. Hence, with inspired CO_2, gas exchange efficiency is drastically reduced, just as Comroe suggested in his "clogging" theory.

This concept of gas exchange efficiency is inherently related to CO_2 production. The metabolic production of CO_2 delivered to the lung ($\dot{V}CO_2$) is related to alveolar ventilation ($\dot{V}_A$) and the inspired (F_ICO_2) and alveolar (F_ACO_2) fractions of CO_2 in the quasi steady-state by

$$(F_ACO_2 - F_ICO_2)\dot{V}_A = \dot{V}CO_2 = (C_vCO_2 - C_aCO_2)\dot{Q} \qquad (36.1)$$

where C_vCO_2 is the mixed venous CO_2 content and C_aCO_2 is the arterial CO_2 content. Using this equation, a small change in alveolar CO_2 fraction is related to a small change in alveolar ventilation by using differential calculus:

$$(\Delta F_ACO_2)\dot{V}_A + \Delta\dot{V}_A(F_ACO_2 - F_ICO_2) = -\alpha\dot{Q}\,\Delta F_ACO_2 \qquad (36.2)$$

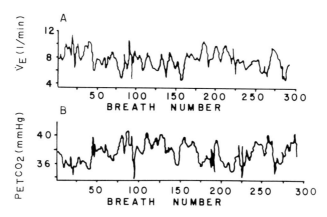

Fig. 36.2 Typical randomlike variation in breath-to-breath ventilation and the reciprocal response of end-tidal CO_2 [Redrawn from Lenfant, 1967 (4).]

where the Δ indicates the small change. Note that the change in arterial CO_2 concentration is assumed to be related to the change in alveolar CO_2 fraction by the solubility coefficient α. Changes in C_vCO_2 and $\dot{Q}$ are assumed to be negligible. Rearranging Eq. 36.2 yields

$$\frac{\Delta F_ACO_2}{\Delta \dot{V}_A} - \frac{F_ACO_2 - F_ICO_2}{\dot{V}_A + \alpha\dot{Q}} = -\frac{\dot{V}CO_2}{\dot{V}_A(\dot{V}_A + \alpha\dot{Q})} \qquad (36.3)$$

Equation 36.3 states that the alveolar gas exchange efficiency is directly related to the CO_2 production delivered to the lung. Thus, by knowing the gas exchange efficiency and the existing nominal ventilation level and the pulmonary blood flow value, $\dot{V}CO_2$ can be determined and used to generate an appropriate ventilation response to both a metabolic CO_2 load and an airway CO_2 load (5,6).

How can the brain monitor gas exchange efficiency and, thus, determine CO_2 production? The natural breath-to-breath variation in ventilation observed in humans may yield the necessary information. Figure 36.2A indicates a typical breath-to-breath variation in ventilation and the associated out-of-phase variation in CO_2 tension for a subject at rest (4). If the brain dictates the changes in ventilation and monitors the changes in CO_2 tension, then it can determine gas exchange efficiency continuously via these signals. With an estimate of the average ventilation and pulmonary blood flow, the CO_2 production delivered to the lung can then be determined continuously.

COMPUTER SIMULATION

To assess the utility of Eq. 36.3 for estimating CO_2 production, a computer simulation was utilized to generate time series records analogous to those shown in Fig. 36.2. The Yamamoto model (16), as modified by Robbins and Swanson (8), was further modified to accept a sinusoidal perturbation in alveolar ventilation of 2.5

l/min. This perturbation yields a sinusoidal envelope for breath-to-breath alveolar CO_2. A Fourier series analysis of the CO_2 time series then yields the fundamental component of the perturbation response and the lung gas exchange efficiency can be determined.

This scheme was assessed at a resting $\dot{V}CO_2 = 0.3$ l/min and at exercise $\dot{V}CO_2$ = 1, 2, and 3 l/min with and without a 30-mmHg airway CO_2 load. Appropriate cardiac output values were determined from the regression equation given by Inman et al. (2). At each metabolic rate, breathing periods of 2, 3, and 4 s were used. Furthermore, at each metabolic rate and at each breathing period, sinusoidal perturbations were 12, 36, 60, and 120 s. Thus, at each perturbation period and each level of inspired CO_2, there are 12 pairs of data (estimated metabolic CO_2 production via Eq. 36.3 vs. actual metabolic CO_2 production). These data at each perturbation period were used to determine the correlation between actual and estimated CO_2 production.

For the 12-s sinusoidal ventilation perturbation, the correlation coefficient r = .995 for an inspired CO_2 of zero and $r = .993$ for an inspired CO_2 of 30 mmHg. In all other cases, $r = 1.000$ (15). These high correlations represent the case where the brain knows the precise value of $\dot{V}A$ and $\dot{Q}$ for calculation in Eq. 36.3. Although the brain, to some extent, dictates these quantities, their actual value may actually be estimated by other means (9,10).

DISCUSSION

A typical experimentally observed time series for minute ventilation and end-tidal CO_2 for a subject at rest is shown in Fig. 36.2 (4). Note the variation in ventilation around its nominal value and the corresponding reciprocal variation in end-tidal CO_2. The frequency content of these signals is in the range of 12–120 s—the range we investigated in our computer simulation.

The purpose of this variation in ventilation around a nominal value may be to provide information to the brain (via the corresponding variation in arterial CO_2) about the level of metabolic CO_2 production. That is, the brain can sense the variation in arterial CO_2 via the chemoreceptors. The frequency content of this randomlike variation can be determined from a neural process analogous to a Fourier transform or Fourier series. The brain must "know" the specific nominal ventilation and the cardiac output. Then by dictating an appropriate perturbation of ventilation (appropriate frequency content and amplitude) and by determining the corresponding frequency content and amplitude of the CO_2 response, the brain can estimate the metabolic CO_2 production via a neural process analogous to the algorithm given in Eq. 36.3.

If the peripheral chemoreceptors are intact, the arterial CO_2 variation indicated in Fig. 36.2 can be sensed without attenuation. Alternatively, if the peripheral chemoreceptors are not intact (as in the case of carotid body-resected subjects; see ref. 5), then this arterial CO_2 variation can be sensed by the central chemoreceptors, although there will be some frequency-dependent attenuation (13). This attenuation would have to be included in the signal processing scheme.

Does the brain actually use this randomlike variation for any specific purpose, or is the variation just a consequence of an imperfect controller? The latter interpretation is well argued in the literature (3). However, we have previously demonstrated that the randomlike variation in ventilation may provide information about dead space (9). Furthermore, an optimal controller scheme requires such variations to determine a cost–function minimum (14). From this perspective, these variations in ventilation may provide information to balance the "cost" of regulation with the "cost" of breathing (7). Finally, motivated by Comroe's "clogging" theory, these variations allow the brain to monitor gas exchange efficiency and, thus, to determine an indirect estimate of CO_2 production delivered to the lung.

We are not suggesting that this variation provides an "exclusive" signal, but rather that it deserves consideration as one of several signals correlated to CO_2 production in a redundancy-type respiratory controller structure (12).

REFERENCES

1. Comroe, J. H. *Physiology of Respiration.* Chicago: Year Book Medical Publishers, 1974.
2. Inman, M. D., R. L. Hughson, and N. L. Jones. Comparison of cardiac output during exercise by single-breath and CO_2-rebreathing methods. *J. Appl. Physiol. 58:* 1372–1377, 1985.
3. Khoo, M. D., R. E. Kronauer, K. P. Strohl, and A. S. Slutsky. Factors inducing periodic breathing in humans: a general model. *J. Appl. Physiol. 53:* 644–659, 1982.
4. Lenfant, C. Time-dependent variations of pulmonary gas exchange in normal man at rest. *J. Appl. Physiol. 22:* 675–684, 1967.
5. Lugliani, R., B. J. Whipp, C. Seard, and K. Wasserman. Effect of bilateral carotid-body resection on ventilatory control at rest and during exercise in man. *N. Engl. J. Med. 285:* 1105–1111, 1971.
6. Menn, S. J., R. D. Sinclair, and B. E. Welch. Effect of inspired P_{CO_2} up to 30 mm Hg on response of normal man to exercise. *J. Appl. Physiol. 28:* 663–671, 1970.
7. Poon, C. S. Optimal control of ventilation in hypoxia, hypercapnia and exercise. In: *Modeling and Control of Breathing,* ed. B. J. Whipp and D. M. Wiberg. New York: Elsevier, 1983, pp. 189–204.
8. Robbins, P. A., and G. D. Swanson. Errors in seminal papers on the within-breath time course of alveolar P_{CO_2}. *J. Appl. Physiol. 57:* 284, 1984.
9. Robbins, P. A., and G. D. Swanson. Irregularities in breathing may encode information for respiratory control. *Biomed. Meas.: Inform. Control 1*(2): 59–63, 1986.
10. Sherrill, D. L., and G. D. Swanson. Application of the general linear model for smoothing gas exchange data. *Computers in Biomedical research,* in press.
11. Swanson, G. D. Overview of ventilatory control during exercise. *Med. Sci. Sports 11:* 221–226, 1979.
12. Swanson, G. D. Respiratory control during exercise. In: *Encyclopedia of Systems and Control: Theory; Technology; Applications,* ed. M. Singh. Oxford: Pergamon, 1988, pp. 4045–4051.
13. Swanson, G. D., and J. W. Bellville. Hypoxic–hypercapnic interaction in human respiratory control. *J. Appl. Physiol. 36:* 480–487, 1974.

14. Swanson, G. D., and P. A. Robbins. Optimal respiratory controller structures. *IEEE Trans. Biomed. Eng. 33:* 677–680, 1986.
15. Swanson, G. D. An optimal controller motivated variation hypothesis. In: *Concepts and Formulations in the Control of Breathing,* ed. G. Benchetrit, P. Baconnier, and J. Demongeot. Manchester, UK: Manchester University Press, 1987, pp. 143–156.
16. Yamamoto, W. S. Mathematical analysis of the time course of alveolar CO_2. *J. Appl. Physiol. 15:* 215–219, 1960.

Index